SHORT SKIRTS and SNAPPY SALUTES

A Woman's Memoir of the WWII Years

Short Skirts and Snappy Salutes
A Woman's Memoir of the WWII Years

ISBN 978-0-9796251-7-6

Library of Congress Control Number:
2007931811

Copyright © 2007 by Caroline M. Garrett

Printed in the United States of America

To order additional books, go to:
www.RP-Author.com/Garrett

Robertson Publishing
59 N. Santa Cruz Avenue, Suite B
Los Gatos, California 95030 USA
(888) 354-5957 • www.RobertsonPublishing.com

SHORT SKIRTS AND SNAPPY SALUTES

A Woman's Memoir of the WWII Years

Caroline Morrison Garrett

For Marti

Acknowledgements

I am grateful to be part of a generation that wrote letters. During the years of WWII, long distance phone calls were expensive and telegrams usually meant bad news. Those of us in the service, even boys who had never before put their thoughts on paper, felt the need to communicate. Mothers saved every scrap of paper we wrote. Mine did – a trunk full of letters and cards.

Through several moves, my mother gave the trunk top priority. "Some day you will want to write a book. The letters will refresh your memory," she said.

Many years later, I had time for such a project, but lacked computer skills. My niece Betsy Morrison came from Colorado to choose equipment and give me a two-day crash course. Eva Tatum took over my computer education, aided by many phone calls to her son Randy stationed with the army in Germany. Marti Henley and Paul Hodges pulled me out of many a crisis of my own making. Without the expertise of all those friends, this work would not have been possible.

Classes with Roberta Moyer taught me the pleasures of memoir writing. Through many enjoyable Tuesday mornings, Lynn Rogers encouraged me and improved my writing skills. The students in her class became loyal friends, who offered valuable suggestions and urged me on. I owe special thanks to Marti Henley, who has been with me every step of the way.

If I mentioned all the people who helped with suggestions and an occasional push to keep at it, the list would be too long. You know who you are and I thank you.

My two youngest fans deserve recognition. Kyle Kucek, starting when he was ten years old, has checked on my progress and encouraged me. Melanece Wesley, from Walpole, Massachusetts, eagerly awaits the adventures of a woman in the army. Thank you.

Table of Contents

Foreword

On August 25, 2005, I was stunned by the headline in the morning paper. "Walter Reed Army Medical Center To Close." I found it hard to believe a Federal Commission had voted to shut down Walter Reed Army Medical Center in Washington, D.C. Surely not Walter Reed. Not the historic hospital where soldiers from America's wars had been treated since 1909. Not Walter Reed where doctors, nurses, technicians and dietitians, including me, had received superior medical training.

I arrived there in September 1944 for a year's internship in dietetics, to be followed by a commission as second lieutenant in the Medical Corps. From the moment the sentry waved me through the gate, I felt the aura of the army's crown jewel — Walter Reed Army Hospital.

Gracious Georgian brick buildings, surrounded by sweeping lawns and wooded areas, offered a respite in the northwest section of the city for hundreds of soldiers recovering from the horrors of battle. At the hospital entrance, staff cars and limousines carrying military leaders, congressmen, and international dignitaries left their passengers by the broad marble steps.

General Pershing, leader of the expeditionary forces in Europe during World War I, lived in a penthouse at Walter Reed. World leaders came there to seek his advice and keep him informed on the progress of World War II. Among others, General Patton had sought General Pershing's blessing before heading for Europe to participate in preparations for the invasion of Normandy on D-Day.

Movie stars, radio comedians, theatre luminaries, and acrobats with trained dogs, all felt privileged to perform for the patients. Mrs. Eleanor Roosevelt strode the halls one afternoon every week to visit "her boys." Even Fala, President Roosevelt's famous Scottish terrier, came to the Veterinary School at Walter Reed for grooming.

My year there gave me a grandstand seat for some of the most important and dramatic events of the twentieth century. The Battle of the Bulge, President Roosevelt's death, victory in Europe, the dropping of atom bombs on Hiroshima and Nagasaki, and Japan's surrender, came with dizzying speed. As those events unfolded, my duties brought me in contact with many key players on the world scene.

When I left for college in 1940, I told Mother I could keep a journal or write to her in detail. There would not be time for both. "By all means write letters," she said. "I promise to keep them."

During the next decade, more than a trunk full of letters, written in fountain pen or pencil, on fancy paper or plain, accumulated in the attic. I also saved many missives from Mother, Dad's weekly "special delivery," and others from my brothers, relatives, and friends. That constant stream of written communication forms the basis for this memoir.

The war years of the 1940's remain inside everyone who lived through that tumultuous period and I am no exception. Here is a picture of life as I remember it during my college years, my army training, and two years in the army.

A highlight was the year spent at Walter Reed Army Medical Center. The training I received there instilled in me the discipline, sense of duty, determination, and fortitude necessary to complete two years in the service. Those attributes have stayed with me throughout a long life. Now the time has come for me, as well as Walter Reed, to be retired.

A sparkling new, modern Walter Reed National Medical Center in Bethesda, Maryland will provide world-class care and, with time, develop its own rituals. I, along with former patients and medical personnel familiar with the history and traditions of the old buildings, will grieve our loss.

Like so many others, I remain proud of my association with Walter Reed Army Medical Center. In my heart, it can never be replaced.

Part I. Woman's College

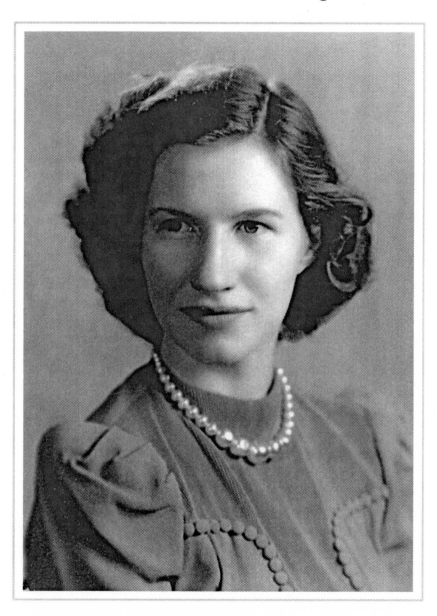

Carol Morrison 1942.

Freshman Year 1940 - 1941

I stood in the shade of the freshman dorm avoiding the hot rays of the North Carolina sun. Determined to keep my composure until my parents drove out of sight, I wondered why I'd chosen to attend the Woman's College of the University of North Carolina in Greensboro. I longed to call out. "Mother, Dad. Take me with you."

To add to my despair, this was my nineteenth birthday, September 10, 1940. I had not felt this alone since I attended YWCA Camp when I was ten. That lasted two weeks. Now I faced four months six hundred miles from my home in Danbury, Connecticut, before Christmas vacation.

As the car disappeared, Mother's last words hung in the air. "Carol, this is the perfect place for you. I know you're going to be happy and make many new friends." I couldn't imagine how, when I couldn't understand a word these North Carolinians said. Southern drawls hadn't sounded this thick in the movies.

Mother and Dad had enthused over the spacious lawns and old brick buildings. They succumbed to the charms of vivacious, red-haired Miss Hathaway, the resident counselor. Dad had expressed his hope that the moderate climate would bring me better health than I had experienced in the harsh New England winters.

As I climbed the long flights of stairs to my room, a wave of homesickness swept over me like a sudden attack of flu. I found my roommate, Nancy Blue, putting on her uniform to go to work in the dining hall. Blonde, pretty and plump, she came from the distant North Carolina Mountains. I knew I shouldn't complain — she had to work to pay her tuition.

That evening, as I studied rules and regulations in the student handbook, I fought to stay awake. Nancy wanted to talk. "This mornin' was so excitin.' T'was the first time I ever rode on a trolley car." Her blue eyes looked enormous. I wondered what she'd think if she knew I easily found my way around New York City by bus and subway.

When we put out the light and settled down on lumpy mattresses, silence hung heavy between our beds. Out of the darkness came Nancy's soft voice, "Do ya lik' ta ride a mule?" I fell asleep thinking this was too much. I'd head for home in the morning.

Sometime during the night, I realized I couldn't quit. If I did that, how would I face Mother and Dad? Few girls had the opportunity to attend college. Woman's College offered me an education with high scholastic standing, a rarity in the South, in a mild climate. My troubled sleep ended with nerves shattered by the shrill alarm clock at 6:00 a.m. Stumbling down the hall to the bathroom, I decided to try one more day.

Registration involved long lines and confusing choices. Skipping lunch, I rushed across campus to meet my advisor, Miss Edwards, head of the Home Economics Department. I'd settled on Home Ec in hopes of going into the new field of restaurant management, an alternative to my dread of becoming a teacher. Miss Edwards proved to be as optimistic as mother, not one to whom I could admit defeat.

Back in the room, I flopped on the bed relieved that Nancy had left for the dining hall. The door burst open revealing a stranger with tumbling locks of chestnut hair dressed in a frilly pinafore. She flounced into the room without being invited and stared at me with hatred in her eyes.

"Ah had a great aunt who said the proudest day of her life was when she shot a Yankee and buried him in the garden." She spun on her heel and left as quickly as she had come. I sat speechless staring at her retreating back. She never again crossed my path, but I did meet others who expressed disdain for Northerners.

In the evening, Miss Hathaway, the resident counselor, invited us one by one to her parlor. While we sipped tea and nibbled dainty sandwiches, she explained all room assignments were temporary. "I need time to get to know you. I try to pinpoint compatible couples. Everyone moves two weeks from today." I relaxed. Perhaps, she'd find someone for Nancy who liked to ride a mule.

When I met Mary Elizabeth Kirschner from York, Pennsylvania, I knew I had found a true friend. Miss Hathaway agreed we'd enjoy living together. We set off on a four-year carefree adventure interspersed with tense days and tragedies of war. Those exciting times bonded us close as sisters.

We wore the same size clothes and the same size shoes, but there the similarities ended. Mary's blonde hair, shapely bosom, and quick wit made her the life of the party. My brown hair, tall lean figure, and practical outlook kept me in the shadows. She had a penchant for getting us into trouble. I figured ways to get us out.

Neither of us had anticipated the animosity expressed by the southern girls over the War Between the States. "I can't believe all this war talk," Mary sputtered. "I don't even dare refer to it as the 'Civil War.' I thought it was something you read about in history books. Guess I'd better not let it be known that I live thirty miles from Gettysburg, Pennsylvania."

I tried to calm her down. "Well, the North was victorious, so we easily forget the war. For the defeated South, the pain, poverty, and shame remain. It's the way they treat the colored people that gets me — separate restrooms and separate drinking fountains. I can't imagine being forced to sit behind the white line on a bus."

It did seem strange to us that the conflict of the 1860s often entered the conversation but the events taking place in Europe in

1940 were seldom mentioned. Perhaps, living on the east coast had given me a broader view of the world.

Mary and I agreed that some of the southern accents sounded like a foreign language. In the North, we'd learned to study hard and were expected to get good grades. Our new classmates talked as though they'd studied only one subject — boys. They resented our academic prowess and blamed their lack of interest in studying on eleven years of schooling versus our twelve.

After the first few weeks, the differences among us faded away. Grits, mustard greens, and sweet potato pie no longer seemed strange fare. Accents, both northern and southern, grew less noticeable. We began to form lasting friendships.

After our hall mates decided Mary and I "would do," the discrimination I felt as a Yankee among the Rebels disappeared. Kathleen, our next-door neighbor said it best. "We'd never seen Yankees before, but y'all turned out to be O.K., even though yuh're still 'damn Yankees.'"

Mary and I laughed. That had become an accolade of the highest order.

The Little Blue Book

During the first semester at Woman's College, the little blue book controlled our lives. The rules and regulations of the Student Government Association dictated our actions day and night — signing in and out, obtaining permission slips from the counselor, 'closed study' for first semester students. We wondered whether we were students or prisoners.

"Listen to this," Mary sputtered. "'Closed study' means we're confined to our room every weekday night from 7:30 to 10:30, unless we go to the library. That's bad enough, but Monday night is 'closed campus night' — no men allowed on campus."

I turned to the page about permission slips. "One must sign a slip to walk off campus or go to the movies. Walking with a young man on campus involves signing out with the hostess and checking in every thirty minutes."

By the time we took the required written test on the rules, we knew them by heart — lights out at 11:00 p.m., a limit of three minutes on phone calls (none between dormitories), smoking permitted in rooms but not in the parlor, room inspection at any time, no typing after 11:00 p.m., no sunbathing.

After three weeks, we discovered how seriously the administration expected us to take the rules. Without warning, a campus check-up took place. Doors to all buildings were locked, while lists were made of all those present. Except for two girls from our dorm, everyone was accounted for. When they admitted they had been off campus riding in a car without permission, their indiscretion brought immediate action — they were sent home within the hour.

On Saturday, classes ended at noon. After checking the little blue book, Mary and I exchanged socks for stockings and jammed the required hats on our heads. As I signed out, I grumbled, "Imagine wearing a hat to go to the ten-cent store." The mile-long walk put holes in the heels of our silk stockings. Replacing ruined hose would put a dent in our limited budgets.

After I wore out another pair on Sunday, I sent an urgent plea to Mother. "Even though the new nylons are expensive, could you send me a pair? None are available here and I think they would be more durable."

That brought a response from my brother Sam. He wrote, "Having by much use of the slide rule concluded that, if you ruin one pair of silk stockings a day for the next year, I'll be unable to continue at M.I.T., I resolved to save myself from impending disaster by saving your hose. Enclosed is a gadget guaranteed to be the perfect remedy."

He sent "Sponge Rubber Heel Clingers." The instructions advised: Use the enclosed sandpaper to roughen the inside of the shoe heel. Follow by moistening the back of the pad with gasoline for one minute. Press the pad firmly in place. Allow it to stand overnight. After I read those instructions, the heel clingers remained in the envelope.

In town we headed for the lunch counter at Woolworth's. The bargain lunch, a grilled cheese sandwich and coke, cost fifteen cents. In 1960 that lunch counter would become famous when a group of colored youths were denied service. They would refuse to leave, sparking a controversial civil rights demonstration.

Not only our lunch, but our purchases, were bargains. "Mary, look at these rag rugs for twenty-nine cents each. No more cold floors by our beds." We wandered through Belks Department Store and Ellis Stone Fine Fashions, but confined our shopping to Woolworth's ten-cent store. The twenty-two dollars I had spent on books, plus the four hundred and sixty-six dollars for the year's tuition, weighed on my conscience.

Back on campus, we dropped by the post office. Mary found an empty box. I had two letters and a newspaper from home. Staying in close touch with family and friends kept letters flying back and forth between North Carolina and Connecticut. Whenever I had a free moment, I wrote. Between classes, late at night, and in the library, I wrote.

Family letters kept me up-to-date with the antics of my youngest brother, Sherman. Now that Sam and I were away at school, Sherman made the most of his role as only child at home. He never took things too seriously and charmed his way through life.

Walking back to the dorm, I read snatches of Mother's letter to Mary. Sherman's first day at Main Street Junior High School had made him indignant. He realized he'd been put in a class with the "dumb ones." He marched into the principal's office.

"I have a brother who goes to M.I.T. I shouldn't be in this room with the dumb kids. I want to be moved in with the smart ones." He got his way, although, as long as he passed, he saw no logic in studying for top grades. Life offered him too many choices to spend hours and hours doing homework.

I lost no time in writing him an indignant letter. "Why didn't you say you had a brilliant brother at M.I.T. and a very bright sister at the University of North Carolina?" After only a few weeks at a Woman's College, I was already asserting my role as an educated woman.

Short on Sleep

After the first six weeks at Woman's College, I felt bogged down by all the work. Three-hour labs wore me out. I dreaded Tuesdays — chemistry lab in the morning followed by compulsory chapel at noon, then clothing lab all afternoon. At least, after chapel, lunch was served family style. Other lunch times we stood in the cafeteria line.

Taking the required physical exam robbed me of precious time needed to study English poets. Moreover, it turned out to be a humiliating experience. After filling out an extensive questionnaire about my health history, the nurse gave me my orders. "Take off your clothes, then wrap this sheet around you. When you're ready open that door."

When I stepped into the next room, I faced four women with pencils poised over clipboards. "Please stand on that circle. Drop the sheet." I stared in horror at the naked body staring back at me from surrounding mirrors. Never before had I seen all of me in my natural state. Now I, and four strangers, saw my pale body many times over.

For the next hour, every part of my anatomy was measured, prodded, pushed, and examined. Expecting that the grim four had found a multitude of defects, it came as a surprise that only my posture caused them concern. Their dire warnings convinced me my backbone might collapse any moment. I left the infirmary with an order for exercises to correct my sagging spine.

Mary returned from her physical questioning why she had to lose weight when I did not. I looked up from my chemistry notes. "That's easy. While I'm on my feet three hours in lab, you sit under a tree and learn French verbs. You need more exercise." I wrote home that I'd lost five pounds but gained beautiful blue shadows under my eyes from lack of sleep. I expected by Christmas I'd be sleek and exotic.

Although the faculty emphasized academic work, our social role as southern ladies was not neglected. All concerts and evening lectures required formal dress. It took much of the afternoon, using my small travel iron, to press the three layers of nylon net on my gown. The red jacket, trimmed with rhinestones and worn over the white skirt, sparkled in the candlelight at the dinner table.

When the Dean and his wife invited us to tea at their home, Mary and I boned up on etiquette. That precipitated a trip to town for gloves. I sat on a stool and watched the clerk stretch a pair of leather gloves by opening wooden tongs in each finger. She placed my hand palm up on a black velvet pad while she coaxed the taut leather over my fingers. The smooth leather felt soft and my hand looked elegant.

"I'll take them." How I regretted my impulsiveness — the gloves cost five dollars. Too embarrassed to admit I could not afford them, I handed over my month's allowance. At the tea, I worked my way down the receiving line shaking hands, some limp, some firm. I remembered the correct protocol — wear the left glove and carry the right.

The University rounded out our education with lectures designed to extend our view beyond the campus to conditions worldwide.

On October, 29 Dr. Frank Porter Graham, President of the University of North Carolina, gave a sobering talk in chapel. He forced us to look at the world situation, something that seldom concerned my classmates in our busy lives.

"You, the members of the class of 1944 have entered college in the midst of a world revolution involving the future of freedom. Our democracy is caught between the two dynamic powers of fascism and communism. Our continent placed between two oceans nevertheless reverberates with the impact of forces in Europe and Asia."

I found it frustrating to live where no one seemed to care about the rest of the world. The radio played hillbilly music interspersed with gospel hymns from morning 'til night. Ma Benson's Home Show plugged the advantages of snuff over cigarettes, but national news would have bored her listeners. At home we'd always joined Dad to listen to the seven o'clock news with Raymond Gram Swing and read the New York Herald Tribune.

The approach of the Roosevelt-Wilkie election did stir up some excitement on campus. The two hundred out-of-state students, mostly northerners, preferred Wilkie. We seldom expressed our opinion among the southern majority of two thousand solidly for Roosevelt.

In Hinshaw Hall, the residents gathered in the parlor wearing pajamas to listen to the results on the radio. It soon became evident Roosevelt would win by a landslide. Mary and I escaped the elation around us by going to bed. Mary voiced our concern. "How can the country survive four years of this man?"

Mary's birthday in November gave us an excuse to forget serious matters for a while and celebrate. Dad had written, "Have a wonderful time, Carol, and once in a while slip down to the King Cotton Hotel for a real meal." Dressed in our smartest wool dresses, pearls and tiny hats with veils, Mary and I stepped into the dark paneled, sedate dining room of the King Cotton.

Soft music, soft light, soft rolls carried us far away from dormitory living. Some of our new friends would have been intimidated by a hotel dining room, but we considered this living the good life. Southerners usually entertained at home, not in public places.

The rare roast beef came from a different animal than the tough, dry roast we ate at college. Lingering over apple pie a la mode and delicious coffee, I asked Mary, fifteen months younger than I, how it felt to be eighteen? She had waited so impatiently for that day. She winked, "I'll let you know after my date on Saturday night."

The following week I explained to Mother and Dad why I had so little time to write letters. "Tomorrow a test on kinetic molecular energy has me worried. Friday — a test in history. Before Monday, I must read a biography, write an autobiography, outline thirty-four pages for English, and baste a dress for Home Ec. I plan to attend three lectures, write six letters, keep up with my regular lessons, and do my washing and ironing. Who has time for men? Not that there are any around here."

I dreaded my first Thanksgiving away from home, until a large box arrived from Mother. She sent a homemade angel cake, crackers, cheese and apples, mints and candy. Dad sent three and a half pounds of cookies — special delivery. With such a windfall, Mary and I planned a late night feed for all our friends.

After a traditional Thanksgiving dinner in the dining hall, we walked uptown to window shop. That evening brought most of Hinshaw Hall to our room for the party. By midnight, except for a few cookies, all the food had disappeared.

The best part of the day had been a letter from Ernie, whom I had dated the previous summer. Betty Urban, my best friend in high school, had introduced me to her brother. Ernie, slight of build, and shorter than I, had charmed me with his sense of humor and interest in my future. I was awed by his dire warnings about the political situation in Europe. He had studied at the University of Budapest and in June had received his Master's Degree in history from the University of Pittsburg.

In September, much to his family's distress, he had volunteered to join the army. His father felt a college graduate with an advanced degree could do better than enlist as a private. Ernie, having seen Hitler march into Austria, recognized the approaching peril and felt compelled to serve his country. He spoke several languages and knew his linguist skills would be useful.

Now, after completing basic training, he wrote from Riker's Island near New York City. "With any luck, I'll be stationed here at Christmas. So eager to see you."

Only a month until Christmas vacation. Only a month until I might see Ernie again. How could I wait that long?

New England Christmas

December 1, 1940. Only three weeks to go until Christmas vacation. My first semester at the Woman's College in Greensboro, North Carolina had opened my eyes to southern culture, so different from the northern way of life. My roommate, Mary from Pennsylvania, and I had learned to adjust to southern drawls but felt distant from the social life due to our northern ties.

Even though I felt fortunate to be in college, the tug of home remained strong. The little blue college handbook emphasized no one could cut class the day before or after a vacation. Lucky me — my Saturday class ended at ten o'clock. I could catch the train from Greensboro at 11:00 a.m. and be in New York at midnight.

Mary's lack of interest in Christmas shocked me. "You mean to tell me you plan to return all your presents for cash? I can't imagine doing that." Soon my enthusiasm rubbed off on her. We walked to town on Saturday afternoons to comb the stores for suitable gifts. That took ingenuity on our meager budgets.

Neglecting an English assignment, I joined the freshmen class in the Y-hut. We turned mountains of shiny magnolia leaves and greens into wreaths and swags to decorate the facades of the dormitories. The old brick buildings took on the charm of English Christmas cards.

Even though no men would be present, we dressed in style for the formal candlelit Christmas dinner. Returning to the dark quadrangle, a lighted candle glowed in every dorm window. Foreign language students strolled the grounds singing carols in Spanish, French, and German. Mary lost her voice singing French songs in the damp night air.

Exhausted on our last night in the dorm, Mary and I struggled to pack. At least, I did. "Mary, you'll never get gifts for eleven aunts and uncles in your bag that way. Put the heavy items in the bottom." For the next four years, I did the packing for both of us. Mary never did get the hang of it.

On Saturday morning, hot sun beat down on the platform of the Southern Railway Station. Weighted down with packages, hatbox and winter coat, I switched Mother's gift book from arm to arm. "Masterpieces of Art" grew heavier by the minute. "Where is that train? I'm so hot in this wool suit I feel faint," I grumbled to Mary.

An hour later, the train to Washington, D.C. steamed down the track. Mary and I struggled up the steps and plopped down in the first two seats we could find. "Let's treat ourselves to dinner in the diner," Mary suggested. I hesitated. After spending fifteen dollars and eight-five cents for the round trip ticket, that seemed extravagant, but I couldn't resist spending seventy cents to dine on fried chicken with biscuits.

In Washington we parted. She headed for the train to Harrisburg, on her way to York, Pennsylvania, and I rushed for the express to New York on my way to Danbury, Connecticut. With every mile my excitement increased. At 1:00 a.m., across the Jersey flats, the lights of New York seemed to shout their welcome. The train plunged into the tunnel and chugged to a halt in Pennsylvania Station.

Snug in my winter coat, I stepped into the wintry air and into the arms of my brothers. "Merry Christmas, Merry Christmas," the greetings from happy travelers resonated along the platform. After Sherman surprised me with a foot-high decorated tree, he grabbed my packages, Sam my suitcase and the heavy book. We raced to the concourse to greet Mother and Dad.

Six hundred miles behind me, only sixty miles to go to home! The car purred along under a canopy of stars twinkling in the dark sky. Mother and the boys dozed. "Dad, has the cold weather shut down the job for the winter?" I remembered the race in past years to pour the last batch of cement before freezing weather brought road construction to a halt. He said this year he'd been lucky and finished ahead of schedule.

At 3:45 a.m., the porch light gleaming in the frosty air marked the end of the journey from North Carolina to Connecticut. Green wreaths with jaunty red bows decorated the windows and the front door. "Oh, Dad, there's no place like home."

Too excited to sleep, I wandered from room to room admiring fresh paint, new curtains, and a remodeled kitchen. In my room, frost pictures covered the windowpanes. I snuggled under a down puff in my birds-eye maple bed, Santa's gift when I was nine. I felt safe, loved, and cherished. Everything was just as I remembered it.

Even Sam and Sherman wanted to continue the tradition of shopping at the Worn Doorstep in New Milford on Sunday afternoon. The gift shop, in a lovely old square house facing the village green, overflowed with embroidered handkerchiefs, jewelry, notepaper, glassware, and knick-knacks.

Miss Fitch, soft and puffy as a marshmallow in a flowered dress, stood behind Miss Starr, sturdy and efficient in tweeds, shirt, and tie. "It would not be Christmas without the Morrisons. We've been waiting for you." While we made our selections, Miss Fitch read Christmas card verses to her captive audience — Dad. The boys found that hilarious.

On the way home, Dad swung by our summer cottage at Lake Candlewood. Sherman and I worked together to free long strands of princess pine held tight by the frozen soil. At home, we wove the fragrant greens around the spindles on the stairs and tied red bows on the banister.

On the day before Christmas, always a strenuous time for cooks, Mother and I started early. We tackled the job she dreaded — preparing the turkey. It took both of us to hold the slippery twelve-pound bird over the gas flame to singe away the pinfeathers.

In a large yellow bowl, the day-old cubed bread took on the pungent fragrance of Bell's Poultry Seasoning. The addition of melted butter, onions, raisins, apples, and turkey broth filled the bowl to the brim. Then came the fun part — stuffing the turkey. After that, it was on to the pies.

Late in the afternoon, at my insistence, Sam suspended a sprig of mistletoe from the hanging light fixture in the front hall. Chores completed, he drove us twenty miles to Betty Urban's in Wilton. Sam had fallen for Betty, my best friend, the day I introduced them two years earlier.

"Sam, I wish you'd let me drive. We'd get there faster." I knew he didn't intend to for that very reason. There had been no word from Ernie, Betty's brother, since his postcard saying he hoped for an army leave for Christmas. It would be a bleak holiday for me, if he did not get home.

As Sam and I walked up the snowy path to the Urbans, those thoughts fled from my mind. In the doorway, erect and proud in his khaki uniform, stood Corporal Ernest Urban. "Ernie, this is too good to be true. Why didn't you let me know you were home?

"Wanted to surprise you. Just arrived last night," he beamed. Without the disapproving scowl of his strict Hungarian father, our kiss would have lasted longer. Bill Urban never approved of any public display of affection.

Betty's mother served piping hot tea and Hungarian pastry, filled with apricots and nuts, to fortify us for the cold evening ahead. Sam and Betty, Ernie and I, joined hundreds of people on God's Acre, the village green in New Canaan, to sing Christmas carols.

Three white churches, their steeples piercing the evening sky, framed the hillside above the lighted Christmas tree. Ernie's arm tight around my waist, our fingers entwined, I ignored the chill creeping through my boots. My happiness blended with the Christmas carols carried aloft by a multitude of voices. ____

In spite of the cold, no one wanted the evening to end. As the final strains of "Silent Night" faded away in the frosty air, the crowd, unwilling to break the spell, dispersed in silence. Ernie's uniform emphasized the feeling in our hearts. We sensed this might be the last Christmas Eve of peace for a long time.

Sam and I tiptoed into the house at midnight and find Mother and Dad sitting by the fire. Dad threw another log on the embers. "You're here for such a short time. We wanted to share some of this Christmas Eve with you. Ever since you were little, this has been my favorite night of the year."

An hour later in my chilly room, one more Christmas Eve tradition remained. I lit the bayberry candles, a gift from my grandmother. Good luck was promised to those burning bayberry candles on Christmas Eve, provided they did not extinguish the flame. When the candles burned themselves out during the night, my good luck seemed assured.

On Christmas morning, the family gathered at the top of the stairs. Laughing, we lined up as of old. Sherman first, although at thirteen he resented being called the smallest, followed by Sam, now taller than I, with Mother behind me. Dad stood at the bottom of the stairs with the movie camera. "Smile," he said. In former years that word had always made Sherman act up for the camera.

Sam clapped Sherman on the shoulder. "Hey, kid, you're slipping. You didn't blast us out of our beds at 3:00 a.m. with a bugle call. Were we ever mad at you, the year you made that racket. Aunt Hannah almost had a heart attack. You insisted it was time to open presents and resented being sent back to bed."

Sherman changed the subject by marching down the stairs into the pine-scented living room. The glittering tree aglow with colored lights touched the ceiling. This year there had been no arguments over the tinsel. I used to hang the strands one by one. My impatient brothers had insisted on throwing wads at the branches.

As we opened gifts, Mother and I smoothed out the paper and made a neat pile of ribbons. The men tore off gift-wrap, making a shambles of the room.

I ran my hand over the hand-planed lid of the antique blanket chest, my gift from Mother and Dad. "A hundred years ago some other girl thrilled over the soft glow of this wide pine board. Perhaps, her father made this box. I bet she loved the lock and tiny key too. Now my treasures will always be safe."

Inside the chest, I found a check for an evening gown, nylons, and a subscription to the New York Herald Tribune. Today my buttons fill the small cedar box that contained notepaper when Sam chose it at the Worn Doorstep.

Sherman had printed personalized stationary on his printing press. "If you like it, you can get me orders from your friends at college." He already had the knack for making money.

Mother and I hurried to the kitchen. By the time our neighbors, the Duryeas, burst in the door shouting "Merry Christmas," breakfast for ten was on the table. Platters of scrambled eggs and bacon disappeared along with mounds of crullers. "They're doughnuts without holes," Sherman explained to little Anne.

As I added three leaves to the table and adjusted the damask tablecloth, I muttered, "Ten for breakfast, twelve for dinner. Mother couldn't do this without me." The boom of the doorknocker sent me scurrying to the front hall. Calling out greetings and laden down with packages, stood Grandma and Grandpa Andrews, Aunt Pauline, Uncle Ed and our three cousins: Polly, five years older than I; Robert, two years older than I; and Ted, my age.

"Here's a present for you, Sam." Polly grabbed Sam and gave him a hearty kiss under the mistletoe. The red flush, which crept up his cheeks to his hairline, made everyone laugh.

At the table, after Uncle Ed gave the blessing, we waited for his next inevitable line. "Sit two inches from the table. Now eat until you touch." By the time Christmas dinner ended with a choice of mince pie, pumpkin pie, or steamed pudding with hard sauce, no one remembered to measure.

While the ladies cleared the table, the men escaped to the living room to watch Grandpa smoke his yearly cigar. I enjoyed washing the good china in hot sudsy water and, at the same time, chatting with Grandma. "At last I'm old enough to take part in the conversation in the kitchen. I used to resent being sent away to play with my dolls." Polly, bored with the conversation, had drifted away to join the men.

Late in the afternoon, everyone gathered round the Christmas tree to open presents. Then came the best part of the day — jokes at supper. Each person received a joke and a silly verse to read. The lace I had sewed on Sherman's shirttails, to remind him to keep them tucked in, proved to be a winner. He took his ribbing with good humor.

Aunt Pauline groaned, "I cannot eat another bite. Well, maybe a piece of mince pie." She was the one who usually broke up the party. "Polly, Robert, Ted, gather up your things, we must get home."

When Robert kissed me under the mistletoe, I enjoyed it. Christmas had been a day of love, good food, good fellowship, and laughter. I wondered whether there would be another to equal it.

Ernie's concern over Hitler's march across Europe made war seem inevitable, but we didn't know our world would be turned upside down before we gathered for another Christmas. The attack on Pearl Harbor would shatter our complacency.

Where Did The Time Go?

Ernie had returned to duty on Riker's Island, a ferry ride away from New York City. On Wednesday, a call from him sent my spirits soaring. "Blue Eyes, I didn't expect to see you again 'til summer but Uncle Sam has given us a break. I have a twelve-hour pass tomorrow. How about you and Betty meeting me at Radio City Music Hall?" Betty had told him Sam was spending three days in Boston supervising repairs at his fraternity house and wouldn't be able to join us.

"You bet we will. We'll take the 6:60 a.m. train and meet you under the marquee about eight. This is the best Christmas present yet. Give my thanks to the army."

Betty and I expected a crowd, but not a line blocking the sidewalk for half a mile. The gray, blustery day did not deter the people determined to see the Rockettes, and "The Philadelphia

Story" starring Katherine Hepburn. The next day the management bragged that six thousand seats sold out for every show from 8:00 a.m. to midnight.

Ernie had staked out a place for us in line. He thought we had a good chance of making the second show. We stood glued to the same messy spot on the sidewalk for two and one half hours. Ernie rubbed my cold hands. "I had no idea we'd have to wait this long. If we don't make it for the second show, we'll have to give up."

Before I could answer, the line began to move. In spite of aggressive New Yorkers trying to break into the line, the momentum of the crowd shoved us along. Ernie wedged us through the bottleneck. Behind us the doors clanged shut leaving the mob outside to wait for the next show.

In the quiet lobby, we stepped into a fantasy world. A soaring staircase led up, up, up past a mural of towering clouds. The raucous scene on the sidewalk had been replaced by warm air, thick rugs and muted colors. My fingers interlocked with Ernie's.

In the cavernous hall, we groped our way to seats. The mighty chords of the organ filled the vast space with layer upon layer of sound. High overhead, pale light grew in intensity, simulating sunrise over the ocean. I whispered to Betty. "I was twelve the first time I came here. The Rockettes wore yellow slickers and danced in the rain. Real raindrops splattering on the stage made the scene pure magic for me."

The red velvet curtain rose revealing the Rockettes, most famous precision dancers in the world, dressed as toy soldiers. In white pants, blue jackets, and tall red hats matching the round red spots of color on their cheeks, their high kicking performance brought thunderous applause.

Next came my favorite part of the program. As if by magic, the symphony orchestra rose from the orchestra pit. The musicians, intent on Handel's "Messiah," ignored the gasp of surprise from the audience. I leaned closer to Ernie. "I can't spot him from this distance, but I once met the piccolo player on a bus. He wanted a date until he found out I was only sixteen."

"Well, he can't have you now. You're mine."

I laughed. "Ernie, you've never faced any competition from that piccolo player."

The orchestra sank back into the floor to be replaced by a manger scene complete with live animals. Near us, a camel waited next to the wall for his cue to appear on stage. After the wise men followed the star to the crèche, the lights dimmed. Only twinkling stars in a night sky remained.

The fantasy world of music, color, and drama came to an end. Higher and higher rose the huge red velvet curtain revealing the giant movie screen. A Loony Tunes cartoon served as buffer between the stage show and the feature film. After the colorful live performers, the black and white film seemed drab until glamorous Katherine Hepburn captured our imaginations. The romantic comedy sprang to life.

When the picture ended, hundreds of people, eager to leave, jammed the aisles. Betty tugged at Ernie's arm. "Let's stay to see the stage show again." As deep rumbles of the organ filled the hall, a new audience rushed into the auditorium. We remained in our seats.

An hour later, hunger forced us into the street. Chilled by a gusty wind, we ran down the street and ducked into an Italian restaurant. Betty, usually a picky eater, wrapped spaghetti around her fork with gusto. Ernie looked at his watch. "Time to go, girls. I'll take you to Grand Central before I head back to camp."

On the train, Betty and I relived every detail of the day. Neither of us spoke of the thoughts uppermost in our minds. Where would Ernie be next Christmas? Was he right that our country could not avoid involvement in the war raging in Europe? President Roosevelt kept assuring us that would never happen.

Betty stared out the window into the darkness. "You are so lucky to be going back to college. You can't imagine what its like to live at home and commute to business school when all your friends are away. It isn't fair that Daddy won't let me go like the rest of you."

Betty's father had immigrated to this country from Hungary at the age of sixteen. After he learned to speak English, he became a professional gardener and often expressed his gratitude for his life in the United States, "the greatest country in the world." However, his old world approach to women had not changed. He believed they should cater to their husbands, remain in the kitchen, and raise sons.

He'd once said, "Mine Gott, Daughter, you are foolish to want to go to college. It's a waste of money to educate a woman. Business school is good enough for you."

Later in the week, Betty and I joined our high school friends for lunch. When the group discussed college life, and bragged about our new self-confidence and sophistication, a pained expression crossed Betty's face. She remained silent.

Sam's return on New Year's Eve revived Betty's spirits. The last night of the year proved a let down for me; Ernie couldn't wrangle another pass. My cousin Ted and I joined Sam and Betty at a movie in Ridgefield. It paid to go with Ted. Having been an usher at the theater, he used his pull to sneak us into loge seats for the price of the balcony.

Out in the street, at the stroke of twelve, Ted and Sam lit four-inch salutes, their contribution to a nerve shattering celebration. In anticipation of this night, they had hidden the dangerous firecrackers in the attic on the Fourth of July.

Ted gave me a peck on the cheek. "Happy New Year, Happy 1941." I tried to smile but the noisy welcome for the New Year seemed all wrong, too much like the gunfire being heard all over Europe. The grim pictures in the movie newsreel remained fresh in my mind. With a sinking feeling in my heart, I wondered about Ernie's future and mine.

New Year's Day 1941 found me in a more positive mood. I did not want to spoil my last days at home. In the evening, the family gravitated to the blazing fire on the hearth. I sat on the floor, my back to the flames, feeling the warmth through the fire screen. Dad spoke for all of us. "All year I look forward to Christmas. Certainly, this has been the best one ever. The sharing, love, and laughter we've enjoyed during this holiday makes the bonds between us grow stronger. We're such a lucky family."

Every December the luster his words gave to that Christmas season come back to inspire me.

Making The Grade

My last day of vacation. That sinking feeling of homesickness struck me on the long drive to Boston to take Sam back to Massachusetts Institute of Technology. Betty's words bubbled up in my mind. "If I ever hear you say you're homesick, I'll never speak to you again." Her resentment over her father's refusal to let her attend college made her incapable of understanding my feelings of ambivalence about home and school.

Dad parked in front of Sam's fraternity, the five-story ATU house on the Charles River, formerly a private mansion. As Sam fumbled with the key, bitter wind threatened to sweep us off the marble steps. He gestured toward the river. "MIT is over there across the ice. To go to class, I have to fight my way across the bridge in snow, freezing rain, sleet, and gale force winds." I was glad I'd chosen the mild climate of North Carolina. I wouldn't last a week in a Boston winter.

The next morning, Mother and Dad drove me to New York to speed me on my way back to Greensboro. By giving me something to look forward to, Dad made it easier to say goodbye. "Mother and I hope you'll bring Mary home with you for spring break." On the train to Washington, my mind overflowed with ideas for vacation in March.

In Washington's Union Station, Barbara Hollister, a schoolmate from Hartford, called to me over the heads of the crowd clustered around the gate. On campus, I seldom saw Barb; she was a class ahead of me and enjoyed being the life of the party. A hearty blonde with the sturdy build of a physical education major, she excelled at tennis and golf.

Companions on the train varied due to train schedules and weather delays. Fifty out-of-state students from Woman's College traveled north on holidays, so I could always spot a familiar face in Union Station. I missed Mary; she'd taken an earlier train. Barb and I ganged up with three other students from Woman's College. Our suitcases bulging with Christmas gifts, we struggled through car after car on the train. No seats.

When the loudspeaker boomed, "Second section, seats available on second section," we were the first ones off the train. Little did we realize we'd have to carry our heavy luggage back the way we had come, up a flight of stairs, across the station, down a flight of stairs to another platform.

We stared in dismay at the second section, two ancient cars hitched to the mail train. On board, too tired to complain, we collapsed on hard wood benches. At the far end of the car, near the potbelly stove, a row of small dirty windows provided feeble light.

Without warning, a jerk sent shudders through the timbers of the antique car. Our odd journey had begun. Jerk, gain speed, jerk, slow down, jerk. Every mile or so, the routine made us grab the edge of the benches. The trainman in his greasy blue uniform stopped long enough to answer our questions.

"Well, we have to slow down at every station to throw the mailbag onto the platform and to snatch the pouch of outgoing mail from an arm extending from a pole over the tracks. That mail is being sorted in the next car right now." We dared not ask how many mail drops lined the tracks through Virginia into North Carolina.

Not only was I tired and cold in the drafty car, I was hungry. On the way to Washington, long lines outside the diner had forced me to miss out on lunch. As I watched the swaying lamp over our heads, the only illumination now that daylight had given way to darkness, I wondered when this trip would ever end.

The trainman appeared at the door, his crooked teeth revealing his need for dental work. "Ladies, put on your coats. Yah'all hurry up now. We're makin' a stop for supper. Twenty minutes ain't long, so git a move on."

The blast of cold air from the open door felt more like Connecticut than Virginia. I peered into the darkness and hesitated. The circle of light from a lantern by the trainman's boots revealed a drop of several feet from the bottom step to the ground. "Jump," he ordered. "I'll catch yah."

One by one, we jumped into his arms, which seemed to give him great pleasure. We stumbled over the tracks to a brick building, where a lone light bulb indicated the door. Inside, several engineers in striped overalls and peaked caps looked up in amazement from their domino games. College girls had never before invaded their male domain.

Our swains treated us like the cotton queen and her court. Seating us at a long red and white oilcloth-covered table, they plied us with hot dogs, potato chips, and ice cream bars. Barb had the foresight to buy doughnuts to keep us energized on the jolting ride ahead.

"All aboard," shouted our caretaker. He seemed to take longer than necessary to boost each of us up to the bottom step. He jumped aboard and the train began to move. Jerk, speed up, jerk, slow down, jerk, gain speed, at snail's pace the train chugged its way to Greensboro. The friendly trainman insisted on carrying our bags into the station. It felt like midnight, but the hands of the station clock pointed to 9:30 p.m.

Mary had reached the dorm hours earlier. She stood at the door holding a two-pound box of Whitman's chocolates sent special delivery by Mother and Dad. What was one more night without sleep? We compared vacations and nibbled chocolates until dawn.

The flu epidemic raging along the east coast proved to be a bonus. Restricted to campus, we studied more hours than usual for lack of anything better to do. Sixty unlucky people ended up in the infirmary and my friend Betty in Connecticut wrote she had been ill for two weeks.

On exam day, the history final, consisting of twenty-two parts, made my heart sink. One section asked for the political reforms in England from 1800 to 1941, listing all the important reform bills. Later, when the history professor called me to her office, I presumed I'd flunked.

Her words made me blush. "Your paper was one of the finest I've seen. If you had done better on the previous exam, I'd give you an A." B sounded fine to me. The final grade in Home Ec was based on the dress I had made. Recognizing its flaws, I hated modeling it in the fashion show and was amazed to receive a B plus. I never wore it again.

My advisor, Miss Edwards, reviewed my grades — A in English and Chemistry, B in History, Home Economics, Spanish, and Physical Education. Not one C. That was a relief. Mary made C in English and Biology, B's in the rest of her subjects.

"Hurrah Mary! For us, closed study is over. We're free to go to the library, walk on campus, and study in other students' rooms. Poor Nancy Blue did not make average, so, she still has closed study." One girl across the hall flunked out.

"Let's celebrate," shouted Mary. Dad's surprise gift of two dollars in his last special delivery made a splurge possible at the King Cotton Hotel. Whenever he urged, "Treat yourselves to a good meal," we headed back to the place we considered the best dining spot in town.

The six of us who stayed in the dorm during semester break relaxed. We stayed in bed 'til noon feasting on claret jelly, crackers, and Nescafe from a package sent from home. While Mary read magazines with as little intellectual content as possible, I wrote twenty-two letters. One went to Sam to thank him for his picture.

"What happened to your wavy brown hair? I hope the new style of short bristles all over your head doesn't last long." I didn't dare tell him his serious expression and jutting jaw line made us refer to him as Mussolini. His expression softened over the years but the butch haircut remains.

Boredom set in. We didn't want to admit it but we were eager for classes to resume on Monday.

Spreading Our Wings

The second semester at Woman's College brought added responsibilities. I became a table hostess serving dinner family style. It took an eagle eye to divide the meager amount of food on the platters into eight equal portions. No solution could be found to the marshmallow problem — seven marshmallows topping the sweet potato casserole for eight people.

In the dorm, Miss Hathaway, the counselor, installed me as proctor on my hall. "It is your duty to keep law and order. At 11:00 p.m. you must check every room for lights out." I found it difficult to be stern with a group playing bridge by the feeble glow of a flashlight.

No one mentioned the Civil War anymore. Much of our conversation centered on the grim possibility of the United States being drawn into the European conflict. In October 1940, passage of the Selective Service Act had forced millions of men to sign up for the first peace time draft. Now thousands of men were being called up for active duty. No longer was I the only one with my man in uniform.

My friends first met Mother and Dad in February when they drove through Greensboro on their way to Florida for their annual winter vacation. Dad rounded up a group of college girls to go bowling, even though I had a three-hour lab and couldn't go with them. Mother went along to keep score. Barb never let on that she cut a class to be included. On subsequent visits to campus, Dad made it a tradition to include an afternoon in the bowling alley for anyone free to go along.

Lecture night gave Mary and me the opportunity to invite Mother and Dad to a special dinner in the dining hall. They said they enjoyed seeing us in the candlelight dressed in formal gowns. After dinner, we walked across campus to Aycock

Auditorium where Miss Kwo from China and Miss Matsui from Japan opened our eyes to the conflict in Asia.

Saturday began at one of our favorite places — the Toddle House. A tiny hole-in-the-wall, we sat on stools at the counter and enjoyed crisp waffles dripping with butter and syrup, served with mugs of strong coffee. Later, as we drove to Durham to admire the beautiful campus at Duke University, a hint of spring filled the air.

"Dad, this is the first time I've ridden in a car since Christmas vacation. You have no idea how I miss that. We never get away from Greensboro to see the surrounding countryside." There was no time that day to take in the quaint charm of Chapel Hill, not if we planned to make it back to Greensboro for roast beef at the King Cotton Hotel.

On Sunday morning, after attending the annual University Sermon in Aycock Auditorium, Mother suggested a trip to Winston-Salem. Miss Hathaway's had recommended dinner at Winkler's Coffee Shop in the old Moravian settlement. The only diners at 3:00 p.m., we sat at a table before an open fire in a cozy dining room. The atmosphere felt more like a country inn than a coffee shop.

On the drive back, Mary asked a favor of Dad. "Could we go through Sunset Hills? That's Greensboro's most exclusive residential area." Our fist glimpse of pillared southern colonial mansions filled us with awe. Only in "Gone with the Wind" had we seen this version of the south.

The time had come for us to get back to work and for Mother and Dad to be on their way. Saying goodbye was easy for we'd see them again in two weeks when they'd stop on the way back to Connecticut. One of our friends, Mary Louise Parks, said it took both sides of three sheets of notepaper to tell her family what a good time she'd had.

Eager to spend more time with me, Mother and Dad cut short their vacation in Florida by a day. They returned from Daytona Beach tanned and refreshed after time with their friends Clinton and Genevieve Hawkins. It had been a novelty to live aboard a cabin cruiser, the *Miome*, but they could not imagine a permanent home in such cramped quarters.

Dad had mapped out plans for the weekend in Greensboro — bowling on Friday and a return trip to Winston-Salem on Saturday to spend more time in the Moravian village.

"Carol, why don't you invite a friend we haven't met to join you and Mary for the day in Winston-Salem?"

I chose Lois, a timid little girl from the mountains. Her eyes glowed. "Ah'd love to go but Ah ain't never been to a fancy place. Ah wouldn't know what to say." Her prediction came true. At Winkler's she ate everything on her plate, but spoke not a word.

We ended the day back in Greensboro with sundaes at Walgreen's, followed by a get-together in the parlor at Winfield Hall where everyone sat around the radio and listened to Edgar Bergen and Charlie McCarthy. Before final bell, my friends gathered on the lawn to say goodbye to Mother and Dad. I whispered to Mary, "Bet not one person here thinks of Garfield and Hazel Morrison as damn Yankees."

March brought cold rainy weather. The coal supply ran so low that we were allotted either warm water for clean clothes and no heat, or cold-water laundry and heat. Only once all week did the radiators grow warm. Mary and I shivered and counted the days until March 24 when she would go home with me to Danbury, Connecticut, for spring break.

Now that we were experienced travelers, we did not intend to weigh ourselves down with heavy suitcases for a ten-day vacation. I sat on the overnight bag, while Mary snapped the catches shut.

She winked at me. "Lucky we can wear each other clothes. My mother would never approve of one bag, plus a small one for shoes, for two of us. What she doesn't know won't hurt her."

On this trip, the train took off on time. In a special car, provided by the Southern R.R. for Woman's College students, we had room to spread out. I was content to watch the falling spring snow blanket Virginia, but Mary retrieved a deck of cards from my purse. A bridge game made the time pass quickly even though we missed our expert, Barb. She had opted to spend her vacation in Atlanta.

By the time we changed trains in Washington, the snow had stopped. With a late meal in the diner, we sped across Pennsylvania into New Jersey. On the stroke of midnight, we stepped off the train in Pennsylvania Station, New York City.

Good Luck in Connecticut

On Mary's first morning in Connecticut, she compared everything she saw to her home in York, Pennsylvania. "I expected the houses to be brick, not wood. I'm used to the open rolling farmland of Lancaster County; I feel hemmed in by the steep rocky hillsides and sharp curves on the roads."

The following day proved an exciting one, the day Mary brought good luck to Dad. I was surprised when he asked us to go with him to a "letting" at the state capitol in Hartford. He had never invited me before. A civil engineer for the Osborne-Barnes Company in Danbury, he prepared estimates for new highway construction. The day the State Highway Commission awarded contracts to the lowest bidders was a tense time for him.

Mary and I were disappointed to miss the opening of the bids, but we were turned away from the crowded room. We wandered the halls of the ornate capitol building and studied the quaint penmanship of the ancient state charter. When we caught up with Dad, his smile said it all.

"Mary, you brought me good luck. Osborne-Barnes was low bidder at a price that will make us money. We're going to celebrate with lunch at the Hotel Bond. Then I'll drive you through Farmington, a really charming old Connecticut town where every house is built of wood."

Mother had her outing with "the girls" on a shopping trip in Bridgeport. When I tried on a pink spring coat, Mary nodded her approval. "Just right for Greensboro weather. Buy the coat and the navy dress with the white collar and cuffs. If you add the navy hat with the snazzy veil, you'll knock the men's eyes out." I doubted that, but I took her advice.

The next day, Mary took her first stroll down New York's Fifth Avenue. We window-shopped until Mary began to limp. "Cheer up, Mary. We'll rest in the theatre." We had tickets to a sold-out matinee performance starring Raymond Massey and Katherine Cornell in "The Doctor's Dilemma."

On the commuter train to Stamford, I slipped off my shoes. Although we felt we had done enough for one day, we were committed to dinner with Sam and Betty. They met our train and whisked us off to my favorite dining place, the Silvermine Tavern. Since stagecoach days, the inn had been noted for good food and hospitality. Part of the fun was saying hello to Abigail, the mannequin in colonial garb who stood by the bar.

On Thursday morning, the shrill alarm clock made Mary groan and hide her head under the pillow. "I can't believe we're going to New York two days in a row. On the other hand, I don't want to miss Fred Waring's live radio show tonight."

"Fred Waring and His Pennsylvanians," his orchestra and chorus, dedicated each performance to a different college or university. Much to our amazement, tonight he was going to recognize the Woman's College of the University of North Carolina.

Our return trip to the City, gave us a chance to see more New York highlights. Radio City Music Hall topped the list. I thought about the long wait for the Christmas show, but lines for the Easter show were shorter. As usual, the stage extravaganza eclipsed the movie, this time Vivien Leigh in "That Hamilton Woman."

"The tribute to spring took my breath away," said Mary. "When thunder, lightning, and rain forced the picnickers to run for cover, I felt I was really outdoors." She said she'd never forget the Rockettes dancing their precision routine under a spectacular rainbow.

The real world offered its own rewards — a ride atop a double-decker bus down Fifth Avenue to the Battery. On the boat ride to the Statue of Liberty, afternoon sun threw a rosy glow and deep shadows on the tall buildings of the skyline. Skeptical of my ability to climb the hundreds of steep stairs to the lady's crown, I clutched the sticky metal rail for support. At the top, the panorama of the New York skyline made me forget the agony of aching knees and racing heart.

The ferry ride back to the Battery seemed slow. Running late, Mary and I pooled our pocket money and splurged on a taxi. As we pulled up in front of the Vanderbilt Theatre, Mary pointed out the cab window. "Look at the marquee. 'Fred Waring and His Pennsylvanians Salute WCUNC.'" She left me to pay the fare.

We joined the crowd of our school friends waiting for the doors to open. The most memorable part of the show came after the broadcast, when Fred Waring put on a fifteen-minute show just for us, the students from Woman's College. Now I understood why Sam bragged about the MIT Glee Club singing with the Boston Pops.

Mary wanted to try a meal in the Automat. The food looked so enticing behind the small glass doors. It made me feel guilty to see so many poor people settle for a five-cent cup of coffee. Too tired to take in another sight, we dozed in the Newsreel Theatre until train time.

Mother and Dad had made certain this vacation ended on a high note. They reserved a three-room suite at The Hotel New Yorker for themselves, Sam, Sherman, Mary, and me. Visiting New York for the third time in a week, made us feel like celebrities. So did dining in the famous Empire Room before attending a theatre performance of "Hellzapoppin."

Our seats, best in the house — front row center in the loge — made us part of the action in the funniest show in town. A new approach to comedy, actors seated midst the audience sprang into action in weird situations. By the end of the second act, the audience had grown weak from laughter.

Early in the morning, Dad gathered the family in the coffee shop for waffles. Mary and I made the train out of Penn Station without a minute to spare. We kept waving long after we could no longer see Mother, Dad, Sam, and Sherman waving back from the platform.

Dreary rain streaked the windows to Washington, but sun burst through the clouds over the Blue Ridge Mountains of Virginia. We killed time by lingering over the sixty-cent special in the diner. Mary sighed. "Just think, last night we ate in the Empire room. Your parents gave us such a glorious week. I hope you realize how lucky you are."

We wrote down every detail of that fun-filled week. We did not want to forget a moment. Such a magical time was not apt to come again.

Carolina Spring

Hand in hand, April and spring arrived on campus. Colorful cotton skirts and blouses, matching the vivid green grass and masses of yellow forsythia, replaced winter woolens. By Easter, April 15, 1941, the air was balmy and mild, even at 3:15 a.m.

Mary and I joined a cluster of students waiting to board the bus in the moonlight. Since our return from Connecticut, we had looked forward to the Easter sunrise service at the Moravian settlement in Winston-Salem.

In old Salem, a large crowd had gathered in front of the stone church. As the clock in the steeple struck five, the service began with Bible readings and hymns. One by one, ten bands, stationed at various points in the city, repeated the same refrain. The notes of the brass instruments, some nearby some far away, echoed across the ancient graveyard.

Half an hour later, the sun, a huge red ball, rose over the freshly scrubbed gleaming marble tombstones set flat in the ground. The worshipers stood in silence moved by the simple service and the sight of row upon row of graves, each one decorated with a colorful bouquet of fresh flowers.

The quiet mood stayed with us on the ride back to Greensboro; the bus left us at the dining hall in time for breakfast. Back in our room, I loosened the green tissue in the corsage box I had found at the door. "Look at this — a corsage of pink roses to match my new coat." For as long as I could remember, Dad has always given Mother and me flowers on Easter. When I was a child, he always chose sweet peas for my corsage.

Mary sighed. "My father would never think to do that. Of course, if he did, Mother would say she was allergic to his choice." I tucked Dad's telegram in my pocket to read later. Mary's father would never have thought to send to her one of those either.

The following week, wisteria, tulips, lilacs, iris, and violets burst into bloom. What a romantic setting for the Freshman Formal. A disastrous time for us — we had no dates. To get in on the fun, Mary and I volunteered to serve the refreshments. Dressed in our formals, we appeared at midnight to ladle fruit punch and pass cookies to those lucky girls with dance partners.

A week later Mary settled for a blind date. She returned early. "I'm disgusted with myself. I never want another blind date. If I'm ever tempted, you remind me of 'the undertaker.' He spent the whole evening talking about autopsies and funerals."

While Mary's evening had fallen flat, mine had been a sobering look at the way events in Europe were about to change our world. Leland Stowe, an ace reporter and lecturer, described in shocking detail atrocities he had witnessed in Greece and France. At the climax of his speech he thundered, "The United States should enter the war. Now!" Caught up in his persuasive argument, most of us jumped to our feet and cheered.

Two days later, Mary and I had a crisis of our own. Mary's mother and her sister, Aunt Alverta, arrived for a visit. "They just want to inspect the way we live," Mary snapped. "We must clean, not only our room but the bathroom. You don't mind the smell of ammonia and I do. It will be your job to remove all the chewing gum from the bathroom floor."

Scraping gobs of chewing gum from the tile of the community bathroom, I wondered why this was necessary.

Mary washed the curtains and bedspreads, then tackled the walls and floor. If she had been less exhausted, she might have been more diplomatic when she greeted her mother in mid-afternoon.

The two ladies appeared at our door tightly corseted in fitted suits, sensible walking shoes, gloves, and hats. Mary's mother, Mrs. Kirschner, wore a smart navy blue straw with turned up brim. Above each temple a plump white pin, two inches long, protruded from the straw, adding contrast.

Mary's first words to her mother made me gasp. "That hat makes you look just like the devil." Mrs. Kirschner set her purse on the desk before bursting into tears. I wondered how Mary could be so heartless. Aunt Alverta rummaged in her handbag for a fresh linen handkerchief, which she handed to her sister.

When Mary tried to explain, she made matters worse. She said she did not mean to be insulting — the pins made her think of a devil's horns. Mrs. Kirschner retaliated by telling us she had never seen such a dirty room. Mary's lack of tact, as well as her Mother's outspokenness, made their relationship a strained one.

The next morning, as I rewashed the curtains before chemistry class, I pondered their harsh words. I gained new appreciation for my mother's light-hearted approach to life. Still angry with her mother, Mary, scrubbing the floor for the second time in two days, banged the scrub brush against the baseboards.

When Mrs. Kirschner arrived for lunch, she took no notice of our efforts. Further inspection brought another cutting remark. "Mary, I am shocked. I peeked in your bureau drawer and could not believe my eyes. You are not ironing your underwear." I wanted to laugh. No one in our dorm spent valuable time ironing rayon panties and silk slips. We just tolerated the wrinkles. Tight lipped, Mary turned away.

Dinner at the Jefferson Roof Garden, atop the tallest building in town, proved a success. Both ladies ate baked ham, sweet potatoes, and lemon meringue pie with gusto. For a few minutes, Mary and I relaxed.

Back at the dorm, we dropped in on an informal dance in the recreation room. Aunt Alverta applauded the dancers. Mary's mother did not. "Alverta, I'm surprised at you. I think jitterbugging is disgusting. Boys throwing girls up in the air like that with their underwear showing." I gave Mary a sly look. It wasn't for lack of trying we hadn't acquired that dancing skill.

The final day brought one more tearful episode. While we were in class, our guests went to a fortuneteller. "Just for fun," Aunt Alverta had said. Later we found them sitting on a bench by the dorm. Sobbing, Mary's mother refused to reveal the dire prediction disclosed by the cards. When she finally dried her eyes, she invited me to visit York in July.

As their train disappeared down the track, I wondered how much fun staying with the Kirschners would be.

Mary's Kin Folk

Relieved to speed Mrs. Kirschner and Aunt Alverta on their way, Mary and I turned to our neglected studies. During steamy days and torrid sleepless nights, we prepared for final exams. Suddenly, our first year at Woman's College was over. The promise of carefree vacation lay ahead.

Mary's final words before we parted in Washington brought excitement and apprehension. "I'm counting on your visit in July." The vacation away from my family would be a first. I wondered what life would be like with Mary's emotional mother.

Rested and relaxed after a month at home, feeling travel-wise and sophisticated, I followed the porter into the parlor car. Only once before had I traveled "first class," going to Atlantic City with Aunt Helen at age fourteen. Then, the porter with a clothes brush in his hand had made me uneasy. Now in 1941, approaching twenty, I appreciated Dad's treat. My long-planned visit to York, Pennsylvania was off to a good start.

After the cool luxury of the train, the sticky humidity on the grimy bus from Harrisburg to York made me miserable. My crisp blue and white seersucker suit grew wrinkled and limp and I wondered whether my shiny straw hat would melt. None of that mattered, when I spotted Mary and her sister, Elaine, standing in the shade of the bus station.

Elaine shared only one feature with Mary, blonde hair. Her skinny frame, sharp features, and high voice surprised me. "We want to take you on a walking tour of York," she enthused. I would have preferred lunch, but instead found myself in the impressive lobby of the library given to the city by one of her ancestors.

Charmed by the old four-story brick buildings hugging the city sidewalks, I forgot about food. We dropped in on Dr. Kirschner in his dental office. He greeted me with a twinkle in his eye. "Glad you could come. You look beat by this soggy weather. What you need is a glass of lemonade."

With that hint from their father, Mary and Elaine skipped taking me upstairs to see their apartment. The family lived in town during the school year. Mary drove us drove three miles to their summer home, a farmhouse half way up Queen Street Hill.

We turned off the highway onto a side road bordering the yard. Towering evergreens softened the outline of the tall fieldstone house, hinting of cool high-ceiling rooms within. To the east, golden fields draped the hillsides like blankets. To the west, far below in the valley, lay the city of York. Mary's mother stood on the steps to welcome me into her sunny spotless kitchen.

The next morning Mrs. Kirschner and I chatted over coffee, while the others slept. She glanced at her watch. "Time for me to be off to the Farmer's Market. I go three times a week for fresh vegetables, eggs, cheese, and meat. Our Pennsylvania Dutch farmers have become world-famous for their industry and high quality products. Come with me."

Driving to town, she chatted about the neighbors — how much their houses were worth and how much money they had. To me, that seemed a strange topic of conversation. No one at home ever discussed money. I had no idea of my father's salary or the cost of building our house. I soon knew that, and more, about the Kirschners and their friends.

At the bustling market in a huge brick building, plump housewives in plain dresses and starched caps stood behind an amazing array of fresh foods. I set our bulging market basket on a counter. "I never knew there were so many kinds of sausage and cheese. What is scrapple? I've never heard of it."

I found out the next morning at breakfast — a mixture of seasoned sausage and cornmeal formed into a loaf, cut in slices and fried. At lunch, Mrs. Kirschner introduced me to another of her favorites — red beet eggs. The longer the hard cooked eggs had been in contact with the pickled beets, the deeper the color.

After a thick sandwich on homemade bread bulging with cheese and cold cuts, she polished off one or two red beet eggs. "Keeping this house clean and cooking for Doc and four children takes energy. I have to eat well to keep up my strength." She was small and compact; I concluded her compulsion for cleanliness burned calories.

Mary and Elaine had gone shopping, which gave me a chance to ask Mrs. Kirschner about her childhood. As the middle child of nine in a German farm family, she had been raised to value thrift and contributing her share. No wonder she worked so hard. Over the years, her father had bought up neighboring farms and raised more crops. With prosperity came a new home for the family, a substantial Queen Anne he built in Dallastown. The older children never forgot the strict upbringing they had experienced.

Until I met Mary's aunts and uncles, I could not keep them straight. Eventually I knew them all, except Uncle Bill, the eldest who lived in Philadelphia. He had escaped the toil of farm life by becoming a perpetual student with degrees in law, medicine, and theology.

Aunt Mary, Aunt Florence, and Uncle Pete came in a single package. One evening Aunt Florence invited Mary, Elaine, and me to supper in the home she shared with Aunt Mary and Uncle Pete. Not a speck of dust ever settled in that parlor. "Girls, take off your belts," ordered Aunt Florence. I wondered why. Later Mary explained that her aunt feared we might scratch the piano.

Compared to her sister, Aunt Mary appeared reluctant to express an opinion. She had been intimidated by a scandal, which tainted her life. After a lavish home wedding, she and her groom departed in a carriage for the railway station. Only then did a neighbor gloat to her mother, "I never did like you, so I didn't tell you before. That man is already married"

When the bride received a telegram on the train, she expected congratulations, not the urgent appeal, "GET OFF THE TRAIN AT THE NEXT STATION. COME HOME." She followed the instructions and abandoned her new husband. She had never regained the confidence to lead a life of her own.

Uncle Pete, youngest of the nine, had not experienced the hard work required of some of his siblings. He flunked the bar exam twice and seemed content to drive his mother around in her limousine. Elaine whispered, "If Uncle Pete puts on a clean shirt, then decides on a different color, Aunt Mary washes and irons it before putting it back in the closet."

Uncle Stacy, former superintendent of schools in Lancaster, now slowed down by a stroke, and gracious Aunt Miriam entertained us for three days at their mountain home near Gettysburg. One evening Mary, her sister Elaine, and I raced down the hill to the main road. We found it great fun to sit on a fence and wave to the soldiers in an endless convoy of army trucks tearing along the dusty highway.

Elaine worried about her mother's reaction to the whistles and shouts we received for our efforts. "That's no problem," Mary assured her. "Tell her we did our patriotic duty." Far into the night, the rumble of the heavy trucks continued — a reminder of increasing preparations for war. Even on vacation, a cloud of uncertainty followed us everywhere.

Three weeks with Mary's hospitable family proved as broadening an experience as the first year of college had been. The emphasis on material wealth, hearty meals, and extreme cleanliness impressed me, but, most of all, I gained a new appreciation of my family and our way of life.

We never stayed home from a Saturday night movie while Mother scrubbed the cellar stairs. My father never bragged about how much money Uncle Will had made in the stock market. My aunts never quizzed me about boyfriends or asked when I planned to marry. Best of all, Mother never cried. She sang while she did dishes.

I felt it a privilege to have been accepted by such a large and unusual family. Mary's relatives became mine adding many new names to my address book.

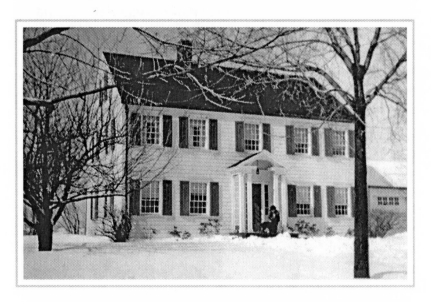

Family Home in Danbury, Connecticut.

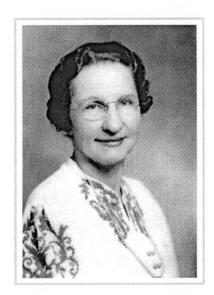 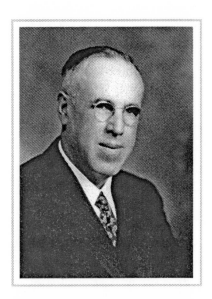

Hazel Andrews Morrison and Garfield Morrison.

Sophomore Year 1941-1942

After my return to Connecticut from Mary's in July of 1941, my thoughts often turned to the truck convoys of soldiers we had seen near Gettysburg. All those eager, young faces whistling and shouting at three young women perched on a fence. The shock of seeing the vast numbers of men training for war haunted me.

Even the movies that summer offered no respite from the ominous news on the radio. Newsreels showed graphic pictures of the armed strength of Germany and Italy, the terror of fleeing refugees and horror of battle. Such scenes were a chilling reminder that only an ocean separated us from the death and destruction in Europe.

Back home, I faced more immediate concerns. When I saw Mother, I blurted out, "What has happened to you?" Usually so full of energy, she had lost weight, grown weak, and taken to her bed. The doctor had no explanation for her rapid heart rate.

Throughout hot humid August, I cooked, cleaned, and shopped. Dad came home on weekends from the highway construction site in Whitehall, New York. Reluctant to leave Mother alone during the week, I felt guilty about returning to college. She refused to be swayed by my concerns.

"I will worry if you stay here. You cannot afford to interrupt your education. It means the world to Dad and me that you're doing so well. I'm sure I'll be better by the time you come home for Christmas."

My last weekend at home. As the family celebrated my birthday, I felt sad. The bad news from Europe added to my worry about my mother. Turning twenty made me feel so old!

My friend Betty Urban's spirits soared even though mine had sunk. She too was going to college, to the University of South Carolina. Her brother Ernie, shocked by their father's attitude that a college education for Betty would be a waste of money, had kept at Bill Urban until he gave in.

Betty had called to give me the good news. "I wish I could go to Woman's College with you, but the University of South Carolina costs less and you know Daddy. I don't dare rock the boat. He might change his mind and make me stay home."

The day of my return to college, Dad and I took the early train to New York. We ran out of time before we ran out of things to say. When he put me on the train to Washington, D.C, I had to settle for a seat in a smoking car. As I eavesdropped on the young couple across the isle, the smoke was forgotten.

Determined to marry before the youth met his draft board, they were eloping to Elkton, Maryland. They hoped no one would question their underage status in a town notorious for performing "quickie marriages."

The train ride from Washington to Greensboro ended after dark. Mary greeted me with exciting news. "Carol, I told you I could change our room assignment. I made a lot of noise and it worked. We've been moved to one of two new dormitories completed during the summer." A week later, the name changed to Winfield Hall giving us a classy new address to match our new quarters.

We liked our sparkling, modern room with a washbasin tucked in the corner. The western exposure gave us a glimpse of sunsets over a tiny lake. That compensated for the room location, opposite the only phone in the dorm.

Concealed in an airless closet, the phone rang until answered by whoever passed by. When the ringing got on our nerves, one of us dashed across the hall to say, "Hello." We became adept at shouting down the hall, "So and so, you're wanted on the phone."

A modern, spacious bathroom meant no more waiting in line for facilities — two tubs and showers, six toilets, a sink for washing hair, and even a chute to send trash to the basement. The pressing room became the busiest place on the hall.

A paneled living room furnished with colonial style furniture set the tone for southern hospitality. From the outside, the pediment over the front entrance and the soft glow of old brick covering the three-story building reminded us of Williamsburg. In such gracious surroundings, sophomore year held great promise.

The buzz on campus concerned army maneuvers to take place in the Carolinas during the fall. The expectation of five thousand soldiers in town every weekend thrilled the students, but not the faculty. Determined to protect us from rowdy young men of unknown origin, they issued a flurry of new regulations to keep us isolated on campus.

"We can no longer leave campus on weekends, except for church?" Mary threw down the instruction sheet. "No strolls to the corner drugstore, no movies, no walks on Sunday afternoon. How can we live like that? Might as well be prisoners"

Being restricted to campus had its compensations. Not a soldier appeared on Saturday, only a few on Sunday morning, but dozens in the afternoon. By evening hundreds of khaki uniforms swarmed the campus. Mary wanted to talk to the men, even though we had not been introduced. We strolled across the grassy quadrangle with Mary's sister Elaine, and Elaine's roommate, Ginny Haynes.

Elaine and Ginny, a welcome addition to our group of friends, were adjusting to their role as freshmen. Ginny, friendly as a puppy, with a North Carolina lilt to her voice, had grown up in Greensboro. An art major, Ginny had moved to the dorm to participate fully in campus life. Her auburn hair, infectious grin, and healthy glow contrasted with blonde Elaine's skinny frame and fussy ways. Ginny had silenced Elaine's complaint about dust under her bed by drawing a chalk line down the center of the room. Elaine swept her half every day.

Returning from milkshakes at the Tavern, a campus hangout, we had not found a way to approach a soldier. A hungry GI took care of that. As Mary nibbled on a Hershey Bar, he broke away from his group of buddies. "Ma'am, would you give me a bite?"

"Sure." She handed him half the candy bar. Elaine, and Ginny looked stunned at Mary's audacity. How dare she speak to a soldier! They drifted away. Mary and I turned our attention to the private and his buddy, who walked with us toward the dorm.

My conquest proved to be a reserved, quiet type from New Hampshire. Two New Englanders, we had much in common. Mary found herself with a fast talker. She giggled when he told her she had beautiful dimples, rolled her eyes when he grew bolder. "Your hair is like a golden shower. Your eyes, your eyes are like the stars." Before she could reply, the final bell sounded. Curfew sent us scurrying to Winfield Hall.

That evening established the pattern for future dates. Mary flirted outrageously while I tried to develop that light touch. Although she often ended up with both men, I never had more fun in my life. Whenever Mary looked my way, I'd say, "Your eyes are like the stars." That private joke always made us laugh.

The last weekend of September, fifteen thousand military personnel swarmed the streets of Greensboro and the Woman's College campus. A surprising sight greeted us on Sunday morning; sleeping soldiers lay under every tree and bush. The men had been ordered south from New England wearing wool uniforms. The intense heat of the previous two weeks had left them exhausted and disgusted. We tried to improve their morale offering them bottles of Coca-Cola.

The realities of army life had already changed the carefree attitudes of our heroes. We listened in horror to tales of paratroopers told to "Jump," who found themselves dangling from high-tension wires. We heard disturbing reports about court-martials, illness, suicide, and the alarming lack of equipment.

The influx of service men soon forced Woman's College to join citizens of Greensboro in planning weekend entertainment for the bored draftees. Six weeks had changed the role of the students. No longer encouraged to avoid service men, we were urged to treat them as our brothers.

Three hundred soldiers and two hundred college girls jammed the college gymnasium every Saturday night to dance. Strict rules still governed our behavior. Once inside the building no one was allowed to leave until the conclusion of the dance.

As the last strains of "Goodnight Ladies" faded away, the men were ordered to line the walls. The women, escorted by college personnel, returned to the dorms. After the last formal gown disappeared from sight, the men boarded buses and returned to Basic Training Center No. 10.

One evening a little fellow from Tennessee told me he wished we could dance all night. He would have been disappointed to know I longed only for a hot bath to soothe my aching feet. Dancing slippers were no match for army boots.

Gold Versus Silver

Our weekends became crowded with dances, movies in Aycock Auditorium, recreational activities, and music under the stars. Sunday morning coffee and doughnuts enticed a crowd to the Religious Activities Center. Sunday evening vespers drew some unlikely participants — their last chance to snag a date for the following weekend.

The weekly campus newspaper, "The Carolinian," offered advice. "So, he's a lieutenant! Can you prove it or is that what he said? He's as clearly labeled as a can of beans. There are several ways you can distinguish him. First, by instinct, which psychologists tell us does not usually exist. Second, by the way he walks -- long, military strides and an extra special ramrod back bone. The third is in plain sight: one shiny bar on each shoulder, gold for second louie, silver for first. Go off the gold standard. This time it pays!"

Mary signed up for a dance, assured the men had been in college before being drafted. She met only one college graduate and spent the evening with a cop from New Jersey. When conversation lagged, she asked, "Is it true that all policemen are flat footed?"

He replied, dejectedly, "Gosh! I wish that was true. Then I wouldn't be in the army."

One Sunday afternoon, Mary and I took two young men from Brooklyn canoeing on the little campus lake. We invited them to stay for supper. Joe shook his head. "Wish we could but we have to hitchhike one hundred miles back to camp before midnight."

Their departure was a lucky break for me. One of my friends told me she had met a first lieutenant from Danbury, Connecticut. I questioned every soldier I could find with silver bars on his shoulders, until I found the right one. That's when I went off the gold standard.

John Zimmerman, First Lieutenant John Zimmerman, tall with the ramrod posture of an officer, told me he had lived on Montgomery Street a few doors from my Aunt Katie. That coincidence made us immediate friends. "John, the south has its charms but I'm homesick for Connecticut. How about you?"

He guided me to a bench under an oak tree. "I was miserable in early October thinking about home and the Danbury Fair. Remember how schools were closed the Friday of Fair week? Early in the morning I joined every kid in town at the entrance long before the gates opened," He laughed. "I probably saw you eating cotton candy. We boys always snuck off to gawk at the rubber man and the hoochie-koochie girls in the sideshow."

Lingering over milkshakes at the Tavern, I found it painful when John told me he had already received orders to go overseas. This one encounter would be our only meeting until after the war, if he had the good luck to make it back. As I walked alone to the dorm, I could still feel his warm hand over mine.

Rumors had spread fast. Back at Winfield hall, my friends peppered me with questions. "Did you really have a date with a tall, handsome officer? How did you meet him?" Someone even suggested I kissed him goodbye. The upcoming chemistry test forgotten, Mary and I talked until dawn.

The following Saturday, Mary and I, having vowed to never spend another Saturday night writing letters, crossed the lawn looking for prey. We snared two soldiers escorted by a civilian youth from Greensboro. I was embarrassed when Miss Hathaway, our freshman counselor, walked by. She could not hide her surprise. Mary had a soldier on one arm and a civilian on the other. I trailed behind holding hands with a private.

"I used to be a corporal," he confessed. "One sad day I got demoted for failing to awaken the cooks until 8:30 a.m. I attended the University of Denver for two years, but now I'm nothing but a private in the army." Mary almost choked, when she heard my date say, "If I ever marry, I want to take my wife to the Shenandoah Valley for a honeymoon."

A special train to take Woman's College students to Chapel Hill for the annual football game between North Carolina State and the University of North Carolina looked like a way to escape campus. At the last moment, due to troop movements, the railroad could not furnish the coaches.

Only 200 bus seats were available. I stood in line for two hours, but the girl ahead of me picked up the last tickets. Frustrated, I agreed to go on a date at 9:00 p.m. That was a mistake.

He turned out to be the worst soldier I had ever met, a radical with a huge chip on his shoulder. He disliked the army, the food, the weather, the people, and everything else. A few like him and I would give up my patriotic duty to men in uniform. Later I found out he was AWOL.

By the second week in November, 359,000 officers and men were assembled in sixteen counties in North and South Carolina.

During weeks of intense field training, their activities increased in severity and resemblance to wartime conditions.

General George C. Marshall, Chief of Staff, arrived to take charge of operations. He was about to test the preparedness of the troops in a mock battle between the Red Army and the Blue Army. He announced these would be the largest peacetime maneuvers ever held in the United States.

Rumors predicted the troops were leaving the area four weeks earlier than scheduled. We would miss the boys but seized the opportunity to plan a shopping trip, only to be told the rumors were false. We remained restricted to campus.

However, a week later not one soldier came in sight. Both the armies had moved farther south to conduct their battle. The students were jubilant. Restrictions were lifted and we felt free at last. In downtown Greensboro, the chatter of college students intent on Christmas shopping replaced the whistles of soldiers. Only three weekends remained before Christmas vacation.

The Southern Railroad boosted our spirits with the promise of special coaches for W.C. girls on December 19. That train would transport us to Washington, D.C., along with some of the 100,000 soldiers heading north for Christmas. From there to New York, we would be on our own.

After the experiences of the past four months, dealing with a few hundred military men on a train would not faze me at all.

December 7, 1941

After the war games ended, tranquility blanketed Winfield Hall. Much as the students missed the soldiers, the majority of us felt relieved to turn our attention to neglected studies. We looked forward to weekends and the freedom to escape the campus. Suddenly, our carefree way of life was shattered by a cataclysmic event.

December 7 began with the persistent ringing of the hall phone opposite Mary's and my room. Irked, I forced myself out of bed to answer. The urgent voice of Dr. Collins, the college physician, asking to speak to Mary, sent me scurrying across the hall to wake her. Mary held the receiver away from her ear to let me listen in on their conversation.

"Mary, your sister is in the infirmary with acute appendicitis. It's imperative I operate at once. I need your parents' permission. Please contact them and ask them to call me. Elaine wants to see you before she goes to the hospital."

With a shaky hand, Mary fed coins into the pay phone and called her father in York, Pennsylvania. She caught him off guard by demanding he give Dr. Collins permission to operate on Elaine. He thundered his angry response. "No jerk is going to operate on my daughter."

Too upset to respond, Mary handed me the phone. I held the receiver at arm's length until Dr. Kirschner paused to catch his breath. I tried to stay calm. "Dr. Kirschner, you don't want to wait until Elaine has a burst appendix, do you?"

After a long silence, he replied with a sigh, "No, Dr. Collins has my permission to operate."

As Mary and I rushed from the room and headed for the infirmary, I grabbed the familiar Western Union telegram stuck under the door. My father never failed to send a telegram or special delivery letter every Sunday. I jammed the envelope in my purse to read later.

We found Elaine calm in spite of her pain. Dr. Collins explained she would drive the three of us to the hospital. She ordered the patient to lie on the back seat under a blanket. She assured Mary and me we could squeeze in the front seat without interfering with her driving. At the emergency entrance, Elaine disappeared on a gurney.

We settled down on a worn-out sofa to await the outcome of the surgery. I withdrew the telegram I had tucked in my purse. The words on the yellow form stunned and shocked me.

MOTHER HAD THYROID SURGERY THIS MORNING NEW ENGLAND BAPTIST HOSPITAL BOSTON. DOING SPLENDIDLY. CAN PROBABLY GO HOME SATURDAY.

I read and reread the message. Why hadn't I been told about her condition? After all, I had cared for her all summer while the doctor had searched for the cause of her rapid heartbeat. Was I being spared the truth of her condition?

When Elaine was wheeled into her room, after successful removal of her appendix, I had to put those worries aside. Dr. Collins told us a shortage of nurses meant we'd have to take on those duties during the day shift. Still upset with her father, Mary announced she was "no nurse" and could not stand the smell of ether. I didn't care for it myself, but I took Mary's place by the bed and held Elaine's head to help her through bouts of nausea. Mary moved to the corner of the room to study.

Suddenly, an agitated young man, carrying a large bouquet and a newspaper, burst into the room. He shook Elaine's arm, "Wake up Elaine, wake up. Elaine! Elaine! Japan has bombed Pearl Harbor." In her groggy state, Elaine did not respond, even when he placed the flowers on her pillow.

He turned to Mary and ran his hands through his hair. "My name is Rep. I dated Elaine last night. How could this happen to her so fast?"

I grabbed the paper and stared at the jet-black, four-inch high headline. PEARL HARBOR BOMBED HUNDREDS KILLED. Shrill voices of newsboys on the sidewalk outside penetrated the quiet room. "Extra! Extra! Japanese Bomb Pearl Harbor Extra! Extra!" I tried to make sense of the meager details in the paper. Surprise attack, severe damage to the fleet, many ships sunk, appalling loss of life, chaos everywhere, and the President to address the nation.

Before he disappeared, Rep mumbled something about returning later. The afternoon wore on. Mary had been right about one thing — she lacked the patience to be a good nurse. Agreeing Elaine would get more rest without her, she headed back to the dorm to study for her Spanish exam. I relaxed in the quiet room and stroked Elaine's hot hand. At last, there was time to reread the telegram.

Upon reflection, I accepted Dad's word that Mother was doing well. My heart sank as I thought about Ernie, now a sergeant stationed in Pine Camp, New York. I wondered how soon he'd be sent overseas. In his last phone call, he had sounded disappointed and disgusted.

"I've been turned down for Officer's Candidate School over lack of a few lousy pounds. I'm ten pounds under weight." He'd sighed, "At least, my new assignment relieves me of dull office work. I'm now the aerial photographer for Pine Camp."

Oh, Ernie! Memories of those Saturday night dates the previous summer took on new significance. Would we ever see another play at The Westport Playhouse? Would we ever again stroll under the stars?

And what lay ahead for John Zimmerman, the Lieutenant from Danbury? Only weeks ago, we'd spent that delightful afternoon together before he shipped out for England. He and Ernie had shared the conviction that our entry into the war was inevitable. They had been frustrated by inaction, but now we faced enemies not on one continent, but two.

The War Games we had witnessed during the fall had not been games. They had been a prelude to War. The men with whom we had shared milkshakes, strolled the campus, danced till midnight in the gym, now faced the grim reality of gearing up for battle.

Elaine's plea for water brought me back to her hospital room. The nurse, who came to check on her, assured me Elaine would have a comfortable night. Visiting hours were over. I must go. In front of the hospital, a lone paperboy still shouted the news. "Japanese Bomb Pearl Harbor." Aware of the scent of ether clinging to my hair and clothes, I breathed in the refreshing night air. My heart remained heavy.

Digging deep in my purse, I found thirty cents for a taxi ride back to campus. An eerie silence lay over the deserted streets. I could guess where all the people had gone. Men, women, and children were glued to their radios listening in fear for further news about Pearl Harbor. Only the stars twinkling in an inky sky had not changed.

December 7,1941. Little did I know that I would be the first among my friends to have my world shattered by World War II.

A Changed World

The morning after the disastrous attack on Pearl Harbor, students, faculty, and employees milled about the campus in a daze. Awaiting the president's address, scheduled for noon, we expressed bitter feelings of shock and fear. Students who never before had paid attention to the news huddled around the radio with those of us who had anticipated war against Germany.

President Roosevelt, in a ringing voice, grave and angry, proclaimed December 7 "a date which will live in infamy." His declaration that America would win an absolute victory in the ensuing struggle aroused our fighting spirit and patriotism. When the president asked Congress to declare war on Japan, members complied in twenty minutes.

Woman's College students noted with dismay the action of Congresswoman Jeanette Rankin of Montana, the only woman in Congress, and the only person to vote against going to war. The severity of the surprise attack united the country. Isolationism disappeared overnight.

The approach of Christmas did not deter draft boards from ordering thousands to report immediately for basic training, much to the dismay of mothers and wives. Those of us with loved ones who already served knew our men would be the first to face the enemy.

Our college counselors emphasized we could best serve our country by studying hard to finish our educations. "Women will be called on to perform jobs and assume responsibilities you can not imagine. The shortage of manpower will give you amazing opportunities. As college graduates, you will be the ones called on to lead."

The Christmas concert by the college choir took place, but the carol sing on the quadrangle was cancelled. No one had the heart for that. One good thing came out of the new government rules and regulations being churned out every hour. Due to the cancellation of all special trains, the dean allowed us to leave for vacation on Friday night instead of after class on Saturday morning.

Mary decided to take her chances for space on a Saturday train. Barbara Hollister and I, bound for Connecticut, shivered on the platform in the damp air Friday night. By the time the train pulled in, four hours late at 9:30 p.m., we wished we had waited until morning.

Barb had come prepared. "Here's a towel to cover that dirty plush so you can keep your hair clean. I have chocolate bars and magazines. Let's relax." When two soldiers asked to join us, Barb made sure they played bridge before saying, "yes."

After changing trains in Washington, we headed for the diner. Steaming coffee, ham, eggs, biscuits, and honey restored our flagging energy. Early morning light outlined the bare branches of the trees foretelling a clear day. Although the train made up some time, we arrived two hours late.

Cousin Ted and Aunt Pauline stood waiting opposite our car. Ted brushed aside my apologies over our late arrival. "We're used to delayed trains now that troop carriers have priority over civilian travelers." He changed the subject. "You look great. How's life as a southern belle?" Same old Ted, always joking.

In some ways, he had changed. He paid no attention when Aunt Pauline complained about his driving. Unlike Mother's sunny disposition, her sister had a sharp tongue. Aunt Pauline's word used to rule. Ted, now a draftsman with a responsible job in a defense plant, felt confident to take charge. He told me his draft number would come up any day. Until then, he was socking away his overtime pay toward college after the war.

Two hours later, Ted delivered me to my front door. He leaned on the horn to announce my arrival. Mother opened the door glowing with happiness, but still pale and thin after her surgery. Dad smiled over her shoulder. When she admitted she needed a nap, Dad swept me off to go Christmas shopping. Snuggling into Mother's new fur coat, I forgot I had been up for thirty hours.

The next morning, I tried to prepare a breakfast equal to that in the diner. Fourteen year-old Sherman buttered a hot biscuit.

"I'm glad you're studying Home Ec instead of French or something. Since Mother's been sick, Dad and I've almost starved." I sensed this vacation would offer few chances to relax.

A phone call from my soldier, Ernie, took me by surprise. "Honey, I'll see you in about an hour. Have only a three-day pass and you take top priority. Once the relatives get hold of me, it will be impossible to get away."

I slipped into my new red wool dress and sat on the stairs. Breathing the woodsy scent of princess pine wound around the banister, I watched through the narrow window next to the front door for Ernie. As he bounded up the front steps, I opened the door wide. His hugs and kisses made my homecoming complete.

He handed me a thin silver box. Nestled in tissue lay a sword shaped letter opener. "So you'll think of me every time you open your mail," he whispered. "How about dinner tomorrow night? I'll make my specialty, chicken curry."

His plans changed. His sister Betty and my brother Sam joined us at Silvermine Tavern three miles from the Urban's home. Sitting by a roaring fire in the taproom, we paid no attention to the fog swirling past the windows. The drive back in a dense curtain of white proved to be a nightmare. A call from Dad made it a Christmas present in disguise.

"The weather is too dangerous for you to drive home. I suggest you spend the night with cousin Mildred." Sam and I saw no point in driving at all. We stayed right where we were, the four of us under the Christmas tree eating popcorn far into the night.

Ernie and I moved to the sofa where we cuddled more than we talked. We did not discuss the hazards of war. He must have felt the same sinking feeling I did. He lifted my hand to his lips. "I hope, when you come home in May, I'm still stationed around here." I could not know then that the glow of that evening would have to last me a lifetime.

In the morning, Sam and I had no problem driving home. We wondered about Mother and Dad's experiences in World

War I. When we asked them, they told us they had truly believed they were fighting a war "to end all wars." They found it hard to comprehend we children now faced the disruptions in our lives they had experienced twenty-five years earlier.

Dazed by events of the past two weeks, the family found strength in time together. Even Sherman passed up some of his parties to spend evenings with the adults by the fire. Christmas day became memorable for its simplicity; only Grandma and Grandpa joined us for dinner that year.

Although Ernie had returned to camp, Sam and Betty convinced me New Year's Eve called for one last fling. I felt lucky I could count on my cousins when I needed a date. My cousin Bob joined us for dinner and dancing at the Hotel Barnum in Bridgeport.

Next to petite Betty, in her black skirt and red jacket, I felt tall and elegant in a chic gold chiffon gown trimmed with black lace. In the crowded ballroom, we discovered many revelers had begun their celebration hours earlier. Sam looked at the tables jammed close together and watched a fellow who was attempting an unsteady highland fling. "Let's go. This doesn't look like fun."

Bob shook his head. "Oh no. We can't get our money back. Where else could we go at 10:00 p.m. on New Year's Eve?" He swept me onto the dance floor, leaving Sam and Betty to fight their way to our table. Determined to enjoy ourselves, Bob and I joined a conga line that snaked around the ballroom.

After a first course of grapefruit, we danced the fox trot. Following the main course of steak, potatoes au gratin, peas, and hot rolls, we danced a two-step. We left the ice cream melting in favor of a dreamy waltz. Sam drained his coffee cup and asked for more. "At last, something to drink. The waiter refused to bring us water but I'm not going to order liquor just to please him."

My brother sent a disapproving glance in my direction; I had shared Bob's bourbon. As more people crowded into the room, the temperature rose to equal the tropics. I felt I was watching a movie when I saw a man slip into oblivion under the table.

We counted down the last seconds of 1941. "Happy New Year." Amid the din of noisemakers in a swirl of confetti and streamers, Bob tipped back my head and looked into my eyes. "Remember the first time I kissed you on your birthday? Sweet sixteen and never been kissed." I remembered.

Many of the revelers missed out on midnight, done in by too much liquor and too many snake dances in a hot room. A photographer, cameras hanging round his neck, stopped at our table. "You're the only sober group I see. How about posing for the Bridgeport Post? Your picture will appear in the Sunday paper." That would send shock waves through Mother. She did not approve of "that scandal sheet."

Bob conferred with Sam. "We'd better get the girls out of here before the manager calls the riot squad." On the drive home, Betty and I thanked the boys for taking good care of us. We agreed New Year's Eve on the town had been disillusioning.

That did not discourage us from enjoying the notoriety of our only appearance in the Sunday Supplement, on January 3,1942.

Spring Break

Mary and I could scarcely believe our good fortune. In April 1942, we were headed to Daytona Beach, Florida aboard the *Silver Meteor* for spring break. Our exciting plans had been the talk of the dorm for weeks.

When Mother and Dad spent their Florida winter vacation with their friends, Clinton and Genevieve Hawkins, they stayed on the *Miome*, Clinton's thirty-six foot cabin cruiser tied up at the Daytona Beach Boat Works. The four of them had come up with a vacation plan for Mary and me. Genevieve wrote to suggest we spend our weeklong break on the *Miome*.

Clinton and Genevieve were like family to me. They spent time at our home every year when they visited friends in the north to escape the summer heat in Florida. Due to the government ban on gasoline for pleasure craft, they could no longer ply the inland waterway or cruise anywhere for the duration of the war.

Mother and Clinton had first met in 1916, when Mother was supervisor of art in the schools of Chicopee, Massachusetts and took china-painting classes from Mrs. Prindle in her home. Clinton was then personal secretary and accountant to the well-to-do widow.

Mother told me the rest of the story in strictest confidence. "Mrs. Prindle was the last of her family. Upon her death, Clinton inherited her imposing home and her money. You can imagine how he shocked the staid New England community when he married Genevieve, Mrs. Prindle's Polish maid."

Of course, I had told Mary, but she did not mention the scandal in her carefully worded request to her parents for permission to make the trip. She emphasized the fun it would be to lie in the sun every day and acquire a tan on Daytona Beach.

Her mother gave a predictable response. "I've been counting on you and Carol coming here. It would be cheaper for you to come home."

Even Mary's Uncle Stacy wrote his disapproval. "Don't you think you are being overzealous to think two college girls can handle a trip to Florida?"

His attempt to dampen our enthusiasm had no effect. I laughed and said, "Your Uncle Stacy would be shocked if he knew, not only did Clinton upset the neighbors by marrying Genevieve, he sold Mrs. Prindle's home and invested the money in his yacht. Naming the boat *Miome*, a contraction of 'my home,' is typical Clinton humor."

Mary's father settled the matter. She read me a few lines from his letter. "I had a hard time convincing your mother she could not deny you the opportunity of a lifetime. The way this war is going, this may be your last chance for a real vacation."

Mary waved a green check in the air. "Here's the money for my ticket. It's all set. We can go."

After an exhausting night sitting up on the *Silver Meteor*, Mary and I arrived in Daytona Beach in mid-afternoon, disheveled, hungry, and six hours late. We has spent much time on sidings watching troop trains flash by on the main track.

At the Daytona Beach station, Clinton, genial and rotund, peered at us through gold-rimmed glasses. Genevieve, tall and friendly, gave us hearty hugs. They rushed us to Howard Johnson's for fried chicken and cokes. Clinton suggested ice cream, but I fell in with Mary's suggestion to skip dessert. "Let's go. We can't wait to see the beach."

Pictures had not captured the beauty of that coast. Under a brilliant blue sky, reflected in the sparkling ocean, a frothy collar of breakers rolled over the hard-packed sand. We drove miles along deserted beach. Vacation no longer existed for men our age busy fighting two wars. Occasionally, Clinton scanned the horizon with his field glasses. As an air raid warden, he had been told German submarines were reported in the area.

When we entered the gate to the Daytona Beach Boat Works, Genevieve told us the shipbuilding program of the Coast Guard continued twenty-four hours a day. Impatient as we were to see the *Miome*, we could go no farther until the Coast Guard issued us identification numbers. We would be required to carry passes at all times.

As we walked along the dock, Clinton pointed out his pride and joy, tied up between two larger yachts. An enclosed deckhouse rose above the white hull. Mahogany trim gleamed and brass fittings shone. When Mary and I stepped from the gangplank onto the deck, we were surprised to see such cramped quarters.

Our indoctrination to shipboard living began at once. Steep stairs descended to forward and aft cabins separated by a tiny galley, a bench, and a fold-up table against the wall. The head took up the space we presumed to be a small closet. We mastered bed making on the narrow bunks, but I forgot to duck and hit my head going topside.

Genevieve amazed us by turning out a delicious meal in her one-person galley. She passed the food up the stairs to us in the wheelhouse, and we made space for the plates on the small table decorated with dyed Easter eggs. As we ate baked ham followed by lemon meringue pie, passersby on the dock peered down at us through the open windows and stopped to chat. Clinton bragged, "Yes, the eggs are my contribution to the dinner."

The four of us lingered over coffee and watched vast fingers of light spring into the night sky, a test by the army of huge spotlights. The searchlights caught distant silver planes, which looked like helpless bugs fighting to escape into the darkness.

In the morning, Mary and I awoke to bright Florida sunshine. Large tumblers of fresh squeezed orange juice awaited us on deck. Clinton must have spread word of our arrival, for several boat owners stopped by to say hello, but he did not allow us to linger over breakfast.

Mary and I learned an unpleasant fact familiar to every sailor — brass fittings must be polished every day. Regardless of plans, top priority went to applying polish and elbow grease to brass rails, cleats, and the ship's bell. That task completed, we received our reward, a refreshing swim in the warm Atlantic Ocean and a picnic on the beach.

The beach picnic did not turn out quite like the relaxed afternoon we had anticipated. Instead of gentle breezes, we fought strong winds and blowing sand. As Mary and I munched on gritty sandwiches, we watched soldiers testing their new vehicles with a new name, "Jeeps."

"Hop in. We'll take you for a ride," offered a brash private in a rumpled uniform.

Mary shook her head. "No thanks." She turned to Clinton. "I like adventure, but I don't trust that soldier or his jeep."

That evening, we sat on deck and watched the sunset. Clinton pulled his canvas chair next to mine. "Carol, you know I think the world of your parents, but there's one part of your education they have sadly neglected. Your mother brags she's so dry her bones rattle. That will not do. I plan to educate you in ways she would not understand." He checked the flags on a passing ship. "I'm going to teach you and Mary how to drink. By the end of the week, you'll be able to handle yourselves in any situation."

That sounded exciting to one who had sampled her first bourbon the previous New Year's Eve. How surprised Mother and Dad would be if they knew the tack this vacation had taken.

As if on cue, a handsome sea captain came sauntering down the dock. Clinton invited him aboard, "Mary, Carol, meet Captain Loring." Lesson Number One was about to begin.

The captain rambled on about his duties on the yacht, the *Carolyn*. Mary and I showed more interest in the tray of glasses Genevieve brought from the galley — our introduction to a rum Collins. Clinton handed Mary and me cold glasses of the refreshing beverage. "Never mix your drinks," he admonished. "Whatever you start with, you stick to that drink for the evening."

With that advice, we began our night on the town. At an arcade on the beach, a penny fed into a machine indicated how "Hot" the person's personality. Only for Clinton, did the needle shoot up to "Naughty" and stay there.

We continued our lesson at The Pier. Mary and Captain Loring danced well together but I stumbled over the captain's feet. The combination of the night train to Florida, sunburn, and more than one rum Collins had made me sleepy. Genevieve said Mary and I looked exhausted. She herded us back to our bunks on the *Miome*.

The next day Mary and I took it easy; we went to see a movie — "The Courtship of Andy Hardy." We were amused by the latest slang expressions of 1942. Girls were "droops" and "zip diggers" in the lexicon of Mickey Rooney.

In the evening, Clinton reported for air raid duty, leaving us aboard the *Miome* to watch the drill. At 10:00 p.m., sirens wailed the first blackout warning. Genevieve, Mary, and I stood on the dock and watched the jeweled lights of Daytona Beach vanish. The boatyard plunged into inky darkness, leaving us in a black void of eerie silence. Overhead enormous stars shone against the black velvet of the night sky.

After five long minutes, bright light once again bathed the boatyard. Government work, supervised by the Coast Guard, could not be delayed. The city remained dark for half an hour. Clinton returned from patrol carrying his loaded pistol. He shook his head in mock dismay. "Not one person came along whom I could shoot."

The drill continued until midnight. Powerful lights on five planes swept the wide expanse of the heavens. As the planes circled, we grew accustomed to the engines' roar overhead. The sound followed us when Mary and I went below. Before she fell asleep, Mary mused, "I wonder how we'd react if this were the real thing."

Up with the rising sun, Mary and I hurried through our stint polishing brass. This day had been set aside for sightseeing.

In St. Augustine we toured the oldest house in the United States before Clinton headed inland through miles of moss draped trees and swampland. Mileposts assured us we would soon reach Hotel Riviera, "The Only Hotel Bar within One Hundred Miles." When Clinton parked near a low building hidden by palm trees, we realized he had chosen isolated Hotel Riviera for Lesson Number Two.

"Never drink on an empty stomach. Nibble on cheese or whatever snack is handy." With those words, Clinton handed Mary a martini. She smiled, twirling the stemmed glass in her fingers.

After one sip she gagged and muttered, "That's too strong for me." Clinton replaced her cocktail with Southern Comfort over ice. Aided by cheese, I finished the martini, including the olive. Secretly, I decided to follow Mary's example and cross martinis off my list.

Mary became so dizzy that Clinton transferred us from the Hotel Riviera bar to Howard Johnson's for hamburgers and black coffee. He assessed her reaction, "Mary, I'm not sure alcohol agrees with you."

She concurred. "I think you're right. No matter what kind of alcohol I drink, it always makes me giddy. I don't enjoy it. I'm switching to coke."

Back on the *Miome*, we found an invitation from another captain friend of Clinton's. Captain Lowrey wanted us to join him aboard his yacht, the *Masquerader*, owned by John Charles Thomas, a renowned opera singer. The captain gave Mary and me free rein to explore bow to stern.

The silver cocktail service and silver serving dishes on the buffet outdid the displays we had seen in jewelry stores. Under the lid of the baby grand piano an electric light burned night and day to counteract the humidity. I stretched out on a chaise lounge in the art deco master stateroom. "Do I look like Rita Hayworth? I wasn't expecting this kind of luxury on a boat."

Mary picked up a perfume bottle. "I can't imagine a yacht costing one hundred and forty thousand dollars. Who could afford to charter this boat for ten thousand dollars a month? Harry said that doesn't include charges for passengers, guests and food!"

Before we went ashore, Mary and Clinton pounded out chopsticks on John Charles Thomas' piano. Captain Lowrey agreed to join us for cocktails on the *Miome*. Genevieve made old fashioneds. I relaxed, at last a drink I could enjoy.

Once again, Captain Loring strolled down the pier, but this time he brought along his girlfriend. Mary turned away, disappointment showing on her face. The first evening Captain Loring had given Mary a rush; now Captain Lowrey showered me with attention. When I complained the names Loring and Lowrey were confusing, the captain grabbed my hand. "Just call me Harry. How about another drink?"

Our glasses empty, the seven of us took off in two cars for Farmer Dan's, a favorite hangout. We ate fried chicken with our fingers. "Care to dance?" asked Harry. As I had so often done in the past, Mary had to sit on the sidelines and watch us join the couples on the floor. I flushed with pleasure now that my turn had come to be the lady receiving the attention.

Tall, lean, tanned, and a touch of gray in his hair, this smooth dancer put me at ease. I could follow him. Perhaps, the jukebox and the informal atmosphere at Farmer Dan's helped. Perhaps, the old fashioneds did. I was enjoying this evening. Clinton drew me aside. "If Harry gives you any trouble, ask him about his grandchildren." The advice proved unnecessary; Captain Lowrey was a perfect gentleman.

The sun reflected off the water before any of us stirred the next morning. I had just dressed when Mary glanced out the porthole. She froze. "Oh, Carol, I can't believe this. Aunt Alverta and Uncle Neiman are standing on the dock. Head them off while I put on my sundress."

Already up the stairs, I called back, "Hurry! I'll stall them as long as I can." I rushed out to greet the visitors, who were scanning the name of each boat searching for "Miome."

"What a surprise to see you," I called.

Genevieve welcomed them aboard. She kept to herself any concerns she had about the glasses in the sink and the unmade bunks. Mary tried to divert their attention by showing off her ability to tell time ship fashion. She insisted they stay to hear the ship's bell strike the hour.

When they had departed, Mary fumed. "Uncle Stacy sent them to check up on me. I know he did. My family is full of busybodies. I can't stand them." Having missed breakfast, we sat down to what had become brunch. Clinton told jokes to lighten Mary's mood. We traded stories and laughed the afternoon away.

Clinton suggested turning in early in preparation for our return trip to North Carolina. My new friend, Harry, came by with a different idea — drinks on the *Masquerader*. On board, I wandered through the butler's pantry, trying to visualize a dinner party using all that silver and china.

Harry served rum and coke on deck, took us out for fried shrimp served with hush puppies, and suggested we go to Farmer Dan's again. That was fine with me.

Harry and I danced under the stars on the outdoor platform. Over and over again the jukebox played "Why Don't We Do This More Often?" When Clinton begged for a change, we switched the record to "Moonlight Serenade."

After hearing that five times, Clinton asked me to dance. I had never seen him dance with anyone. "I had to ask you." He confessed, "It was the only way I could choose the music." The evening came to a hilarious close when Harry and Clinton danced the hula.

Back on the *Miome* at 3:00 a.m., Clinton reviewed the lessons he'd taught Mary and me. "One — Never mix your drinks. Two — Eat snacks, including cheese all evening. Three — Know your limit. Never get talked into 'just one more.' Four — Don't forget the water! All evening and, most important, before you go to bed, drink water."

Over mugs of coffee, he gave us Lesson Number Five. "Before you turn in, stir one teaspoon of baking soda in a glass of water. Drink this to avoid a hangover." His remedy worked. Five hours later, we awoke feeling refreshed and ready to polish brass until it gleamed.

In the evening, as we waited for the *Silver Meteor*, fatigue descended like a cloud on all four of us. To everyone's relief the train arrived on time. Standing outside our coach, Clinton and Genevieve managed only a half-hearted wave. Looking too exhausted to wait any longer, they left before the conductor shouted, "All aboard."

All the way to Jacksonville, I gazed out the window at rows of orange trees and stately palms. I wondered when I'd see them again. How I wished I could sleep on a train as Mary did. In the middle of the night, the temptation to speak to her proved too strong to resist. I shook her arm, "Mary! It's 3:00 a.m. Want some coffee and scrambled eggs before we climb in our bunks?"

"Sure," she giggled, "But don't tell Uncle Stacy." She settled down for another nap. I thought about how much to tell Mother and Dad about spring vacation — certainly nothing about the drinking lessons or the many dances in Harry's arms.

We returned to college bragging about life on a cabin cruiser, older men, and five rules to follow when drinking alcohol. We mesmerized our friends with tales of our one-week adventure on the golden sands of Daytona Beach.

Mary hinted at romance with a ship captain, intrigued by his blue eyes. I described dancing until 4:00 a.m. and staying up to watch the sun burst out of the Atlantic Ocean, and how we turned day into night by falling into our bunks at 8:00 a.m. to snatch a few hours sleep.

In the quiet of the dorm room, Mary and I talked about how lucky we were to have shared such a wonderful vacation. Well chaperoned, protected, and safe, we had experimented with a way of life alien to that of our parents.

Just as Clinton predicted, his "Five Rules for Drinking Alcohol" became as valuable to me as anything I learned in college. When I became a lieutenant in the army, his advice became essential for my survival. Mary's conclusion she should stick with Coke would serve her equally well.

The Home Stretch

Vacation in Daytona Beach faded into the background. With final exams approaching, playtime ceased. The spring heat intensified, making it hard to concentrate on term papers, lab reports, and pop quizzes.

April had brought a surprise — a change in rank from sophomore to junior. We had expected that advance to come in September. In Aycock Auditorium, our new status entitled us to trade our chapel seats in the distant balcony for those on the main floor. Dad's telegram, "I am so proud of my Junior," made me realize how quickly the college years were slipping away.

Still confined to campus, Mary and I strolled the grounds on weekend dates with soldiers. They complained about everything — army food, long marches, inexperienced officers. We figured their griping was a way to cover up their nervousness about the uncertainties awaiting them overseas.

Letters from home made us aware of shortages and restrictions that made life difficult for our families. Dad expressed concern over the lack of new tires. They seemed to have disappeared overnight. His car had remained on the lift at the Texaco station for a week until two tires became available.

The uncertainty of finding gas had made driving to Florida for a winter vacation impossible. He and Mother rode the overnight sit-up train to Daytona Beach. They found rooms plentiful but rental cars in short supply. A red convertible, the only car available, came at an exorbitant cost. Mother said the envious glances cast their way by other drivers almost made the high price worthwhile.

Sam thought it clever to write me on coal-black paper using snow-white ink. When the ink made untidy globs, he decided "blackout" paper proved more trouble than it was worth, even for a joke.

My cousin Ted, declared 1A by his draft board, expected to leave for the air corps any day. Bob, his older brother, wrote me a depressed and angry letter over his classification of 4F. He saw no reason why a childhood bout of rheumatic fever made him unfit for military service.

Some mothers were relieved by the 4F classification, but young men felt humiliated to be rejected to serve their country. They wanted to be patriotic and join a branch of the armed forces along with their friends.

Only my brother Sherman, now a high school student, remained free of worry and responsibilities. His antics relieved the pressure for my parents. Dad wrote of the afternoon his homeroom teacher kept him after school for laughing so hard he had disrupted the class.

As driving rain beat against the window, he approached the teacher's desk. "Miss Rowley, would you like to meet my father? I think he's getting soaked standing out there in the rain waiting for me." Miss Rowley fell for Sherman's line and excused him.

One evening, I called Mother in despair. "I feel so guilty. I just spent my last dollar on nylons. It's the government's fault for making us shorten our skirts. How much material is that going to save? The shorter the skirts, the more noticeable the runs in the rayon hose. I've had ladders running up my legs for two weeks."

In 1939, one of the sensations of the New York World's Fair had been the DuPont exhibit of their new product, nylon. Nylon hosiery made its appearance nation wide on May 15, 1940. Women charged into department stores to buy three quarter million pairs that first day. Now we faced giving up our precious nylons for the war effort. The manufacture of parachutes meant dwindling supplies of nylon to make hosiery for college girls, matrons, and movie stars.

Dad expressed increasing concern over the dim prospects of completing the highway in Whitehall, New York. He sent me a letter from the steel company with the comment that the first sentence should win a prize.

Gentlemen:
    Due to the fact that we have been requested by the war department to manufacture badly needed defense items on the welding machines which we contemplate using for the manufacture of welded fabric covered by the subject contract, and to the further fact that we are at the present time unable to secure rods from our mills with the priority rating available on this job, and to the further fact that we are unable to purchase materials from any other welded fabric manufacturer with the priority rating available, we are obliged to advise you that it will be impossible to begin shipment of this welded fabric prior to the last of June or the first of July.

Dad reported the state inspector wanted to eliminate the use of steel to reinforce the concrete by increasing the thickness of the pavement from eight to nine inches. It seemed doubtful such a roadway would be strong enough to hold up under incessant truck traffic.

While awaiting a decision, Dad drove home to Danbury, Connecticut, one hundred and eighty miles on Route 22. He described the ride as "really spooky." He saw few cars and only one gas station open for business.

The day before gas rationing went into effect, Mother drove my grandmother around town to call on her friends. There might not be another opportunity for the elderly ladies to get together. Over teacups, they bemoaned the lack of sugar. Mother suggested I send them recipes using substitutes — molasses, marshmallows, and honey.

After five months at war, shortages of steel, tires, gasoline, medicine, sugar, shoes, and nylon had become acute. Each day brought new restrictions to the civilian population. Everyone shared fears about rationing, high prices, new taxes, and long working hours.

To complain was to show disrespect for the thousands of draftees shipping out to Europe and the South Pacific. Unspoken lay the growing realization that huge losses of life and years of struggle lay ahead before the United States could win the war.

On campus, Mary and I were isolated from many of the tensions our parents experienced at home. We concentrated on entertaining the soldiers on the weekends. The prospect of a bleak vacation — no dates, no gas, and no shopping — led us to bend the rules when we met a group of six carefree Marines.

For the first time, we missed curfew.

This Summer Will Be Different

On the last weekend before exams, Mary and I risked a reprimand, or worse, by leaving campus with six service men. We caved in to their invitation to drive to a lake on a dreamy spring afternoon. Eight people crammed into a wreck of a Ford, did not deter the driver. He careened along the narrow road with the verve of a true Marine.

My precarious perch on the lap of a long-legged new acquaintance allowed him to clutch me in an iron grip. He encouraged his buddies to recite ribald versions of nursery rhymes all the way to a picnic area near Guilford Battleground, site of a battle in the Revolutionary War. All of us were surprised — we considered North Carolina Civil War territory.

Sitting on a blanket under the delicate spring-green trees, no one wanted to break the magic of the peaceful afternoon, the last these Marines might ever know. They were reporting to their ship on Monday headed for an unnamed battle zone. When I looked at my watch, I panicked. "Mary, we're going to miss curfew."

Our reckless driver jammed the pedal to the floor but the overloaded jalopy poked along at a lethargic pace. At the entrance to the campus, we left our dates and their incriminating car. Half an hour late, we fled on foot toward Winfield Hall.

Mary laughed at my fears about being caught. "Carol, you have too much conscience. I'm not worried. If someone reports us, the penalty will be light for a first offense." I relaxed when our tardiness went unnoticed.

On Sunday night, soldiers from Fort Bragg staged a rousing performance at Aycock Auditorium. The men wanted to thank us for entertaining them on campus every weekend. Some of the best talent from the big name bands now wore khaki instead of tuxedoes. The swing we heard that night made the girls jump up and dance in the aisles.

Mother and Dad's letters kept me counting the days until summer vacation. Dad suggested Mother and I should visit him in Whitehall, New York. The farmhouse where he boarded had plenty of room. He described the wholesome meals and the restful way of life, except for a crowing rooster.

Mother tried to prepare me for the summer ahead. "Every day we hear about more things we'll have to do without, but given my eyes to enjoy the beauty of each day, my hands with which to do work, and feet with which to walk, I am sure I can make my own happiness."

She anticipated we'd be housebound all summer but assured me we could be contented. "Already our valley is just beautiful. We'll sew and have some teas and relive many of the

wonderful times we have had other years. I think we will love
it."

Looking ahead, I scribbled her a hasty note. "Will you meet
me in New York, or shall I hurry home in time for Joy White's
evening wedding? Either way suits me. With only two exams to
go, I'm looking forward to glorious days of freedom and lots of
sleep."

Mother answered that I should take trains all the way to
Danbury.

The second year of college ended. Mary and I hated to part
from friends we might never see again. Three girls in our hall
had told us they would not return in the fall. In such uncertain
times, others would marry, volunteer for war work, or join the
WAC. As we dashed off to catch the midnight train, I could
think of one consolation. "Mary, you and I will be back in
September. We can look forward to that."

Now pros at traveling, we joined forces with soldiers who
were not the rowdy type. Our protectors kept us amused with
jokes, wild stories, songs, and a game of bridge. In Washington,
D.C., the soldiers carried our bags, forcing us to run in our
spectator pumps to keep pace with their army boots.

Mary headed off to York, Pennsylvania. I settled down on
the train to New York and reread the postcard received the day
before from Ernie, recently promoted to staff sergeant. "Keep
your fingers crossed and let's hope this time I am accepted for
Officer Candidate's School. I'd be eligible for leave — a chance to
see you after five long months apart."

As the train pulled into Penn Station, Barbara Hollister, my
schoolmate from Hartford, stopped by my seat and suggested
breakfast at the Automat and some shopping to kill time until
the noon train to Connecticut. On Fifth Avenue, we admired the
window displays, a fanciful world away from Belk's Department
store in Greensboro. We doubted the glamorous gowns were for
sale due to shortages but everyone could dream.

Happy to be in New York, my heart sang. How suddenly
life can change!

No Words Could Prepare Me

This must be the way a movie star feels, I thought. Swinging my hatbox, I stepped from the train in South Norwalk, Connecticut, on June 3, 1942, planning to catch the next train to Danbury. A soldier at my side lugged my heavy suitcase. In spite of crowds of service men, the grimy tiring overnight train ride from Greensboro had been uneventful. My second year at the Woman's College of the University of North Carolina complete, I looked forward to vacation.

Surprised to see Mother and my brother Sam standing in the shadows of the South Norwalk station, I rushed toward them. Their expressions of grief and sadness slowed my pace. The hatbox bumped against my knee. My heart sank.

Sam could not speak. Mother gave me a tearful kiss before saying, gently, "Why don't we get in the car? It will be easier to tell you what has happened away from all these people." She held my hand, as she said, "Carol, there are no words to prepare you for what I must say."

She took a deep breath. "Ernie died in a plane crash three days ago. He was on duty making aerial photographs of Pine Camp when the plane went down. Both he and the pilot, a man married two weeks ago, lost their lives." She struggled to continue. "Dear, we know you will want to attend the funeral. The service begins in half an hour at the Congregational Church in New Canaan."

Too shocked to feel anything, too stunned to cry, I could not respond to Mother's attempt to console me. I reached into the hatbox to replace my jaunty chapeau with the navy straw. Mary had urged me to buy that hat to wear with my pink coat. I had not anticipated needing it for a funeral. Not for Ernie's funeral!

Approaching the church, the white steeple piercing the brilliant blue sky seemed to give me strength. Through misty eyes, I stared across God's Acre, the village green, at the dark pine tree. Ernie and I had huddled under its branches at the carol sing on Christmas Eve. How warm his hand had been holding mine.

I took a deep breath, squared my shoulders, and stepped into the crowded sanctuary. Pew after pew of mourners formed a dark mass before the brilliance of the flag-draped coffin. The scent of roses and lilies hung heavy in the still air. I kept my eyes on the flag.

When I glanced at Ernie's family sitting before the casket, I felt too numb for tears. Ernie's mother and father seemed to have shrunk in their grief. Betty, my dearest friend, whom I had never before seen wearing black, appeared small, pale, and vulnerable.

Opening my purse to find a hanky, my fingers curled around Ernie's postcard. The last words he had written to me, just two days before he died. Someday, I would share the message with Betty. "It's been five long months since I held you in my arms. We'll soon make up for that."

The shock was so overwhelming that afterward I remembered little of that day. Only the strains of "Abide With Me" played softly on the organ and, later, the slow notes of "Taps" echoing over the fresh grave stayed with me. Those refrains ran round and round in my head for months.

My test of courage came the next day when Sam and I paid a visit to the Urban family. Seared in my memory is the anguished cry of Ernie's mother, "I wanted my son to go with you."

Ernie's father, Bill, a proud stern demanding Hungarian sat in a distant chair, defenseless and subdued. Even at 11:00 a.m., I could not refuse his request to share a drink "in memory of mine son." The strong whiskey served in a tiny glass burned my throat. For the next sixty years, whenever we met, regardless of the hour, Bill and I drank a toast to Ernie.

Two days later, the family's emotions were battered anew. A letter from the army congratulated the parents of Ernest Urban on the selection of their son for Officers' Candidate School. Ernie never knew he had attained the goal for which he had worked so diligently.

Over the summer, Betty found her comfort with Sam. As their dependence on each other grew stronger, I stood alone, constantly reminded of the days when I was part of a foursome. Black coffee became my solace. Cup after cup of steaming black coffee kept me going day and night.

Betty and I consoled each other during a long week with her parents at Fairfield Beach. We tried to appear brave for their sake. Our attempts to use Ernie's complicated camera failed. During walks on the beach, Betty talked incessantly about Sam. Planned as a respite, the change the scene did nothing to ease the ache in our hearts. The four of us were relieved to return home.

Mother tried to lift my spirits. "Let's take the train to Whitehall to visit Dad on the job. I'm concerned he's working too hard. The boys can get along without us for a week." The reinforcing steel had arrived, making it imperative Dad put in extra hours to supervise completion of the highway.

During the long jolting train ride, I wondered what life on a farm would be like. Mother had stayed on her Aunt Katie's farm when she was young, but for me this would be a new experience. The two-story house with its steep pitched roof appeared overpowered by the imposing barns. Beyond the vegetable garden, fields of corn stretched to the distant woodlot.

My room under the eaves had one small window and a ceiling so low I bumped my head. Next morning in the sultry heat, I watched the cook stoke the kitchen range with coal. Unfazed by the climbing temperature, she turned out biscuits, pancakes, fried eggs, and bacon. My compliments were for her strong coffee poured from a huge enamel pot.

On Sunday, Dad gave up his day of rest to take me to Fort Ticonderoga. I heard him tell Mother he thought I'd forget my troubles at the historic fort. He was right. On the strenuous climb up many flights of stone steps to the cannon placements overlooking Lake Champlain, I thought of the soldiers stationed there in the 1750s during the French and Indian Wars.

The eventual defeat of the French had put the fort in British hands. The story of the capture of Fort Ticonderoga in the early days of the Revolutionary War by Ethan Allen and his small band of Green Mountain boys from Vermont enthralled me.

The week in Whitehall came to an end. Aware that Dad relaxed with Mother at his side, I suggested she stay on. What I did with my time mattered little to me. I could at least be useful by going home to keep house for my brothers.

The next morning, I boarded the train under a blazing sun, which proclaimed another hot day. Through my tears, I glanced out the window. To my surprise, I saw Dad waving from the ladder on the side of the water tower. He had climbed several rungs up the ladder to wave goodbye to me.

Tested Again

I had come home not a moment too soon. Stacks of plates and cups stood in the sink. My brothers had decided to put off dish washing until the cupboards stood empty. Sherman's first words made me feel someone needed me.

"Boy, am I glad to see you. Sam thinks his summer job in Norwalk has promoted him from middle son to top dog. He may be a draftsman at Norwalk Tank Company but I'm not his slave."

I plunged the glasses and silverware into soapy water. "Grab a dishtowel and tell me about it." He said he'd looked forward to summer vacation but so far, it had been "dull, dull, dull." By the time he had poured out his frustrations, we had restored order to the kitchen.

"Jock and I are mad. We want to help win the war, but everyone tells us we're too young to work. We even had to prove to the girls we could knit scarves for 'Bundles For Britain.'" He showed me the neat rows of knit and purl on a scarf near completion.

After lugging several baskets of laundry to the washing machine in the basement, I grabbed Sparkle, the cocker spaniel. Usually, he tried to run from a bath, but this time he seemed grateful for the attention. It was a family joke that his baths were my responsibility because his tail belonged to me.

The distant ring of the telephone sent me dashing up the cellar stairs to talk to Grandma. Next came a call from Aunt

Pauline, followed by one from Aunt Hannah. I had been home only a few hours and wished these people realized how much I had to do. By night, too exhausted to eat much supper, I climbed into my own bed and fell asleep. For the first time since Ernie's death, the cycle of sleepless nights broke.

The next day, order prevailed in the house. I doubted Sam had noticed until he said, "I couldn't believe it when I saw four clean shirts hanging in my closet. Last week there were none." After some coaxing, the boys agreed to help with the chores. I posted a schedule on the Frigidaire before relaxing with a magazine on the shady porch.

Within two minutes, the phone rang. Annoyed, I ran into the house. "Carol." The somber tone of Aunt Hannah's voice told me something was wrong. "Carol, I don't know how to tell you what I have to say."

Every muscle in my back tightened. Was I again hearing those chilling words Mother had used the day of Ernie's funeral?

"I just heard from your mother. Your father suffered a severe heart attack this morning."

I tried to concentrate on her words. She said the next three days would be critical. Dad was too ill to be moved from the farmhouse but the doctor would drop in several times a day. A nurse was not available — Mother would care for Dad round the clock. She could not leave his bedside to go downstairs to the phone.

"Try not to worry," advised Aunt Hannah.

Not worry? Not worry? Ernie and now, perhaps, Dad! Not worry? Heartsick, I wondered why Mother had called Aunt Hannah instead of me. Mother and I had grown so close during the past month. Hearing her voice would have been reassuring. On reflection, I realized she could not bear to give me more bad news. Talking to me would have been too emotional for both of us.

My sleeping problem returned, but I had to carry on. One of my new responsibilities involved money. Clutching Dad's checkbook and Mother's instructions, I climbed the marble steps to the First National Bank. Intimidated by the vast marble interior, where customers spoke in hushed tones. I felt everyone was staring at me.

The teller's steely eyes behind her wire rimmed glassed deflated my resolve to appear at ease. I managed to say in a whispery voice, "May I please speak to Mr. Jost? He's a friend of my father's and I need his help."

She motioned to a guard, who opened the brass rail surrounding the huge mahogany desk of the bank president. The man in uniform indicated I should sit on the straight chair. A man's hand, wearing a gold signet ring, reached across the desk to shake mine. As if by magic, Mr. Jost had appeared.

"I was sorry to hear of your father's heart attack," he said. "What can we do for you?" His eyes were kind, his manner friendly. He no longer appeared to be the unapproachable figure I had always pictured from the other side of the brass railing. By summer's end we had become good friends.

My busy days fell into a routine. At 5:30 a.m. on my way to the kitchen to make sandwiches for Sam's lunch, I pounded on his door to warn the sleepyhead to hurry. Some days, late for his train, he had no time to eat the hot breakfast I had prepared.

Occasionally, I freed an afternoon to spend with my Grandmother. Her calm reassurance proved an antidote for Aunt Hannah's dire predictions about Dad's future. I turned to Aunt Pauline for practical advice to lift my spirits. " Let's surprise your mother by making clothes for you to take back to college," she suggested. In the fabric store she steered me to simple patterns and materials suitable for a beginner.

My frank talks with Mr. Jost in the bank had made me aware of the financial burden of Dad's illness. I was pleased to report to him I was doing my part to keep within budget by making my fall wardrobe.

In Whitehall, six weeks passed before the doctor allowed Dad to sit up. Day after day Mother had remained by his side in the small sweltering room under the eaves. When Dad dozed, she wrote me brief notes. I appreciated her compliments about the job I was doing, but felt depressed by her suggestions of a dozen more things I should do.

"Dear, tomatoes are at their best now. It is time to make the catsup. Buy a bushel of tomatoes. You will find the bottle capper in the cellar. Follow my recipe, exactly. Your results will be just as good as mine."

In desperation, I called Grandma. She gave me instructions I lacked on how to sterilize the bottles, dip the tomatoes in boiling water to make the skins slide off, and use the bottle capper. "It might be best to let Sam do that," she warned.

Sam, walking home from the evening train, followed the aroma of tomatoes and spices, which grew stronger and stronger near our door. "The whole neighborhood reeks of catsup," he complained. He expected supper, not bottles, capper, and caps lined up on the counter.

Grabbing a tablespoon, he dipped a sample of the tomato mix from the kettle. He clutched his throat and gasped, "Water! Water! Quick! Give me some water! What did you do?"

I had not thought to taste the foolproof recipe. Now I tried a cautious sip. Too much cayenne pepper brought tears to my eyes and burned my throat. My long day of hard work had resulted in a disaster.

Next morning I added several cans of tomato juice to the spicy mixture. Two kettles of catsup sat on the stove with no improvement in flavor. I could not handle this emergency. For the first time I called Mother in Whitehall. She must have been alarmed to hear the distress in my voice. When I explained my problem, she burst into laughter.

"Dear, I am so sorry. I truly am. I forgot to tell you to add only one-fourth of the cayenne pepper called for in the recipe." After I hung up the phone, I gave in to a few tears. She had enjoyed a much-needed laugh, but it wasn't funny to me. What was I going to do with gallons of peppery catsup?

Sam made the decision — bottle the stuff and forget it. The balky capper kept him busy all evening. He had to admit the rows of red bottles made an impressive display in the cellar cupboard. When Mother came home, she did not mention the bottling caper. I suppose she eventually sent the bottles to the dump. I've never cared much for catsup.

Later that summer a different condiment played a part at Sherman's fifteenth birthday party.

Learning From Experience

Sherman wanted a dance for his fifteenth birthday on July 27. Determined to do what Mother would have done, I assured him that was a great idea. On the red-letter day, we moved the porch furniture to the yard to make room for twelve couples. He turned down my suggestion to put the record player in the corner.

"No. Let's put in the center under the balloons and streamers. That way we can dance in circles and everyone can hear the music." He was right about that — every man, woman, and child in the neighborhood heard the songs of Frank Sinatra.

The warm July evening was not compatible with frosting on a three-layer cake. Hoping it would not melt, I heaped waves of blue icing around a toy sailboat similar to the boys' catboat. The fruit punch needed ice. Plop! Ice cubes, cherries frozen inside, splashed into the lobster pot, the largest kettle I could find.

Although Sam had said he was too busy to help with the party, he wandered into the kitchen eager to taste the refreshments. The drink looked refreshing, worth my effort squeezing dozens of oranges and lemons. As Sam dipped a sample, ashes from his pipe drifted into the colorful drink. I wanted to hit the novice pipe-smoker.

Grabbing a bottle of Worcestershire Sauce from the cupboard, he teased, "That's nothing. How about adding some of this?"

To my horror, the bottle cap flew off. Large dollops of hot sauce sank out of sight in the punch. Still holding the Worcestershire bottle, Sam fled. There wasn't time to go after him. I'd deal with him later.

At break time, the thirsty dancers clustered round the punch bowl. They said they had never tasted punch quite like it, a most unusual flavor. They emptied the bowl twice and finished off the cake before returning to the dance floor. When the records played out, no one noticed. A rising moon had replaced loud music with romance.

Some couples had claimed the rattan furniture on the lawn. Others retreated to the branches in the apple tree. Alarmed to see the party getting out of hand, I had to act fast. Switching on the floodlight, I announced, "The party's over. Its time to go home."

Concerned over what the parents might say, I was relieved to hear from only one irate mother. She accused me of serving spiked punch to fifteen-year olds. I had to confess. "Yes, the punch was spiked but not with liquor. Worcestershire Sauce put the kick in it.' I laughed to myself. Sam had contributed to the party after all.

July had been a discouraging month. August began on an optimistic note. Mother found time to write a long letter.

"With all my heart I know how hard this summer has been for you but it makes me happy that you have not become cynical. I have always noticed since my days at Pratt that hard and disappointing experiences made my friends either cynical or very much sweeter. When one has in their heart the faith that we both do, that God knows the reason why and cares, every experience contributes to making us finer women."

August 21 became a red-letter day. The mailman brought the first letter from Dad. We sat on the front steps while I read the good news to Sam and Sherman.

"Surely it was a great stunt I played on all of you to go and get sick and so keep Mother all to myself most of the summer. Now I am improving so rapidly that I really think our trip home is not too far away. Bless your hearts! The doctor is not coming today for the first time. He says I can try taking a few steps."

A week later Mother wrote that Dad could sit up until he felt tired. He signed his next letter, "Love to all the family, our lady of the house, our engineer and our plane builder." Sherman spent his evenings working on model planes.

The heat of August gave way to the chilly mornings of September. Dr. White took Dad for a long drive before giving him the word we had waited so long to hear. "You are ready to go home."

Aunt Hannah and Sam pooled their gas rationing stamps for the eight-hour trek to Whitehall. We needed no alarm clock to wake us for that trip. We found Mother and Dad waiting for us on the porch of the old farmhouse. In spite of appearing pale, thin, and weak, Dad's optimism and sense of humor reassured us he was going to be OK. Through her fatigue Mother radiated happiness.

Seeing home again brought tears to their eyes. The freshly mown lawn, the trimmed bushes, and the gleaming windows all proclaimed "Welcome Home." They wandered from room to room. Mother admired the crisp, starched bedroom curtains, which had taken me hours to iron. Dad exclaimed over the clutter free garage and neat cellar, a transformation brought about by the scrap drive.

Over supper, we lingered in the candlelight, each person eager to take part in the conversation. The expressions of love and pride on the faces of Mother and Dad, told me all I needed to know.

I had passed the test of that difficult summer with flying colors.

Time to Celebrate

The summer of 1942 ended on a more optimistic note than it had begun. With Mother and Dad back home, tensions eased for all of us. In previous years, we had held a joint party for my birthday on September 10, and Mother and Dad's anniversary on the eleventh. This year Dad declared September 10 "Carol's Day."

After the grief, anxiety, and responsibilities of the past months, I felt old beyond my years. I kept those feelings to myself and tried to face the future with confidence equal to that of my parents'. If Dad could remain optimistic, I'd try to follow his example. As a family, we found strength in Mother's sunny outlook, Sam's love for Betty, and Sherman's ability to keep us laughing.

No trip to New York, no theatre tickets, no new clothes, and no Blue Grass perfume this year. Such luxuries had lost their appeal in wartime. Now, Dad's recovery had become vital to my happiness.

Luxury on this birthday meant sleeping in until 9:00 a.m. A twenty-five dollar war bond from Mother and a ten-dollar bill from Dad seemed a fortune. Sam surprised me with a make-up box covered in fake alligator to carry on the train. Sherman had cut lawns to earn money for Elizabeth Arden bath powder.

Aunt Pauline presented me with a length of flowered organdy and a pattern to make an evening dress. Aunt Hannah found a red sweater and Aunt Helen came up with two pairs of rayon stockings. Grandma's gifts were best of all. She rode two buses and walked a mile to bring me an artificial flower for my hair and two hankies.

At my evening party, a colorful arrangement of yellow chrysanthemums and fall leaves reserved our table at The Spinning Wheel Inn in Redding. I lifted the napkin covering the breadbasket. "This is a birthday surprise. Rationing hasn't done away with the hot sticky buns." The varied menu of previous years had been replaced by fruit juice, creamed chicken on biscuit, peas, parsley potatoes, tossed salad and chocolate cake.

Mother regaled us again with her story of my birth one day too soon. She and Dad had hoped I'd be born on their first wedding anniversary. Perhaps, that would have happened, had she not decided to climb Hoyt's Hill two days before. She and her friend, Grace Sherwood, climbed higher and higher picking the first colored leaves of fall.

When Mother tired, they took a shortcut across a farmer's field. Soon they found their way blocked by a stone wall. "Grace, there is no way I can climb over those boulders, but I think I could roll under that gate."

Rolling under proved easy. Stopping did not. Like a bouncing ball, Mother's bulky form tumbled down the hill. She averted disaster by grabbing a small sapling. In spite of the strain on the young tree, the roots held firm in the ground. As she struggled to her feet, her carefree laughter echoed across the hillside.

That adventure brought me quickly and easily into this world the following morning. On viewing their fair little daughter, Mother and Dad forgot their disappointment the baby had made her appearance the day before their anniversary.

Sherman said he'd heard that story so often he felt he'd been there. He kept up the carefree tone of the evening. "Now, you've reached twenty-one, I'm going to call you 'Old Lady.'" I could not respond to his jest. He did not realize how old I felt.

Between May and September, the loss of Ernie and the responsibilities thrust upon me had changed me. I was entering a new phase in my life. I would return to college, no longer a starry-eyed girl, but an adult.

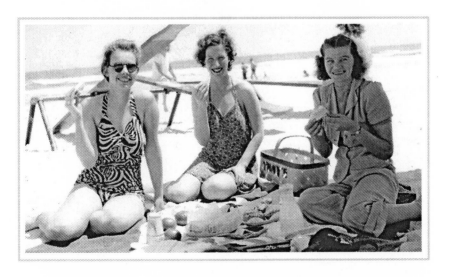

Spring break in Florida, 1942. Mary, Carol, and Genevieve.

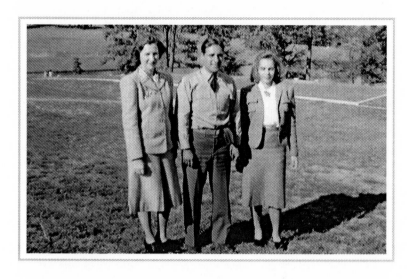

Mary and Carol with a soldier from Brooklyn in 1942.

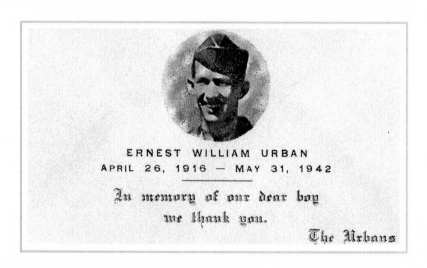

ERNEST WILLIAM URBAN
APRIL 26, 1916 — MAY 31, 1942

In memory of our dear boy
we thank you.

The Urbans

Junior Year 1942 - 1943

No tears when leaving home in September 1942. I had done what I could to help the family; now I looked forward to my junior year at Woman's College. The refrain, "Nothing Could Be Finer Than to Be in Carolina" kept running through my head.

Mary, tan and slimmer, greeted me at the door to our new room. "You're going to love this location at the end of the hall. It's great to be away from the telephone." We agreed it would take many late-night chats to catch up on three months separation. She began by describing her fling with summer romance. While I had struggled with serious matters, she had flirted the time away.

"Mary, how could you manage four proposals in twelve weeks?" She said it was easy when working in her father's dental office. Although she insisted, "they didn't mean a thing," I noticed a gleam in her eye when she described her first glass of champagne with Dave Monroe before he left for basic training in Wyoming.

Registering for classes, the three "P's" dominated my schedule — Physiology, Psychology, and Physics. I wondered how I'd find time for projects in Home Furnishings. My first assignment, on a scorching September day, almost made me change my major from Home Economics. A damp towel covering my face, I thought I'd smother stuffing chicken feathers into a casing to make pillows for a daybed.

The origin of cording had never entered my mind, until I cut yards of material into bias strips. After the strips had been sewn into tubes and turned right side out, white cord had to be threaded through. That tedious process made me late for physiology lab.

That evening, determined to finish the pillow project, I tackled the tricky part — turning the pillow corner while sewing the cording between two layers of material. I never wanted to do that again. Mary had been smart to major in French, I thought dejectedly. She had no three-hour labs. I had three every week.

Back at the dorm, wailing sirens caught me off guard for the first practice air raid drill in Greensboro. Officials insisted the city was vulnerable to sabotage because the natural gas line ended there. Slumped down on the cold tile in the dark hall, my plans to study for a physics quiz evaporated.

Mary and I became pros at dealing with drills. At the shrill blast of the siren, we grabbed sweaters and blankets as well as snacks. During the uncomfortable hours on the chilly floor, we never knew whether a real attack was taking place. That never happened. Forbidden to study by flashlight or talk, only the lonesome whistle of the distant train broke the silence. We dozed until the "All Clear" signal sent us to bed.

On the Fiftieth Anniversary of the founding of the Woman's College, Lieutenant Commander Mildred McAfee, head of the WAVES and president of Wellesley College, spoke at chapel. She challenged us to meet the responsibilities of becoming intelligent and capable leaders for the post-war world.

"I hope the demonstration in war-time of the versatility and adaptability of American women will be sufficient evidence to shatter some of the myths about feminine inadequacy. If that hope is fulfilled, it will follow that women will continue to merit the opportunity to be educated." Her snappy blue uniform impressed the students as much as her words.

At the lecture series in Aycock Auditorium, Ruth Mitchell, sister of Billy Mitchell the flier, electrified the audience. She painted a graphic picture of the mistreatment of the Serbs by the

Germans. Her description of capture while serving with the Chetniks, and her mistreatment in prison, aroused our passion to help the half-million Chetnik orphans. Upturned open umbrellas passed overhead from student to student brimmed with dollar bills for orphan relief.

No more seconds at dinner! Mary and I made up for scanty meals by indulging in doughnuts and cupcakes from the bakery. We even fell for the favorite treat at the corner hangout — fried doughnuts with ice cream. A sugar-glazed doughnut heated in the sandwich grill, topped with ice cream, and washed down with cherry coke stemmed appetite for hours.

Rumors kept us agitated. We might not be allowed to graduate. There might not be transportation for travel by Christmas. The dean announced it would be too expensive to keep college open for out-of-state students if they could not get home. Mary and I decided to get away for a weekend before the crackdown made it impossible.

Our counselor waited until Friday evening to sign our permission slips for a weekend with my friend Betty Urban at the University of South Carolina We packed one suitcase, one hatbox and one make-up box, proof we had learned to travel light.

At closing bell, we headed for a late movie with Mrs. Haynes, mother of our friend, Ginny. She treated us to barbecue before leaving us at the train station at midnight. We finally escaped the overheated waiting room, to board the train at 2:30 a.m.

The man seated ahead of us said he, too, was going to the state capitol. Soon after the sun rose in a cloudless sky, the conductor bellowed "Columbia." The sleeping passenger in front of us did not move. As Mary and I passed his seat, I shook his shoulder and reminded him this was his stop. Mary scolded me for being too bold but he ran after us on the platform to thank me.

The walk to town proved to be more than we had anticipated — twelve blocks. Waffles, bacon, and coffee in the

Wade Hampton Hotel Coffee Shop restored our energy. On the way back to the station to retrieve our bags, we toured the state capitol and saw where General Sherman's Union Army men had shot a corner cornice off the building.

Betty had class until noon. Looking for her room, we wandered down a corridor. "Here we are, Mary. My picture is on the bookcase and Sam's is by the bed." On Betty's return, our gabfest began. We ate Hungarian pastry her Mother had sent and called it lunch. After a tour of the campus, we took in a movie.

I was upset when Betty told us she had a date with a soldier and had arranged blind dates for us. Mary and I had sat up all night to visit her, not go out with two men we'd never see again. Returning to Betty's dorm after another movie and cokes with our escorts, Mary and I agreed South Carolina men surpassed their North Carolina brothers in flattery.

Betty did not come in until we were in bed, although she said she had had a dull evening. I could not stay irked with her for long. We talked so late we missed church on Sunday Morning. The day passed quickly. When the dorm closed at 11:00 p.m., Mary and I were forced back to the station.

For the second time in three nights, we waited for a 2:00 a.m. train. I had the good luck to sit with a charming second lieutenant. We chatted like old friends all the way to Raleigh. Mary struggled with a burly sergeant who insisted on sleeping with his head on her shoulder.

By 10:30 a.m. our adventure was over. We agreed this was our best weekend so far. My birthday money had made it possible.

There was also good news from home. Dad had taken a job overseeing the building of an airstrip at Westover Field in Massachusetts. He and Mother were staying with her friend, Alice Chapin, in Chicopee. Sherman remained at home with neighbors. His study hall teacher found a way to keep him from disrupting the class. She brought him a sheet of writing paper and a stamped envelope. At the end of the period, he had to turn in a completed letter to Mother and Dad.

Dad's job proved to be a challenge seven days a week. He wrote that he faced opposition greater than our army experienced in North Africa. He felt the planning had been done by boys rather than trained engineers, but he tried to see a funny side to the nightmare.

When he requested ten men, seventy-five showed up. Trucks dumped off French Canadians, who spoke no English. After waiting two hours for picks and shovels, one gang started taking off forms surrounding the new pavement. They were so rough and inexperienced that they broke out huge chunks of concrete.

"I thought I would die laughing when the inspector sent word that, if the general superintendent did not have an interpreter around in twenty minutes to stop those men removing forms, he was going to call out the army guard and shoot them!"

Dad's return to work and his upbeat letters relieved my mind. In spite of my fears, he had recovered from the heart attack he had suffered in July.

Serenade In Blue

November 15, a red-letter day for Mary — her twentieth birthday. Dave, her champagne date in August, called from his army base in Cheyenne, Wyoming. The extravagant call lasted thirteen minutes. Mary's eyes sparkled. "I have a guilty conscience, but in spite of the cost, I enjoyed flirting with Dave."

I insisted she write him a thank-you letter. She soon ran out of ideas and asked for my help. Dave would have been surprised to know much of the letter was not in her words but mine.

Determined to find dates for the Junior Prom, we invited paratroopers from Fort Bragg. As I slipped into my blue taffeta gown, my confidence sagged at the thought of a blind date. I did not anticipate a tall blond sergeant with the romantic name, Raoul Martell. When we stepped onto the dance floor to the strains of "Serenade in Blue," theme for the blue and silver decorations, Marty's charm put me at ease.

Not all escorts equaled mine. The girls passed on the word about a corporal they nicknamed "Disaster." No one wanted to spend time with an older man lacking a few teeth and most of his hair. We each took a turn letting him stumble over our feet for just one dance. Marty broke down and confessed he had borrowed a sergeant's coat. He understood only officers would be admitted to the dance.

He changed the subject to a graphic description of his first experience in a plane when he had been ordered to "Jump." After that scary descent, he learned to enjoy the exhilaration of falling through space.

"No alcohol allowed on campus? How can you put up with that?" Marty's buddy shook his head in disbelief. During intermission, our dates had to settle for coke or grapefruit juice. In the parlor after the dance we offered them tomato juice and crackers. The paratroopers left early, probably, desperate for stronger stuff.

My brother Sam's description of his prom was in sharp contrast to mine. A fraternity man at M.I.T., he wore tails to escort his date to the Statler Hotel in a horse and carriage. She probably did not know how lucky she was to dance with a man wearing shoes instead of weighted paratrooper boots.

Mary and I laughed at the gaff of one of the patronesses. Overcome with fatigue, she introduced Sam as "Miss Morrison." The name followed him down the receiving line. He wished his fraternity brothers would stop calling him "Miss."

After our Junior Prom, Mary and I looked forward to Thanksgiving Day. Parishioners from the Presbyterian Church had invited all the college girls for breakfast in the church hall. The men of the congregation hustled to cook fried apples, sausage, grits, biscuits, and coffee for two hundred college girls. Their enthusiasm made up for their lack of expertise.

After a Thanksgiving service in the sanctuary, Mary and I worked off the hearty breakfast in a brisk walk to the National

Theatre. One of our hosts, owner the theatre, treated us to a preview screening of, "White Christmas" starring Bing Crosby and Rosemary Clooney. By the last scene we sensed that picture would be a hit.

Worried we might miss Thanksgiving dinner in the dining hall, we hurried back to the campus humming "I'm Dreaming of a White Christmas." To our amazement at dinner we were offered all the food we could eat with no war restrictions to mar the day. Even so, sweet potato pie did not equal pumpkin in my estimation.

Late in the afternoon, Mary, her sister Elaine, Ginny, and I walked to Ginny's home for supper. We fixed our own sandwiches followed by a favorite southern dessert, ambrosia, a delicious concoction of oranges and fresh coconut.

Back at school, Mary and I could not resist opening Mother's box at midnight. We invited our hall mates to gorge on cheese, crackers, cinnamon jelly, and caramels. Our one-day splurge of good eating might have to last us until the end of the war.

Betty wrote an amusing account of her holiday at the South Carolina home of her roommate, Margaret. Margaret's father, too old to be drafted, had enlisted in the army as a private. After her mother had invited neighbors, two lieutenants and their wives for Thanksgiving dinner, her father insisted army regulations forbid him from socializing with officers. Much to the family's embarrassment, he ate alone in the kitchen.

Dad's weekly letter brought the good news that he and Mother were back home. The Boston company, who had hired him to supervise construction at Westover Field, had run into financial trouble and could no longer afford his services. His letter included a check for my Christmas ticket to New York, twenty-two dollars round trip. A rumor that the Southern Railroad would ration tickets before the holidays proved false.

Christmas vacation began at noon on December 18. I felt guilty when Ginny's father used a gas ration stamp to drive Mary, Elaine, and me to the station. The radio reports indicated no gas would be available for cars indefinitely. To our delight, seats to Washington were plentiful. We found the "rule of one" had been imposed in the diner — one cup of coffee, one teaspoon of sugar, one pat of butter per passenger. Worst of all — no ice cream!

As the lights of Washington came in view, we gathered our belongings. The train lurched to a stop on the bridge over the Potomac River. For an hour, before the train proceeded to the station, we sang every Christmas carol we knew.

Mary and Elaine had plenty of time to catch their train to Harrisburg. I had to sprint for mine to New York. In Philadelphia, the train entered a dim-out area. The government required all shades be lowered to the sill. Passengers boarding in North Philadelphia grumbled at finding standing room only in cramped aisles in the murky gloom.

In Pennsylvania Station, I spotted my classmate, Connie Bradley. Although we had ridden in separate coaches from Greensboro, she, too, was headed for Connecticut. She clung to my arm as we groped our way through the deserted dark waiting room. The taxi ride to Grand Central Station gave us an eerie glimpse of the dimmed-out city. We had missed the midnight train by an hour. "Connie I'll call Mother, then we'll settle down to spend the night. We'll have this huge waiting room all to ourselves."

In the ladies room, the scrubwoman, a fat jolly Irish, "God Bless You" type, was carrying on an animated conversation with a plumber. While he repaired washbasins and a gangly colored boy filled soap dishes, the floor sweeper and I stopped to listen to the conversation.

The scrubwoman smoothed her apron. "Oi tell you. People never think of us and 'ow 'ard we work. If they didn't pull out two sheets at a time, the terlet paper wouldn't go so fast." Three heads nodded in agreement.

After I saw Connie off to Bridgeport at 3:45 a.m., I sat alone in the gloom of the shadowy station.

Two hours later, I was among the few passengers who boarded the early train to South Norwalk. I had planned to take a nap but dawn breaking over a bleak landscape held my interest. When I left the train to board a bus for Danbury, my nylons offered no protection from the bitter cold. The frigid air took my breath away.

"Ten below zero," remarked a passenger through the muffler covering his face.

I laughed to myself. I had gone to North Carolina, where the temperature seldom dipped below freezing, to escape days like this one. Now this frosty morning seemed perfect. It represented home, only an hour away, and Christmas with the family.

No Place Like Home

The sight of Mother and Dad huddling close together on the platform at the Danbury station made me forget my freezing feet. Often I had cried when leaving home, this time I cried for joy to be back. Soon a blazing fire in the fireplace warmed my toes. After coffee and cinnamon toast, I regaled the family with my mishaps and adventures.

Before lunch, I toured the house savoring each familiar scene. Storm windows had been added to insulate the chilly kitchen. Dad looked at the frost on the outer glass. "I'm so lucky to have kept a high school friend like Bernie Dolan. He promises he'll never let us run out of fuel oil. He's allotted us seventeen hundred gallons for the winter. We really have to conserve. Last year we used twenty-two hundred."

The dining room had been closed off. We ate around a crowded card table in the small room off the kitchen. Although we had not played there in years, we still called it "the playroom." The luxury of an open fire in the living room would last only through the holidays. After New Year's that room would be closed off until spring.

In the bedrooms, frost made feathery designs on the windowpanes. When we complained of the chill, Mother laughed. "When I was a child there was frost on the floor under our beds every morning all winter. Of course, Father did not have to worry about freezing pipes as we do now. We had no bathroom."

Sam's arrival from M.I.T. interrupted the tour. The night before, Betty had waited seven hours in New York for the delayed arrival of his train from Boston. He had spent the night at her house in Wilton.

The family wanted to spend every possible moment together. Sam and Sherman tagged along to John McLean's Department store to watch me buy a warm coat. Sherman said my camel hair selection made the shopping spree worthwhile.

"Hey, Sam, get a load of Carol's new coat. She has the nerve to wear a color called 'nude.'"

Sunday morning we dressed in our warmest woolens for church. The thermometer registered twenty degrees below zero and the car would not start. Getting a taxi took time, but I didn't mind being late. Walking down the aisle to our pew in the third row, I hoped the congregation made note of my stylish new coat.

Swags of evergreens added color to the stark white church walls. Pine sprays tied with red ribbon hung in every window. Outside the small panes, bare branches of the trees stood silhouetted against the pale blue sky. As we sang, "Hark the Herald Angels Sing," I tried to forget the past year by pretending Ernie stood by my side.

In afternoon Sherman had a chance to shine. Playing his bass, he made his first public appearance with the high school orchestra and chorus. Fifteen years old, wearing Sam's tuxedo, he appeared quite grown up until he spoiled the illusion. When his nose visibly twitched, he drew the bow across the strings, across his nose, then across the strings. He never missed a beat.

"Sam can you believe what we're hearing? Our little brother now plays Bach and Mendelssohn. Our lover of swing and jazz has added classical music to his repertoire. While we've been away, he's been growing up."

Biting cold and lack of gasoline kept us close to home. Dad's frequent plea, "Who's ready for a game of bridge?" usually found volunteers. Mother and I took turns playing cards, cooking, and wrapping gifts. The numerous games made us all better players.

On Christmas Eve a crackling fire on the hearth warmed the living room to a tolerable degree. None of the bustle of other years intervened. As the five of us ate supper from trays, Sherman remarked, "This is the best lukewarm meal I ever ate."

When I dashed from the warmth of the fire to my icy room, I did not give up my Christmas Eve tradition of lighting bayberry candles. Burning them to the socket in nineteen forty-one had not brought me the promised good luck for the following year, so, this time I blew out the flames after twenty minutes. This pair might have to last years.

On Christmas morning one thing had changed. Sam and Sherman slept until after 8:00 a.m. Our greatest Christmas gift — heat! Dad turned up the thermostat a few degrees. Sun streamed through the windows of the dining room opened for that one day. By the time we finished breakfast, the traditional box of raised doughnuts made by Mrs. Magersuppe, once Mother's helper, stood empty.

Reluctant to leave the sunny room, we poured more coffee and brought gifts to the table. When the men left for fresh air, Mother checked on the turkey in the oven. I gathered up the discarded wrapping paper and ribbon on the floor, took the good china from the corner cupboard, and set the table for twelve.

So far, we had been spared the wartime separation experienced by many families. Grandma and Grandpa Andrews, Aunt Pauline and Uncle Ed, and our cousins, Polly, Robert, and Ted, arrived for dinner. Highlight of the meal for me was the cut glass bowl of hard sauce dusted with nutmeg. Grandma had saved enough butter to make my favorite topping for the steamed pudding.

In the days following, the weather moderated but vacation remained low-key. Sam was pleased when Aunt Hannah loaned him her car with a full tank of gas. He invited me to drive to New Canaan to see Betty. Seven months had passed since her brother, Ernie, had been killed in the plane crash. It felt like seven years to me.

Sam and Betty were looking ahead to a future together. Betty's parents and I still grieved. Was it only a year ago Ernie and I had spent the evening sitting on the floor by the Christmas tree listening to the symphony?

On New Year's Eve Mother whispered, "Would you please play bridge tonight? Dad is so blue." She seldom let us see her concern for Dad since his heart attack. In all probability, this would be the last Christmas in our childhood home. The doctor had told Dad he must live in a warmer climate. Determined to make our holiday special, he had not let us see his worry over a job.

We played the old year out, made a hilarious evening of it, including a ginger ale toast at midnight. I wondered whether deep inside the others experienced the overwhelming sadness I felt. This might be our last Christmas and New Year together.

We smiled, clapped, and cheered. "Happy New Year. Welcome, 1943."

The Home Front 1943

Back at Woman' College after Christmas break, news from home took priority over alarming headlines about the war. In a phone call, Dad told me he felt strong and ready to work seven months after his heart attack. "Although I do not feel old at fifty-one, I fear my age is against me in the job market. The doctor insists I find a less stressful occupation than engineering."

My impetuous, impractical, artistic mother, inspired by an article in "Woman's Day" magazine, thought she had the answer to Dad's dilemma. Not only would she supplement their income, she could do her part to win the war. She planned to care for eight toddlers, from 8:00 a.m. to five 5:00 p.m. to free their mothers to work at the Barden Corporation, a defense plant. The plant manager assured her there was a "crying need" for her service. It seemed so simple to her. Just move three large rugs downstairs from upstairs to protect the living room floor and have Dad knock together some small tables.

Eager to give me the details, her excitement was palatable over the phone. "I am very much pepped up about this project. One mother is coming to see me tonight. I hope to start with eight children at one dollar each per day and will take more after I get organized. What do you think of my venture?"

I pictured the chaos when eight little ones needed to go "potty," but I couldn't find the words to tell my mother she would be doomed to failure. "Well, more than one pair of hands will be needed. I wish I could be home to help you."

Before I could call back with a more persuasive response, the bubble burst. None of the mothers could transport the children three miles out of town to our house. She received only one inquiry. Wasting no time on the failed project, she turned her talent to making blackout curtains.

I recognized her determination to work as a sign of the anxiety she and Dad felt. I tried to boost their morale with amusing letters. Writing of a gala midnight party to try out the hot plate sent by Aunt Hannah, I did not mention hot plates were forbidden in the dorm. Lacking sugar for tea, Mary and I had substituted cinnamon jelly and called the hot drink, "Russian Tea." Our dorm mates loved it.

Dad's letters sounded less optimistic than usual. He had followed up job leads in Philadelphia and Cleveland to no avail. In February, he planned a trip to Florida to investigate a hotel for sale in Cocoa. That sounded good to me — on his way home he planned a stopover in Greensboro.

A train reservation became available on such short notice, he left on Monday minus a shave and trim from his barber. Barbershops, beauty parlors, stores, and most businesses were closed on Mondays to conserve fuel. Banks and schools remained open.

Walking back to Winfield Hall on February 26, Mary and I saw Dad stepping from a taxi. After a hug and a kiss, I stepped back. "Let me look at you. Florida sun has given you a healthy glow. You look years younger than you did at Christmas."

"Dear Heart, I never felt better. The good news is I have found a wonderful opportunity for our future. I've seen an orange grove, where I'm convinced Mother and I could make a living. How would you like to step out the door and pick an orange off the tree for breakfast?"

That evening Dad treated Mary and me to steaks at The Mecca, the first time Mary and I had tasted meat in weeks. We plied him with questions about Florida. I fell in love with his description of Bonita Grove in Homestead, thirty miles below Miami.

The business sold hand picked, tree ripened fruit, packed in gift boxes to be shipped north. A charming, two bedroom house surrounded by green lawn and towering palm trees stood separated from the road by a low coral rock wall.

Next morning Dad and I settled down to talk. He showed me clippings of job possibilities he had investigated. He had ruled out the hotel — too far from town. Gas restrictions limited taxis to twenty-five miles round trip. I ruled out the fishing camp and the tearoom. "Dad those would never work. If Mother ran the kitchen, you'd lose your shirt. She'd feed the guests so well you'd go broke."

Dad looked relieved. "You think the grove is the best bet?"

"I do. You would be taking on a new challenge and working outdoors. You and Mother would be sharing a way of life you'd both love. Moreover, she could find plenty of outlets for her energy."

"That's what I hoped you'd say. Let's round up your friends and celebrate tonight with steaks at The Jefferson Roof." Steak twice in two days! I must be dreaming.

When Dad arrived home, excited and exhausted, Mother thought the grove an answer to their prayers. Before Dad could catch a night's sleep, the realtor called to say he had another offer on the property. Since Dad had first refusal, he had twenty-four hours to decide whether he wanted to buy Bonita Grove.

Dad's conservative sister, Margaret, expressed her doubts. His sister Hannah thought the grove a once in a lifetime opportunity. She took him aside and offered him help. "Bob, I have some money in the bank. You're welcome to it, either as an investment or a loan."

Due to Hannah's generous offer, raising the funds moved quickly. Two days later Mother and Dad left for Florida on the *Orange Blossom Special.* On Sunday morning, one week after Dad had told me about the grove, I received a telegram.

NEXT WINTER YOUR ORANGES WILL COME FROM MORRISONS' BONITA GROVE. Signed: Mother and Dad

Breaking the Rules

In the spring of 1943, Dave made progress in his "on again off again" romance with Mary. When he invited her to attend his graduation ball from Officers' Candidate School at Camp Lee in Petersburg, Virginia, she scrapped her plan to never date him again. Without asking her parents permission, she accepted his invitation.

When she confessed to her father, he refused to send money for her ticket. Her lack of tact had made her request sound like a command and her father made it clear he would not change his mind. It took her mother to come up with a solution. "You may go to the dance, provided Carol goes along to chaperone. Someone has to keep an eye on you."

Mary and I found her mother's reasoning a huge joke. "That's fine with us," we chorused, giving Mary's father no time to think up another way to stop us. We planned to spend the remaining vacation days after the ball at Mary's home in York, Pennsylvania. Convinced nothing could stop us, we turned our attention to travel plans and clothes.

I had my heart set on a gown I had seen at Belk's — a soft shade of yellow, just right for spring. The sweetheart neckline and delicately embroidered bodice enhanced the billowing skirt, which flowed over many layers of nylon net. When Mother surprised me with a check for the trip, I threw my shabby white formal in the trash and rushed to town to claim my treasure.

One serious hurdle remained — the rule in the student handbook stating students were not allowed to cut the last class before or the first class after a vacation. Mary's last class ended one and a half hours after departure time for the train to Richmond.

An unbreakable rule was not about to stop Mary. She dragged me, reluctant and tense, to the office of the Acting Dean, Annie Beam Funderburk, who had taken over for Dean Harriet Elliott. Dean Elliott spent most of her time in Washington, D.C. serving on President Roosevelt's brain trust.

Annie Beam Funderburk, a middle age woman of ample proportions with a no-nonsense air, appeared as forbidding as her name. She sat behind an imposing mahogany desk in a room filled with the scent of roses and lemon verbena polish. "Sit down and explain why you are here," ordered Mrs. Funderburk.

Mary had rehearsed her speech. She wanted to make every second count.

"My fiancé graduates from Officers' Candidate School in Virginia the day our vacation begins. He's heading overseas and I may not see him again for years. Maybe never. He could get killed." Her voice rose. "The only train to reach Richmond in time for the ball leaves Greensboro at 10:30 a.m. My mother will not let me go unless Carol goes with me. This means we must cut our last class."

If Mary and Dave were engaged, it was news to me! The more she talked, the harder I pressed my feet on the floor. Mrs. Funderburk peered sternly over her glasses. All seemed lost. "You do realize this is a rule which cannot be broken?"

"Uh-huh." Mary's nervousness began to show.

"Do not say 'uh-huh,' say, 'Yes, Mrs. Funderburk.'"

"Yes, Mrs. Funderburk."

"Do you want me to call Dean Elliott in Washington?"

Mary's bravado returned. "Yes, Mrs. Funderburk. I would appreciate that."

"Come back in a week for my decision," snapped suspicious Mrs. Funderburk.

As we left the office, I accused Mary of holding out on me. "Why didn't you tell me you and Dave were engaged?"

She laughed. "Dave doesn't know it either. How else could I get Annie Beam to cave in? You pressed the floor so hard I could feel the floorboards give under your feet."

One week later Mary and I became the first students ever granted permission to cut class before vacation. At 10:00 a.m. on March 19, we hailed a taxi. Mary slammed the door. "To the railway station and please hurry."

Like Cinderellas, we were off to the ball.

The Graduation Ball

The train for Richmond, Virginia left Greensboro forty minutes late. Mary and I didn't care. Her determination to attend Dave's graduation ball from Officers' Candidate School at Fort Lee, Virginia had overcome all obstacles.

Uncomfortable in our wool suits on a warm March day, we stowed suitcases, hatbox, make-up box, and coats on the overhead rack. To lighten the load we ate our box lunches in mid-morning before changing trains in Danville, Virginia. Six hours after leaving Danville, we reached Richmond, grimy and hungry.

In front of the train station, I guarded the luggage, while Mary stepped to the curb to hail a taxi to take us to the bus station. When she put her hand to her eyes to shield them from the sun, a carload of sailors squealed to a halt.

"Want a ride? We'll take you anywhere you want to go."

She glared at them and said, "My fiancé is getting his car from the parking lot." Mary knew how to squelch a bunch of rowdy sailors.

The driver of a decrepit taxi banged our luggage into the front seat and left us to scramble into the back seat on our own. The reason for his surliness became evident when the bus station turned out to be only a few blocks away. He unloaded the bags, grabbed his fare, and took off before we had a good look at our surroundings.

Mary stared at the small building in need of paint. "Is this a bus station?" We were standing next to a single gas pump in front of a converted garage. Inside, a few wooden benches stood on an oily floor before a pile of old tires.

Two girls in tawdry evening dresses, one dressed in blue, the other purple, looked out-of-place in the late afternoon sun. Their long skirts trailing across the greasy floor were edged in black grime. When the bus arrived, the blonde refused to board the bus until she finished painting her nails scarlet.

The jolting bus ride seemed to take forever. Mary's excitement at the thought of seeing Dave was matched by my apprehension over the thought of another blind date. Dave had described O.B. English, called Obie, as "tall, blond, fun, not a drinker."

Our arrival at the Petersburg Bus Station caused a sensation. A hundred new second lieutenants, all awaiting the arrival of their dates, shouted a noisy welcome. Dave rushed out of the crowd to give each of us a hearty kiss. That brought forth a rousing cheer from his buddies.

Dave, still painfully thin, had gained in stature and confidence. He appeared taller in a well-tailored green uniform than he had in rumpled khaki the last time I had seen him on campus. He pointed to the gold bars gleaming on his shoulders and grinned. Mary gave me a wink. I had helped her select them in a Greensboro jewelry store.

Dave grabbed a suitcase in each hand. "I'm supposed to keep my right hand free to return salutes but I'll take a chance. We can get away with anything today. The hotel is only a block away." In the lobby, he let out a shout, "Hey, English." A green uniform stepped forward — my first glimpse of my date, Obie.

He appeared as Dave had described him — tall, blond, charming. His first words gave me a clue the evening might not be what Dave had promised. "Glad to meet ya'. I'm from Texas.

Like all Texans, I like to drink. Dave and I'll wait in the bar while you gals change."

Mary and I stepped into the elevator. The pimply-faced young operator inquired, "Aren't they going up, too?"

Trying to act sophisticated Mary replied in a chilly voice, "Not now."

In our haste to change, a blizzard of clothes from our suitcases landed all over the room. Stepping into the shower, I forgot to remove my watch. Mary's shaking hand could not get her lipstick on straight. A call from Dave had slowed her down. "Mary, I just wanted to hear your voice," he whispered.

When we joined the men in the bar, Dave studied his watch. "It's almost eight now. The dance starts at nine and we have a long cab ride to get there. We must hurry." In the dining room white tablecloths, damask napkins, fresh flowers, and an extravagant menu set the scene for a leisurely meal. We had no time for that kind of evening.

Obie insisted on ordering plank steak for me. I had no idea what that might be. However, the last item listed under entrees on the menu, the most expensive at two dollars and fifty cents, it had to be special. I kicked Mary's ankle so hard that she got the message. Both she and Dave ordered plank steak. Obie then sent my self-confidence to a new low by ordering a ham sandwich and a bottle of beer.

The sizzling steak arrived on a two-inch thick plank, surrounded by mounds of Duchess potatoes, baby carrots sprinkled with mint, radishes turned into miniature roses. Such a work of art seemed too beautiful to eat but the late hour left little time to relish it. We still had to dress for the ball, a feat we managed in ten minutes.

During a taxi ride, at breakneck speed, to the Officers' Club, Mary and I pinned on our corsages. The men had chosen fragrant gardenias, mine tied with green velvet ribbon, perfect on my yellow gown, and Mary's tied with tawny ribbon to complement her chartreuse formal.

We arrived and found the party in full swing. To my disappointment, we had missed the receiving line. I realized that was a faux pas, but Obie's smirk made me suspicious he had planned it that way. He had to admit the elegance of the surroundings was impressive. The ballroom appeared endless. Mirrors on every wall reflected the high-ceiling room from floor to chandelier. French doors opened onto a terrace where borders of spring flowers flanked an enormous swimming pool. Dashing uniforms, pastel ball gowns, soft lights, and romantic music cast a spell over the dance floor.

Obie immediately took me downstairs to the informal club. Uniforms three deep jammed the longest bar I had ever seen. As I sipped Scotch and soda, I nibbled on cheese. Clinton's rules on how to drink were being put to the test. After Obie had consumed a couple of drinks, I insisted we appear at the ball. Much to my surprise, we danced well together. When we changed partners, I struggled with Dave. I needed a firmer hand on my back to direct my steps. As long as I talked about Mary, Dave didn't seem to notice when I stepped on his feet. He grew uneasy when Mary and Obie disappeared.

I knew where to find them — downstairs in the bar. Obie introduced us to his friend Bill. I figured Bill's comments about a mutual friend of theirs described many of the officers at the ball.

"George is like a setter. He points at a girl, then goes after her."

Eager to enjoy the spring evening and avoid another drink, I coaxed Obie outdoors to stroll around the swimming pool. The balmy air, the strains of music floating over the water and the starry sky made me long for a date interested in me instead of the liquid refreshments.

The dance ended at midnight. After the band played "Goodnight Ladies," we tried to make up for the missed receiving line by paying our respects to the Major and his wife at the door. The graduation ball of the Eighteenth Class, Officers Candidate School, Fort Lee, Virginia had given Mary and me a glimpse of the social life enjoyed by officers on some military posts.

Two years later, when I received my second lieutenant bars at Walter Reed Army Medical Center in Washington, D.C., the event took place without fanfare. Members of my class ate dinner in the staff dining room for the first and only time. Before sending us on our way, the chief dietitian presented us with roses and wished us successful careers in the army.

Vacation In York

Shivering in the damp night air outside the Officers' Club, Mary, Dave, and I joined the long line of revelers waiting for taxis. Obie had dropped out of sight. Undoubtedly, he had returned to the bar for a nightcap. Dave was furious his friend had stood me up. I assured him Obie's disappearance didn't bother me and I meant it.

Outside our room, I thanked Dave, said "Goodnight" and slipped through the door. Mary followed a few minutes later. Too excited to sleep, we compared notes on our dates and the ball. We paid little attention to the melee in the hall, although the sounds of breaking glass, screams, and laughter continued until daylight.

At checkout time, I asked Mary for the room key. "What key?" she replied dreamily. After searching the room to no avail, I opened the door and found the shiny room key sparkling in the lock. Luckily, the rowdy crowd in the hall had not noticed it.

"Don't tell your mother," I warned. "She'll never let me chaperone you again." Mary wagged her finger at me and giggled.

When we told Dave each of us had presumed the other locked the door he scolded us for our negligence. Later, he gave me a key-shaped wooden pin for my lapel and suggested I wear it as a reminder to always check the door.

By the time we boarded the noon train for Mary's home in York, Pennsylvania, Dave had already returned to duty. The only women in a car of enlisted men, we could have used the protection of Mary's lieutenant. Frustrated that their duffle bags had been left behind on the platform when they were being transferred to an unknown destination, the soldiers began to raise hell before the train left the station.

One fellow, who had been "rolling the ivories" all night, fell asleep. A buddy tried to give him a hotfoot. One lighted match, two lighted matches, finally, three sent thick smoke curling around the sole of his boot. A small flame flared up. The soldier slept on.

In Washington, D.C. we left the train, glad to be rid of our unruly traveling companions. When an April shower dashed our plans to see the cherry blossoms by the Tidal Basin, we gave up sightseeing and caught the 5:00 p.m. express for York.

Ahead of us, a burly sergeant sat next to an anemic college boy. The young man dressed in the latest style — pork pie hat, plaid jacket, tight pants, and saddle shoes — slouched in his seat. The sergeant glanced at him with disdain before producing a pint of whiskey from his pocket. "Care for a drink?"

The poor fellow tried to be a good sport. After he gulped a large swallow, he could not hide the tears running down his cheeks. A soldier across the aisle added to the civilian's discomfort by pouring bourbon in paper cups for his friends, all belting out a ribald song. Three privates, who sat on the floor at my feet doing card tricks, ignored the caterwaul rendition of hillbilly music ricocheting through the coach.

Mary unwrapped a Hershey bar. "This is like the circus, so many acts to watch."

As the train pulled into York, the setting sun broke through the clouds and illuminated the Pennsylvania hills with a golden glow. Mary, irked that no one had come to meet us, called home. Her sister, Elaine, answered the phone.

"Thank goodness you called. You just broke in on my conversation with Daddy. I am trying to explain how I wrecked a fender on his car this morning. You'll have to take a taxi."

Mary's mother waited for us in the kitchen. Determined to show off the changes in the remodeled farmhouse, she grabbed my arm and steered me toward the stairs. Not until I had admired every room and the stored clothes she had purchased on lay-away, did she allow me to join the others by the fire in the living room.

Revived by the soothing warmth of the burning logs and an audience, Mary and I gave a colorful account of the ball to an appreciative audience — Mary's parents, her brother George, and her sister Doodle. Later that evening, Elaine and her roommate, Ginny, joined us. They had traveled directly to York while Mary and I had detoured to Richmond. Mrs. Kirschner's brother, Uncle Pete, kept us answering questions until midnight.

The following evening, Mrs. Kirschner showed us off at the Woman's Club. Mary and I tried to stifle our laughter at the "Spanish Fiesta," featuring a chorus line of senoritas well passed their fortieth birthdays. Spanish shawls looked ridiculous on overweight, gray-haired women, particularly, the mistress of ceremonies. Throughout the program, she fidgeted with the fringe on the shawl slipping from her ample shoulders.

Dave's arrival on leave added some spice to our vacation. He requested Mrs. Kirschner's permission to take Mary and me to the Hotel Yorktowne for champagne. Her Mother's response stunned Mary.

"Well Dave, I guess a new lieutenant deserves a celebration. Yes, you can treat Carol and Mary to champagne. I know I don't have to worry when Carol is chaperone." She did not understand why we laughed so hard.

To Dave's surprise and mine, Mary balked at the location. "I will not go to the Yorktowne." Dave pleaded; Mary set her jaw. "I'm not going where everyone in town will see us. Word will get back to my aunts and uncles and I'll never hear the end of it."

Dave shook his head. "It's not as if we planned to do anything wrong."

Mary refused to consider the hotel but agreed to celebrate at Ye Olde Valley Inn. The run-down stone building close to the highway had once been a stagecoach stop. We stepped into a dimly lit room reeking of smoke and stale beer, the accumulation of the past two hundred and three years.

"Champagne! You want champagne?" The waiter looked surprised. "That'll take a while." He did not exaggerate. When Dave questioned the long delay, the waiter confessed, "Nobody orders champagne here. We had to send out for it."

The wait proved worthwhile, even Mary drank two glasses of the expensive vintage. After we left the inn, she demanded Dave stop the car so she could take a brisk walk to clear her head. We all needed fresh air — the aroma of Ye Olde Valley Inn had permeated our clothes.

At 5:00 a.m. I awoke to find Mrs. Kirschner standing by the bed with a flashlight in her hand. "What are you doing here? You girls can't be here. I didn't hear you come in." After we sat up in bed to convince her we were Mary and Carol, Mary settled back to sleep. Lured by the aroma of coffee, I tiptoed downstairs.

As Mrs. Kirschner handed me a delicate white cup, Pete, her youngest brother, barged into the kitchen. Still wearing his overcoat, he berated his sister.

"How could Dave take those girls to that disreputable roadhouse? He must have been out of his mind. Ye Olde Valley Inn! Not a fit place for a niece of mine."

I sprinted upstairs to prepare Mary for the storm brewing below. "Your aunts and uncles already know about our champagne drinking escapade. Uncle Pete is telling your mother everything."

"How did Uncle Pete find out?" She groaned. We never solved that riddle.

In the eyes of his eight siblings, Pete had never buckled down to hard work. The time he spent on street corners listening to the complaints of workingmen had led him to support their cause by joining the Woodworkers Union.

His first assignment had been to organize the workers in the furniture factory owned by his brother-in-law Neiman, husband of his sister Alverta. That audacious act caused a rift in the family, although Mary's mother remained loyal to Pete.

Spring break ended none too soon. Dave's leave had lasted only three days. Lack of sleep, too much hearty food, too many relatives, and too much shopping had worn us down. Before we left, Uncle Pete gave each of us a present — a gold edged card making the bearer a member for life of the Allied Woodworkers Union of America.

Back at college, Mary and I were astounded to find small leather-covered boxes in registered mail from York, Pennsylvania. We had thought Uncle Pete was joking when he said he would send each of us a surprise. Boxed like jewels, in blue velvet, lay blue enameled pins. A circle of initials, those of The Allied Woodworkers of America, surrounded a crossed hammer and saw outlined in gold. As I pinned Mary's new jewelry on her collar, I laughed. Certainly, I was the first union member in my family.

"Mary, how soon do you think we can turn up at a union meeting? When we flash our cards stating we, as lifetime honorary members, have the right to vote with the consent of all members present, we should create quite a stir."

Two years later Uncle Pete was forced out of the Allied Woodworkers Union of America. Mary and I remain members in good standing.

Along with the registered package, my mailbox contained a permission slip signed by Dad.

To the Parents of Woman's College Students:

Due to the presence of the Air Corps Basic Training Center Number Ten in Greensboro, student government has passed a series of regulations as a protective measure for students.

Does your daughter have your permission to have an unchaperoned date off campus with a soldier whom she had met at a chaperoned function on campus, provided she had had at least three dates with him on campus?

The situation is by no means alarming, but it is our desire that you have a complete understanding of the precautionary steps we have taken. May we request that you reply at your earliest convenience so that we may have your opinions at hand when college resumes after the Spring Holidays?

Parent's signature: Garfield Morrison "Yes"

Very sincerely yours,

Mrs. Annie Beam Funderburk

Acting Dean of Women

Our vacation ended as it had begun. Annie Beam Funderburk had the last word.

Saying Goodbye

After spring break, lab reports, pop quizzes and term papers blurred days and nights into one. Junior year had brought my heaviest workload and prepared me well for finals. They were a cinch. On the last night before summer vacation, the dorm threw a graduation party for Barbara Hollister, the only senior on our floor.

Barb and I relived our adventures of the past three years on train trips between New York and Greensboro. We remembered plush seats in air-conditioned cars before hoards of service men and faulty equipment made our wartime travel an exhausting ordeal.

I found it hard to say goodbye. "Barb, I'll always remember those bridge games, particularly, your flashing bright red nails as you dealt the cards." Barb's graduation made the rest of us aware of the uncertainties we would face in one more year.

Mary and I were impatient to leave the campus. She was going home with me for two weeks. Her mother said Mary's visit was my reward for acting as her chaperone. Mary and I joked about that on our way to the station where we joined hundreds of passengers milling about in the steamy heat.

When the gate to the tracks opened at 9:00 p.m., soldiers on duty had first priority. Mothers with babies, soldiers on leave and old people followed them. The rest of the seats went to the fastest sprinters. Slow movers were left behind.

Mary and I felt smug to make it aboard even though we found no unoccupied seats. We lugged our suitcases through the stuffy cars into the only air-conditioned coach. Little did we realize we'd still be standing seven hours later when the train pulled into Washington, D.C.

In the middle of the night, only halfway home and exhausted, we limped in high heels on swollen feet through Union Station. "Let's try for the express," I gasped. "That makes only five stops to New York. At this bleak hour, we may be lucky and find seats." We found adjoining ones and Mary fell asleep before the train left the station.

In New York, an argument erupted outside Pennsylvania Station between our cab driver and one of his buddies. Our request to go across town to Grand Central Station made the belligerent cabbie shake his unlighted cigar in our driver's face.

"Yah can't do dat. Dat's a short trip and we ain't supposed to take fares on short trips. Let 'em walk."

"Hop in, ladies." As our man shifted into gear, he stuck his head out the window. "I ain't goin' to leave dese young ladies stranded here with all dis luggage." That time our heavy bags proved an asset.

In early afternoon, Mary and I stumbled off the train in Danbury, Connecticut. The family had always met me, but this time the platform stood deserted. A call home brought a common response. "We have no gas. You'll have to take a taxi."

An hour later, we hobbled up the steps into Mother's waiting arms. Soon we were sipping lemonade on the screened porch and soothing our swollen feet in pails of warm water and Epsom salts. As we pulled ourselves up the stairs to the twin beds in the guest room, Mother called, "Don't get up until you feel like it." Two days later, our sore feet still puffy, we limped downstairs.

I was eager for family news. Mother told us my cousin Polly, flush with big wages earned in a drafting room, was treating her family to a week in a rented cottage at Compo Beach in Westport. Even her brother Ted, granted a one-week vacation from his essential job at a defense plant, was going along. At the mention of Ted's name, Mary's eyes lit up. She had met him on her previous visit and, obviously, she wanted to see him again.

She drew me aside. "Wouldn't it be fun to surprise Ted? Do you think we could stay at Aunt Hannah's cottage? You've always told me about the fun you had at Compo Beach before the gas shortage left the cottage sitting empty."

I told her that was impossible. "Number one — How can we travel twenty-five miles without gas? Number two — The storm shutters are still on and the water turned off."

Mary looked at obstacles as challenges. She called for a train schedule and informed me we could get to Westport with one change. She decided we could walk five miles to the beach, if we had to. If we opened one bedroom at Aunt Hannah's, we could spend the rest of the time with Ted's family.

A five-mile walk did not appeal to me, but Mother went along with Mary's plan. She assured us Aunt Pauline and Polly would welcome unexpected visitors. Two days later we hit the road.

From the Westport Railway Station we struck out on foot under a sun, hot and relentless. "We'll travel light and live in our bathing suits," Mary had said, but after a few blocks, my overnight bag weighed a ton. Within half a mile, the first car we'd heard pulled up beside us.

A gray haired man lifted his hat. "Where are you girls headed? Perhaps, I can give you a lift."

Mary gave him a dazzling smile and handed him the same line she'd found successful with Annie Beam Funderburk, the Dean of Women back at school. "My fiancé has a week off before he heads overseas. He's staying with his family at Compo Beach. We want to surprise him."

"Well, Little Lady, that's out of my way but let's just say it's my patriotic duty." We arrived at the cottage in time for lunch.

Polly, Aunt Pauline, Uncle Ed and, most of all, Ted, were delighted by our surprise visit. Aunt Pauline would not hear of us sleeping in the closed-up cottage. Ted moved to the daybed on the porch; Mary and I took over his room. As we made the beds, Mary hummed a happy tune. "Didn't I tell you this would be fun?"

We did enjoy carefree days like those of my childhood — swimming at high tide, racing across the sandbars to collect shells at low tide. We ate clam chowder made from clams we had dug on the flats and gorged on lobsters from Captain Allen's Clam House.

After supper the family gathered round a lantern on the porch to slap mosquitoes and play pinochle, Uncle Ed's favorite. Mary and Ted would slip away to walk on the moonlit beach while the rest of us played on. Sun, sand, waves, and laughter gave us a respite from the realities of war.

Mary wished she could spend the summer with me, but she had signed up for a job in July as a counselor at Y.W.C.A. Camp. I had to keep my promise to Aunt Pauline to help her teach canning for the Red Cross.

The government had encouraged the populace to plant Victory Gardens. Front yards, side yards, and back yards yielded a surplus of vegetables, which had to be preserved for winter use. Soon hardware stores ran out of Mason jars and rubber rings to seal them. I found it tedious work to stand over a hot coal range in the heat of July and explain the steps necessary to sterilize canning jars.

A distressing call from Mother ended my job in the Red Cross Training Program. The strain in her voice made me hurry home. "Carol, Grandma's illness has been diagnosed as cancer. Caring for her leaves me no time to pack for the move to Florida. I need your help."

She went on to say the prospective buyers of our home could not come up with enough cash. Dad had found a couple willing to rent the house for two years starting in September. That gave us six weeks to remove our possessions.

After I worked out a plan, I recruited my reluctant brother Sherman to be my assistant. When he heard my ideas, he said our brother Sam was lucky to escape all this work. Sam would be at M.I.T. all summer in an accelerated navy course leading to early college graduation.

"Sherman, we'll start by making tags — red for Florida, blue for the sale, green for storage in Aunt Hannah's barn, and white for Aunt Pauline's living room. Let's start with the attic and work our way down." We found the heat in the attic unbearable after ten o'clock. The summer sun beating on the roof sent the temperature soaring.

I didn't know it was going to be so hard to say goodbye to family treasures — relics of Dad's army days, portfolios of Mother's artwork, Sam's models, Sherman's Tonka toys, my dolls. As I leafed through Life magazines, I wept and let go of the past.

Three weeks later, an advertisement appeared in the Danbury News-Times. "SALE! Household - Toys Kitchen Utensils Furniture Rugs. 21 Ridge Road. Saturday 9-5."

The impatient crowd of people swarming over our lawn at dawn caught us unprepared. When Dad opened the front door two hours early, a stampede of determined women rushed past him. They snatched the pots and pans in the kitchen, had a tug-of-war over blankets, and fought over my doll buggy.

"I'll give you twenty-five dollars," shouted a man in a tattered shirt.

"Sold." I replied. Perhaps, someone would have offered more but I sensed he was making a sacrifice for his little daughter. Mother would be amazed. She had thought my asking price of ten dollars exorbitant.

I held the crumpled bills in my hand. That unexpected windfall did not soften the blow when I saw a young fellow lug the birds-eye maple headboard to my bed down the driveway. I had longed to keep my bed, a gift from Santa Claus, but decided it must go.

The sale ended soon after the original starting time. Eager buyers had snatched up everything in sight. The lack of available goods, plus the dearth of metals due to the scrap drives, had made even our mundane items valuable. Before we had time to tally the results, a large truck rumbled up the drive. Sherman helped load furniture headed for Aunt Hannah's barn and the Victorian sofa going to Aunt Pauline's living room.

Sherman and I had made a good team. As we had tried to spare Mother and Dad the emotional impact of dismantling the house, our relationship had grown closer. Only he knew the tears I had shed and the sadness I tried to hide.

Harder than disposing of possessions, was the helplessness I felt as I watched Grandma suffer and grow wearier after her surgery for breast cancer. She lay in Mother's four-poster bed wan and uncomplaining. There was no way to ease the anxiety her illness caused Mother.

I forced myself to pack my trunk and concentrated on my return to college for my senior year. There seemed to be a family crisis whenever I had to tear myself away.

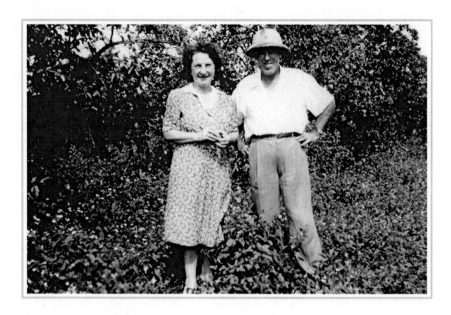

Hazel and Garfield Morrison at Bonita Grove.

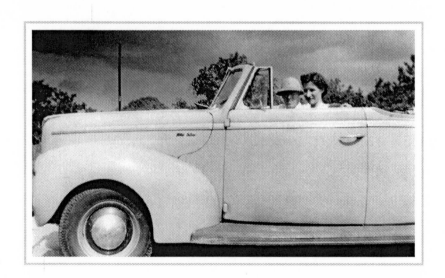

Carol with father in Florida 1944.

Senior Year 1943 - 1944

When I returned to college for my senior year in 1943, I felt out of place. My friends chatted about soldiers and clothes, while my thoughts turned to my beloved grandmother. Saying goodbye to her had been heart-rending, for I knew she was dying.

I was losing not only Grandma but probably our home as well. Although the house was to be rented for the next two years, Mother emphasized that she and Dad planned to make Florida their permanent address.

I felt confused by Mother's seeming lack of concern over leaving the place the family called "Home." I failed to recognize circumstances beyond her control had forced the move to Bonita Grove. She preferred to look ahead, not back. She and Dad, involved in the disruption in their lives, appeared unaware of the uncertainty hanging over my head like a cloud. Graduation was approaching and I had no plans for the future.

Back at school, a hectic schedule left little time for worry. Classes emphasized practical experience over theory, which brought new responsibilities. Cafeteria Management meant writing menus, ordering food, supervising employees, maintaining sanitary standards, and dealing with customers on the food line.

Our class met our first test the day the cooks and line workers were given time off for an employee picnic. Miss Tansil, our supervisor rubbed her forehead. "I'm sorry, girls, I'm too sick to stay. Confident you're capable of managing on your own, I'm going home." She didn't look sick to me.

We attacked our assigned tasks with an eye on the clock. After I had breaded fish and more fish, one hundred servings, I had new respect for the cook. The cafeteria line opened only five minutes late. Service ran smoothly, until Dean Harriett Elliott, Dean of Women, sampled the hot food.

"Who is in charge of this operation?" Not waiting for an answer, her voice grew louder. "Something is wrong with this fish. The flavor is very bitter. Take it off this counter at once. Do you want to give people ptomaine poisoning?"

Dean Elliott threw down her napkin, left her plate of food uneaten and stomped out of sight. The three of us responsible for the hot food were stunned. In the kitchen, we stared at the offending pan of fish. None of us wanted to be responsible for poisoning the customers but we had no substitute.

"Let's taste it," someone suggested. We each grabbed a fork and took a speck from a separate fish. "Does anyone detect anything strange?" No one did. "Shall we return the pan to the line?" The yes vote was unanimous.

After reheating the pan, we doused the fish liberally with lemon juice and added sprigs of parsley to each serving. Not one customer complained.

The next morning Miss Tansil complimented us on using common sense. "Dean Elliott always finds fault. Any bitterness she detected in the fish came from iodine. That's nothing to be concerned about."

In November, an invitation in my mailbox boosted my morale. At first glance, I thought the printed card must for someone else. I read my name again before the message sank in. I found it hard to believe I'd been chosen to join The Alpha Kappa Chapter of Omicron Nu, the national honorary Home Economics Society.

In a secret candlelight ceremony, the officers of Omicron Nu inducted four of us, two faculty members, another senior, and me, into the chapter. A pink carnation corsage pinned on the shoulder of my white sharkskin dress, could not save me from feeling tongue-tied in the receiving line. I found it exhilarating to have faculty members shake my hand and compliment me on my work.

The following day, our class went on a field inspection trip to the kitchens of Greensboro's new army base, Basic Training Center #10. No one had told the sentry that twenty of us would show up at the gate at 9:00 a.m. He invited us into the guardhouse to keep warm while he called for the major in charge of food service.

The major arrived in a cloud of dust in a jeep. He gulped at the sight of a group of college girls wearing stylish clothes and high heels. Elated at the thought of seeing hundreds of men, we had dressed in our best. He scratched his head.

"Well, you can't walk. It's three miles to the kitchens. I'll try to get a truck for you to ride in." After a long delay, our transportation arrived, the biggest truck we had ever seen. The floor of the truck was at least four feet off the ground. I wondered how he expected us to climb that high. He proved the army had a solution for any problem.

He climbed into the truck and reached down to take a firm grasp of the hand of the first girl in line. After he pulled her up, he told her to to grab the hand of the girl below. He jumped to the ground and gave the next girl a boost by pushing on her rear. Her classmate hauled her into the truck.

My green corduroy suit posed a problem. The straight skirt made it impossible to lift my foot up to the floor of the truck. The major lowered me to the ground. After I hiked my skirt an immodest height above my knees, his second boost was successful.

On a bumpy ride, our heads bounced against the canvas top causing us to slide off wooden benches into a heap on the floor. We discovered we could stay seated, if we braced our feet on the opposite bench. That way we could wave to the surprised soldiers we passed. Their whistles followed us all the way to the butcher shop.

The butchers cut meat in a refrigerated windowless room. Like the sentry, they had not been notified of our planned visit. They put down their knives to gawk at us, while we stared at the twenty-four thousand pounds of beef looming before us like a mountain. They cut up that amount every day. No wonder it took three years to become a butcher!

They told us each man was entitled to ten minutes outside in the fresh air every hour. No one took his break until time for our departure. All thirty butchers, dressed in white aprons and caps, lined up against the wall to give us a royal sendoff. We could see them snickering, as they watched the sweaty major boost us one by one into the truck.

Our next stop — the mess hall. Going in the back door, we passed a private on K.P. duty washing mops. He looked tired, forlorn, and discouraged. Shaking his head he mumbled, "This is a hell of a place to come sightseeing."

The immaculate kitchens surprised us. We stood single file watching the food preparation. Cleaners, who scrubbed everything — pots, pans, walls, windows and floors, outnumbered the cooks. Nothing escaped the scrub brush. When the major offered us doughnuts, a private followed us with a broom to sweep up any sugar spilled on the floor.

The field trip gave the class insight into food preparation in an army facility. We forgot the discomfort of the truck, remembered the whistles of the soldiers. We forgot the chill in the refrigerators, remembered the friendly butchers bidding us farewell. For us the day had been a grand adventure, but not for the overworked major.

We bet he put in for a transfer.

Christmas 1943

Shivering, I watched the dim headlight on the engine grow larger. As the train slowed, I buried my nose in the collar of Mother's borrowed fur coat. The dreary hour, 2:00 a.m., and the subfreezing temperature, twenty degrees, could not dull my spirit. I was impatient to leave Raleigh, North Carolina for Miami, Florida to celebrate Christmas.

My desire to see the family had overcome my reluctance to spend the holidays in the balmy south rather than the snowy north. There would be no carol singing in the snow, no flickering flames in the fireplace, and no cousins for Christmas dinner. Instead, Sam, Sherman, and I would pick oranges at Mother and Dad's new home, Bonita Grove.

Mother's enthusiasm had sparked my interest. "We'll not forget the old traditions and we'll have fun making new ones."

Dad's heart attack had precipitated the move to a warmer climate, but I could not picture him as a fruit grower. He was still a civil engineer to me, although he insisted he enjoyed the challenge of growing and shipping tree-ripened handpicked fruit. Mother had taken to packing gift boxes like a pro.

Mary Haynes, mother of my friend, Ginny, had driven me to the Greensboro bus station. Before she saw me off to Raleigh, she pressed a five-pound fruitcake in my hands, a last minute gift for Mother.

In the crowded Raleigh station, I had mingled with service men, mothers with crying babies, and a scattering of grandparents. We'd been packed together as tight as sardines in a can. Jammed against a sputtering steam radiator, I'd perched on my suitcase balancing the fur coat and the bulky boxed cake in my lap.

Three hours later, a squawking announcement had ended my long hot wait. "*Silver Meteor* for Miami arriving on Track One." Dad had bought two tickets for the all-reserved-seat train in July. In my purse, I had the seat number of my brother Sherman, who had boarded in New Jersey.

Wrapping myself in the warm coat, I adjusted my fashionable pale blue felt hat, shaped like a huge pancake, and gathered up my awkward belongings. Only one passenger had followed me out into the frigid gloom. Weak light cast by a pale moon outlined the pine woods beyond the tracks.

As the engine slowed, the whoosh of steam from the air brakes almost knocked my hat off. That style had looked glamorous on Barbara Stanwyck, when she strode across a hotel lobby in a movie, but she had not had to cope with an approaching train. Only the slim elastic stretched under my hair from ear to ear kept my chapeau from flying away.

The long train hissed to a halt. A conductor, appearing no larger than a doll, jumped to the platform at the rear of the last car. I ran toward the dim arc of his swinging lantern, my heels clicking on the frosty pavement. The suitcase grew heavier, the fruitcake grew more slippery, and the make-up box and purse banged against my thigh.

Without warning, a large warm hand covered mine on the handle of the suitcase. "Need some help?" A knight, clad in khaki not shining armor, had come to my rescue.

I released my grip on the bag. "I certainly do."

As we sprinted toward the impatient conductor, my rescuer whispered in my ear, "You can help me, too."

Alarmed, I tried to remain calm. "What could I possibly do for you?"

"Just let me do all the talking."

I jumped up the high step on the last train car. At a wave of the lantern, the train began to move. My benefactor ran along side pleading with the conductor who stood at my side.

"Sir, my wife has a reservation on this train. I have no ticket. My unit is shipping out for overseas in a few days. My woman and I need to spend this last weekend together in Miami. No telling when we'll see each other again. Help us out and let me aboard."

I looked down, worried to see my suitcase still in the soldier's hand. The train gained momentum, he ran faster. At last the conductor growled, "Hop aboard." I ducked but could not avoid the firm kiss my "new husband" planted near my ear.

We plunged into the dark car and groped our way through several more coaches to my assigned seat. I shook the sleeping form next to the aisle. "Sherman, Sherman, wake up. Merry Christmas."

"I ain't Sherman," growled a sleepy voice.

We retraced our steps to find the conductor. "Lady, every seat on this train was sold at least three times. You're lucky to be aboard. Sit anywhere." My escort spotted two unoccupied seats. The passenger across the aisle told us the couple had gone to the diner. I shed the warm coat, removed the impractical hat, now precariously perched on the side of my head, and placed the fruitcake on a ledge with a steam pipe running through it. The suitcase remained in the aisle, the make-up box balanced on top.

Two MP's appeared at the end of the car checking military passes with a flashlight. My hubby froze. "Don't move. I'm AWOL." As the looming figures drew closer, he ran his left hand across my shoulder blades. He slipped his right hand around my waist pulling me closer. "Look at that moon. Isn't that romantic?" His face close to mine, he nuzzled my ear.

MP's could see only the back of his head. They passed silently by. When the door slammed behind them, I tried to pull away. "You're safe now. You can stop the act." After a few more squeezes, he let go.

Back from the diner, the legitimate occupants of the seats waited for us to gather coat, hat, purse, fruitcake, make-up box, and suitcase. We stumbled down the aisle until we found another temporary place to sit.

I must have dozed off. The soldier shook my shoulder. "Thanks, this is where I get off." Somewhere in Georgia, my "husband" left the train and disappeared into the night. I did not even know his name.

When dawn streaked the sky, I resumed my search for Sherman. This time I awoke the right person. "Merry Christmas, Sherman. Merry, Merry Christmas." Suddenly, Christmas in Florida looked exciting. Mother, Dad, my brothers Sam and Sherman, and I would be together.

That wartime Christmas of 1943, many families could not gather in one place. We counted ourselves among the lucky ones.

Turning Point 1944

By 1944 the soda shop, called The Tavern, had lost its standing as the hub of the campus. That distinction now belonged to the post office. Twittering and chattering like a flock of birds, girls jammed the basement room at all hours of the day. Mail provided the link to soldiers, sailors, marines, fathers, and brothers stationed thousands of miles away.

Some students shrieked with joy at the sight of the blue tissue-thin stationary used by all military forces overseas. Others gasped in disbelief peering into empty boxes. No one moved. They stood rooted in place, unmindful of the crush behind them.

I elbowed my way through the crowd, twirled the combination lock on the small brass door. After the familiar click, the door popped open revealing a long, white envelope. Late for chemistry lab, I glanced at the return address and was surprised to read "War Department Official Government Business." The contents would have to wait until after class.

Three hours later, striding toward Winfield Hall in the chilly dusk, I pulled the letter from my notebook and read the three short paragraphs. I could not believe what I was seeing. The signature seemed to jump off the page. Helen C. Burns, Major, A.U.S.

> This is to inform you that you have been selected for assignment as a student dietitian at Walter Reed General Hospital, Washington, D.C. for the course beginning September 1, 1944. This course is of six months duration, followed by a six months' apprentice course.
>
> Upon successful completion of the course and if found physically qualified, you will be expected to accept an appointment as Medical Department

Dietitian. You will be expected to remain in the service for the duration of the war and six months thereafter.

Further instructions will follow from the Commanding General, Army Medical Center. Please advise immediately whether you wish to accept this appointment.

Yours very truly,

Helen C. Burns, Major, A.U.S.

Director of Dietitians

Was this the result of the civil service exam taken in December? The message gave no hint. Miss Tansil, our instructor in Institutional Management, had made it mandatory for the class to take the exam for student dietitian. She had said, "In wartime everyone will be required to take a civil service exam sooner or later. This will be a good experience for you."

On a cold dreary Saturday morning, twenty grumpy students had trudged along dark streets to the basement of the post office. Some of the class had studied all night, which seemed silly to me. After eight hours sleep, I felt alert and eager to get this behind me. Sitting on a hard chair under sweating steam pipes in a stuffy room, I raced through hundreds of multiple-choice questions. After three hours, I put down my pencil and rushed off to go Christmas shopping with Mary. The test was soon forgotten.

Now, that exam had come back to haunt me. The words, "Advise immediately" sent shivers down my spine. I enquired whether any of my classmates had received a similar communication. No one had.

Frantic days and sleepless nights followed. Everyone seemed elated over my appointment but me. I was scared. Miss Tansil and Dean Funderburk emphasized my acceptance would benefit Woman's College. They reminded me I'd be doing my patriotic duty. The dean predicted women would soon be drafted and I would be an officer — that I should feel lucky.

Mother and Dad offered congratulations, but no advice. They assured me I'd make the right decision. My friends teased me about becoming a lieutenant. Deep inside I knew I had to do this, I had to complete Ernie's mission. He had died for his country and I could do no less than serve in his place. I put off making a commitment by writing Major Burns for further information.

A follow-up letter from the War Department forced my hand. "This is to inform you <Caroline Morrison> that you are required to report to the nearest army facility within <10> days for a physical examination. Return the enclosed form signed by the examining physician. You must comply with this order."

Eight days slipped away before I found the courage to follow up on the "You Must Comply" order. I cut phys ed. class and called a taxi.

"I'd like to go to Basic Training Center #10."

The driver looked surprised. "You want to go to Basic Training Center #10?"

"That's right. To the hospital."

"Halt!" At the gate to the army base, the ramrod stiff sentry barked his order at the cabdriver. The cabbie slammed on the brakes sending my purse skidding across the floor. I handed my letter to the serious young private stationed at the guardhouse. He glanced at it, shrugged his shoulders, and pointed in the direction of the hospital.

The dilapidated taxi looked out of place next to the line of jeeps parked in front of a long, low building. Mounds of dirt surrounded the unpainted structure. Like hundreds of army bases throughout the south, basic Training Center #10 had been thrown up almost overnight — pine forests leveled, barracks hastily constructed. Often draftees arrived for basic training before buildings were complete.

No one questioned my letter from the War Department. The young corporal at the reception desk read it and summoned a nurse. A stern middle-aged woman, she expressed no surprise at the sight of a female seeking a physical in this bastion of masculinity.

"Follow me," she snapped. I studied her starched brown and white striped seersucker wrap-a-round uniform. She wore a matching cap set squarely on her head and sturdy brown oxfords made for marching. Unlike the sweet civilian nurses dressed in white I had known, she appeared tough and devoid of compassion.

Marching down a long corridor past closed doors on either side, I hurried to keep pace with her firm, military stride. She opened the last door on the left, tossed a sheet in my direction, and issued a one-word command. "Strip."

The door slammed shut. I felt abandoned in a room as forbidding as the old battleaxe had been. Pine pitch seeped from the raw boards paneling the walls. An examining table and a lone chair faced a wall of windows. Glancing outside, I faced hundreds of recruits trying to follow the drill sergeant's orders. GIs within a few feet of the window! I felt as though all eyes were staring in at me.

Only one place offered me privacy — below the level of the windowsill. Sitting on the floor, I removed my blouse, skirt, shoes, and stockings. Reluctantly, I struggled out of my slip, bra, and panties. Wrapped in the scratchy sheet, I warded off my nervousness by making a neat pile of my clothes covered by my jacket.

The thud of footsteps in the hall forced me to my feet. The door flew open. Garbed in only a sheet, I faced a tall handsome blond captain. "What the hell?" He began again, "What the heck are you doing here?"

"I'm not sure, Sir. President Roosevelt sent me." I handed him the letter.

Suppressing a smile, he read a few lines.

"I have no way to give you a physical. You're the first woman to turn up here." He hesitated, "Tell you what I'll do. I'll take your blood pressure."

My cold feet gripped the splintery floor. My heart pounded. Embarrassed but amused, I tried not to shake when the captain felt for my arm beneath the drapery. How I wished I were meeting him under less humiliating circumstances.

"Perfect." he declared. "Absolutely perfect." PASSED. He printed the word in bold, block letters on the form, signed his name with a flourish. "I predict a great career for you in the army." Before I could thank him, he disappeared.

The next morning another War Department envelope lay in my mailbox. Major Burns stated in three days she would be flying from Washington to Greensboro to answer my questions. She concluded her letter, "I am eager for you to be one of the sixteen student dietitians in the class starting September first."

For months, I had worried about a job after college graduation. If I accepted the appointment to Walter Reed, the problem would be solved for the duration of the war plus six months. However, one question remained, which no one could answer.

How many years would it take to win the war?

Dinner for the Dean

At the beginning of our last semester at Woman's College, most seniors thought they could coast toward graduation. My biggest hurdle lay ahead — six weeks in the home management house. Designed to put Home Economic majors to the test, the rigid schedule and long hours would make it difficult to keep up with regular classes.

The gracious, brick home on a residential street housed eight students and an advisor. My partner, Doris McRoberts, spoke with a New Jersey accent, which amused me. We discovered we had the same fondness for New York City. As we toured the house, I remarked, "Doris, this is the cleanest place I've ever seen." She reminded me it was now up to us to keep it that way.

Mahogany furniture gave off a faint aroma of paste wax, windows gleamed, hard wood floors shone. Artistic arrangements of fresh flowers graced the entrance hall, the living room mantel, and the majestic dining room table, which seated twelve.

Much as I missed Mary, my roommate back at Winfield Hall, Doris and I got off to a good start. We found our large bedroom, furnished in Swedish modern, a luxury compared to our cramped dorm rooms with scarred furniture. The bathroom provided privacy we had never experienced at school.

The kitchen reminded me of a magazine advertisement for modern appliances. Our advisor told us we were lucky to draw the toughest assignment first and get it over with. For the next two weeks, we'd be cooking for nine people. It would be our responsibility to maintain a budget, plan menus, buy food, and prepare three meals a day.

She emphasized we must maintain strict sanitary conditions in the kitchen at all times.

After she left, Doris flopped down in a chair. "Let's forget sleep. How can we do all this and keep up with our other classes in only twenty-four hours a day?"

"By not wasting a minute," I replied. "Let's get started." Doris always lagged a few steps behind.

According to the Department of Agriculture, food for the average family, based on low, medium, or high income levels, cost thirty-two, fifty, or seventy-five cents per person per day. As luck would have it, Annie Beam Funderburk, Acting Dean of Women, came to dinner the Thursday night we served a low-income meal.

Doris and I agonized over the menu. Not beans for the Dean! Chicken? Too common. We appealed to the butcher. "I have just the thing, beef heart. With meat so scarce, you're lucky I have one." The price was right, thirty-eight cents. We bought it.

"Doris, do you know how to cook this thing?"

"No. I'll ask Miss Tansil in the cafeteria. Let's make a deal. If I cook it, will you carve it?" We shook hands to seal the bargain.

When Dean Funderburk arrived at 6:00 p.m. sharp, our housemate Marge, hostess for the week, offered her a chair in the living room. Marge served the guests fruit juice and crackers. When I checked the dining room across the hall one last time, I heard her attempting to make conversation.

The silverware lay exactly one inch from the table edge. The open corner of each napkin faced right, the lower edge in line with the silver. Individual salt and peppershakers stood squarely between the bread and butter plate and the goblet. Not a chair wavered out of line.

Stepping to the living room door, I announced, "Dinner is served."

I took my place at the head of the table, with Dean Funderburk seated to my right. Doris, a starched white apron over her blouse and skirt, came through the swinging door carrying a tray of covered vegetable dishes. She arranged the dishes within my reach and returned to the kitchen. When the door swung open again, all conversation ceased.

Doris, hesitating in the doorway, held a heavy ironstone platter in her outstretched hands. On the cold white dish, rising from a sea of carrot tops, towered the beef heart. She gave me a weak smile before positioning the main course before me.

As I stood and seized the carving knife and fork, my hands shook. The first jab with the fork failed to pierce the hard skin of the beef heart. A second attempt lower down sent the heart skidding across the platter in the direction of Dean Funderburk's lap. Only a swift block with the carving knife averted disaster.

I changed tactics. With the broad knife blade balanced against the stubborn organ, I aimed the fork at the center and stabbed with all my might. Two small holes resulted, an opening where I could insert the tip of the knife. I exhaled but relaxed too soon. Hacking through the middle of the heart, I watched in dismay as the stuffing popped out in all directions, splattering the white damask cloth.

To my chagrin, someone snickered, followed by Dean Funderburk's hearty chuckle. Laughter ran from person to person round the table. Trying to ignore the merry diners, I sawed the meat into odd sized pieces. Doris quickly camouflaged the unsightly jumble with gravy.

Doris and I made no apologies for the insipid gelatin topped with whipped evaporated milk served for dessert in pink glass dishes. On a budget of thirty-two cents a day, we had done our creative best.

Back in the living room, Dean Funderburk sipped demitasse. "Girls, I want to compliment you on your efforts. This has been a meal I shall never forget." Doris and I sighed with relief when she left without asking to inspect our messy kitchen.

As we washed the china, my humiliation faded away. "Doris. I bet our acting dean is on the phone to report to Dean Harriet Elliott in Washington. When President Roosevelt meets with his 'brain trust' in the morning, Dean Elliott will probably tell him about this dinner."

We hoped the president would tell his wife. Mrs. Roosevelt would approve of serving beef heart to 'make do.' "We did make one mistake," Doris noted. "We should have done the carving in the kitchen."

We moved on to high-income meals. Steak, asparagus, and pie with ice cream brought compliments but none of the hilarity of the night we introduced Dean Funderburk to beef heart. After our stint in the kitchen ended, our assignments as hostesses and house cleaners were child's play.

The March day I moved out of the home management house, the bright daffodils leading to the front door could not lighten my mood. My grandmother had died two weeks before. I had accepted the appointment to Walter Reed but worried about joining the army. A painful wisdom tooth had been disrupting my sleep.

Back in my room at Winfield Hall, I told Mary I lacked the energy for the planned trip to her home in Pennsylvania for spring break. She decided she'd prefer to stay in Greensboro with me. Her mother wrote an explosive response to our change of plans. Her words made Mary furious.

"It is certainly gratifying to slave for years to bring up children and then have them turn out to be Columbuses who never come home, if they can help it, and never stay after they get there."

Mary gave in but I did not change my mind. Mary left for York with her sister Elaine and Elaine's roommate, Ginny. I stayed in town with Ginny's parents, Mary and Bryan Haynes. In a peaceful room under the eaves, I slept and slept. Mr. Haynes cooked his specialty, lump bread, just for me. Mrs. Haynes took me shopping and 'visitin' with her relatives. We loafed, laughed, and drank wine with dinner.

By the time classes resumed, I felt refreshed, relaxed, and ready for the activities ahead. Only a month remained before graduation.

A Night To Remember

All too soon, graduation crept up on the class of '44 at the Woman's College of the University of North Carolina. Mary and I had worked toward that goal for four long years, but the thought of saying "Goodbye" to friends we might not see again made us wish that day could be postponed.

Eager for a final fling at the senior ball, we wondered where we could find dates. Men in our age group, including Mary's friend, Dave, had disappeared to fight a war. He had been denied leave from his base in Mississippi. Determined we would not miss out, Mary came up with a plan. "Why don't you ask your brother Sherman and I'll ask my father?"

Dr. Kirschner, Mary's dentist dad, sent her an instant reply. "I would be honored to escort my daughter to the ball."

Her mother expressed disapproval. "I don't see why Doc should go to the expense of having his tux altered for one night." Mary ignored her mother's remarks and made her mother promise to attend the graduation.

Would Sherman, sixteen, want to be with us "older women"? I wrote him anyway. His enthusiastic response made us laugh. "Sure, Sis, I'll come, provided you line me up with a good looking blonde for every dance."

The problem of dates solved, we turned our attention to final exams. The hottest April in years made studying almost impossible. Only at midnight did our stifling dorm room cool down a few degrees. We sipped cold water, flavored with lemon juice, and tried to concentrate on our notes. After half an hour, I gave up and went to bed.

Mrs. Haynes invited both sets of parents to stay at the Haynes' home graduation week. She called to read me the replies she received from Homestead and York.

My mother wrote, "Dear Mary, Bob and I would be delighted. You and Bryan have done so much to add to Carol's enjoyment of college."

Mary's mother wrote, "Dear Mrs. Haynes, I am very sorry. We cannot stay with you. I have to have my own bathroom."

Tension, laughter, and tears built to a crescendo during the last week Mary and I spent in the dorm. We had shared a room in Winfield Hall for three years. Exams, not as difficult as we anticipated, came to an end. We sold our furniture, packed our trunks, and put our cares on hold.

Along with the arrival of our parents came a crisis — a call from Dave. "Mary, I can't miss your ball. Pulled some strings to get leave. I'll arrive from Mississippi Friday morning ready to dance the night away."

Mary wailed, "What am I going to do? Dad's tux has been altered. Mother will be furious if he doesn't go with me."

This time I came up with a possible solution. "Do you suppose he'd take Nancy Davis? Let's ask her if she'd go with him."

Mary, although skeptical, had no better idea. We had felt badly that, although Nancy's twin sister, Barbara, had a date for the ball, Nancy remained dateless. I crossed the hall to sound her out. "Mary has a problem. Dave is coming after all. Would you consider going to the ball with Dr. Kirschner?"

Nancy did not hesitate. "If he's game, so am I." Dr. K's response echoed Nancy's.

Eager to meet his date, Mary's dad arrived early at Winfield Hall. When no one greeted him at the reception desk, he opened the parlor door and ambled down the hall.

"Man on the hall. Man on the hall," someone shrieked. As the alarm spread, doors slammed shut. Hearing the fuss, the dorm counselor, led bewildered Dr. Kirschner back to the parlor.

He tried to explain. "I have three daughters. I'm used to hair in curlers."

Mary, Nancy, and I floated into the parlor on a wave of perfume. Mary had daubed all three of us with Chanel Number 5. Dave had brought her the largest bottle on display in the PX. She could have splashed some on every girl in the dorm and had plenty left over.

We found our escorts huddled in the corner telling jokes. Dave, thin and pale in freshly pressed khaki, his army lieutenant's summer uniform, held an orchid in his hand. Speechless, he stared at Mary, draped in her pale blue jersey ball gown. "You look like a golden Roman goddess," he whispered.

Dr. Kirschner, trim and distinguished in his tux, bowed to Nancy, dressed in a plaid taffeta skirt with black top, and presented her with a gardenia. "Nancy, you make me feel so young."

Sherman, eager and assured in cadet blue, handed me a camellia. "Sis, even though you're not a blonde, you look beautiful in that yellow gown."

The graduation ball was going to be a night to remember, after all.

The six of us strolled toward the Alumnae House where golden light streamed across the lawn from the tall windows. The brick building radiated southern charm with broad marble steps leading to a portico supported by tall white columns. Inside, we stepped into a dream world of flowers, pastel gowns, uniforms, tuxedos, music, and romance.

Sherman did not let the receiving line intimidate him. He had a word for each lady and a hearty handshake for the governor. The band swung into "I'll Be Seeing You." My sixteen year-old brother, a smoother dancer than I, put his hand around my waist and glided me across the floor.

In spite of the open windows, the heat became oppressive. At intermission, we gathered around the punch bowl, although the small punch cups of lime sherbet mixed with ginger ale did not quench our thirst. Stepping out into the warm night, Dr. Kirschner sank down on the marble steps. "Nancy, forgive me, I have to take off my shoes."

From our perch on the top step, we glanced down at Bryan and Mary Haynes, Dad, Mother, and his wife, strolling toward the Alumnae House. They had promised to look in on us at intermission. Mrs. Kirschner looked up from the sidewalk with disapproval. "George, George, you come down here."

Dr. K slipped on his shoes. "Come on Nancy." He took Nancy's arm and guided her back toward the ballroom, calling over his shoulder, "Goodbye." Mrs. Kirschner turned without a word and strode toward the car. Mother, Dad, Mary, and Bryan could not suppress their laughter.

Back in the dorm at 1:00 a.m., Mary, Nancy, and I kicked off our shoes and lay across the bed in our ball gowns. We agreed the commencement ball had lived up to our expectations. Mary said she felt pressured by Dave's insistent plea to marry. She wanted to travel, not settle down. Nancy and I teased she had chosen the wrong age group for her date. Nancy's escort had been too old, mine too young to force us into difficult decisions. All we had done was have fun.

Only the baccalaureate service and graduation ceremony remained. In two days, our college years would be over.

June 6, 1944

The following day, Mary and I could not stop talking about the ball. Dr. Kirschner, soaking his sore feet at the tourist home, sent word the evening had been worth the morning after. Dave had already left on his long journey back to Mississippi. The rest of us relaxed and looked forward to an evening picnic in the Haynes' back yard.

Mary's sister Doodle and brother George had tagged along from York, Pennsylvania with their parents. Doodle, fourteen, cast longing eyes at my brother Sherman. He, a man of the world after his popularity at the ball, paid no attention to her. George, fifteen, looked uncomfortable and talked to no one but his family.

When the shade of ancient oaks spread across the lawn and shielded the guests from the warm rays of the setting sun, twenty of us gathered at the picnic table. Mary Haynes' sumptuous meal included platters of fried chicken, ham with raisin sauce, grits, juicy sliced tomatoes, Bryan's famous lump bread, slabs of watermelon, and pitchers of ice tea. She surprised us with homemade ice cream — a rarity in wartime. Even Mrs. Kirschner relaxed. She knew how to enjoy good food.

After the Baccalaureate service on Sunday morning, Mary and I rounded up ten of our classmates to accompany Sherman to the station. We wanted to give him a big send-off for his trip back to Admiral Farragut Academy in New Jersey.

As we waited on the platform, a troop train stood on the opposite track. Hot, bored soldiers hung out the windows. When the shrill whistle indicated an approaching train on our side, Sherman lined us up and gave each college girl a farewell kiss. The soldiers went wild. To our surprise, the engine thundered by without stopping.

The approach of the next train gave Sherman an excuse to make his kisses more passionate for the benefit of the soldiers. Their shouts and whistles showed their appreciation. That train did not slow down. By the time the third one came in sight, Sherman had perfected his technique. We groaned when that engine ground to a halt.

"Sorry to leave y'all," Sherman shouted, his face smeared with lipstick. After he jumped aboard, we lingered until the last car flashed by. The frustrated soldiers on the stalled troop train deserved our final waves and blown kisses.

Back on campus, I sat with Mother and Dad on a bench in the shade. At last, we could talk face to face for the first time in months. Only then could I let down and admit how traumatic the events of the past few months had been.

"Deciding to accept the appointment to Walter Reed almost did me in. Everyone put pressure on me — the army, the faculty and my friends." I put my hand on Dad's arm. "Only you and Mother insisted that I must make my own decision. You trusted me to make the right choice."

I turned to Mother. "It's scary to commit to a year's training followed by army service for the duration of the war plus six months. That could be years. But duty calls and I must go. Now that I've signed up, I'm looking forward to my adventure."

I didn't want to sound discouraged. They had faced problems worse than mine in the past two years — Dad's heart attack, the move from Connecticut to the orange grove, Grandma's death, and Florida's worst drought in thirty years. I didn't mention I'd been devastated by the sale of the cottage at Candlewood Lake, although I realized they needed the money to drill wells to save the orange trees.

Dad cleared his throat. "Carol, we thought it better to wait until we saw you to tell you our latest news." His serious tone warned me to expect something disturbing. "We have an offer on the Danbury house. It has been a wonderful home for eighteen years but now we must let it go. Drilling the wells has cost more than I estimated."

I could not hide my despair. Hot tears ran down my cheeks. He put his arm around my shoulder. "Carol, I'm so sorry. We'll still make it a good summer. Mother and I will be in Connecticut. We plan to stay with Grandpa and you can stay with Aunt Hannah. That way we can do things together."

Mother tried to soften the blow. "I have always said I would never be married to a house. Of course, you will miss the only home you've known, but you're about to spread your wings and fly. We love our little Florida house. That is where our future lies."

After a sleepless night, I tried to concentrate on dressing for graduation. I could not put the sale of our home out of my mind. It seemed like a nightmare that would not go away. As I fastened the hooks on my black robe, Mary adjusted the tassel on her cap.

We raced across campus to find our assigned places in the procession. The front of the column began to move, a wavering line not the orderly march we had rehearsed. On a steep decline in the sidewalk, the pace increased. Taken by surprise when my high heel caught in a crack, I was thrown forward. I found myself sprawled full length on the cement walk.

In danger of being trampled, I scrambled to my feet and struggled to catch up with my partner. My ruined nylons concerned me more than the blood trickling down my leg — my gown would hide that. I had hit the gritty walk, scraping a layer of skin from the palms of my hands. Nothing could be done about the searing pain.

I sat in Aycock Auditorium, unable to pay attention to the speeches. Finally, my turn came to cross the stage and receive my diploma from the governor. A large, well-fed politician, he seized my hand in his beefy paw. He looked startled by the tears running down my face. He did not know he was crushing my bruised fingers, fingers that had lost a skirmish with a cement sidewalk.

Back at the dorm, a dozen long-stem red roses from my brother Sam made me forget my pain. Mary and I distributed the flowers to our friends before we took the last group picture. No one had colored film. We felt lucky to have a role of black and white.

Mary and I had planned to top off the morning with a special celebration. For this rite of passage, Nancy and Barbara Davis joined us. Champagne glasses waited on the bookcase. A bottle of champagne, a small one from Dave, lay amongst melting ice cubes in the washbasin. Mary divided the contents of the bottle, about an inch of pale liquid for each glass. As she proposed a toast, her hand shook.

"Here's to the last four years, probably the best we'll ever know. Here's to the end of this damn war."

We clicked glasses. Nancy choked on the first tepid sip. Her words broke the tension. "This is the worst stuff I've ever tasted, reminds me of antifreeze. I'm glad Dave didn't send you a magnum."

Barbara, Mary, and I laughed. "Nancy when did you taste antifreeze?"

We agreed the weekend festivities had exceeded our expectations in spite of the flat champagne.

On Tuesday morning, the euphoria of graduation was swept away. A radio newsflash shattered the morning calm. "D-Day!" Mary turned up the volume. "Our troops have landed in France. Today is D-Day." Unable to tear ourselves away from the announcer's excited words, we lingered. "The largest expeditionary force ever assembled, led by General Eisenhower, stormed ashore at Normandy at dawn. Allied troops under heavy enemy fire. Strong German resistance."

An hour later, Mary and I stood in front of Winfield Hall locked in a final embrace. Plans for our summer in Mexico had gone awry. I could not ask Mother and Dad to pay for a vacation. Mary was going alone to summer school in Mexico City. We found ourselves overwhelmed by the prospect of leaving each other for life in the real world.

We wept for ourselves and for the end of life, as we had known it. The war was changing everything. Most of all we cried for the men landing on the beaches in Normandy.

June 6, 1944, D-Day — a day no one would ever forget.

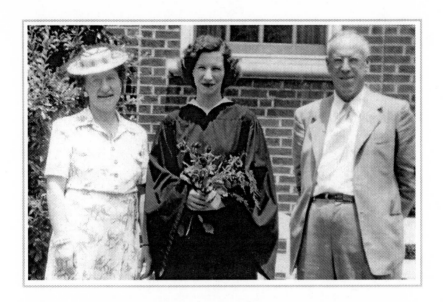

With parents at Graduation 1944.

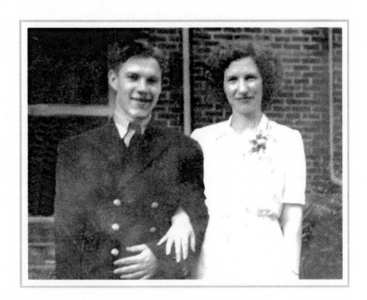

With Sherman at Graduation.

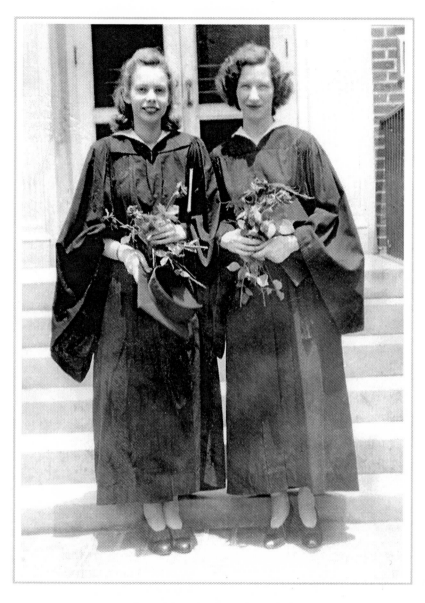

Mary and Carol, best friends, at Graduation.

Part II. Walter Reed Army Hospital

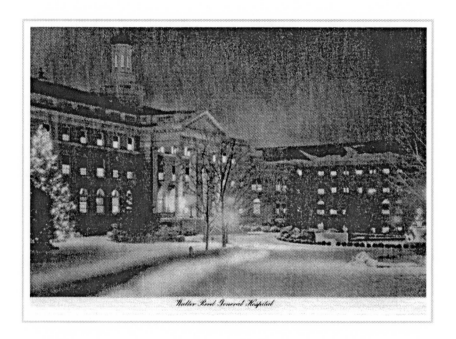

Walter Reed General Hospital

Doing Things the Army Way 1944 - 1945

Washington, D.C. slumbered in the sultry heat of late summer on the last day of August 1944. Excited and apprehensive, I had arrived by train from Connecticut for my internship in dietetics at Walter Reed Army Medical Center. Words from an army directive kept running through my mind. "Upon completion of a year's training, you will be expected to serve in the army for the duration of the war plus six months."

Now only a five-mile taxi ride stood between Walter Reed and me. I knew nothing about hospitals or army regulations. My life had taken this unexpected turn after I passed a civil service exam, a requirement for one of my courses at the Woman's College of the University of North Carolina.

Driving along 16th Street, the cab driver pointed out marble embassies and modern hotels. When he swung through the gate to the Medical Center, lush green lawns, lofty old trees, and gracious Georgian brick buildings surprised me. I had not expected a military installation to resemble my college campus.

The driver jolted me back to reality, "Here we are. Delano Hall. The Nurses Quarters."

He set my bags on the curb in front of a three-story brick building. I took a deep breath before walking up the marble steps past tall white columns, which supported a portico topped by a cupola. The building was a magnified version of the Alumnae House, where I had danced at the Commencement Ball four months earlier.

As I stepped into a parlor, furnished with mahogany tea tables and wing chairs, a tall, erect lieutenant, dressed in a brown and white striped seersucker uniform and cap, came forward. She smiled and gave me a firm handshake.

"Welcome to Walter Reed. I am Lieutenant Childress in charge of your class." She led me to quarters in the basement where two of my new roommates were unpacking. "Girls, we'll meet in the parlor at 1800 to go to supper. After that you'll begin your indoctrination into army life."

Outside a row of windows, a green lawn and towering oak trees stood in contrast to the stark white room. White tile rose half way up the walls. Separated by washbasins, six beds, covered in white bedspreads drawn taut, stood in a line on the white tile floor. Six students were housed in a similar room next door, four lucky ones in a suite across the hall.

Lieutenant Childress had introduced me to Emma Penhallegon and Marie Lanou. Within minutes, I knew they would be life-long friends. Emma's curly brown hair, rosy cheeks, and steady blue eyes radiated good-health and charm — the first Mormon I had ever met. Marie, tall and thin with straight dark hair matching her piercing brown eyes, ran on nervous energy like a colt. She came from Burlington, Vermont.

I chose the bed next to Emma. "Beware," she warned, "the mattress is hard as a rock."

Marie pointed across the beds. "Know why this room has so many washbasins? It used to be the nurses' beauty parlor. The partitions came down to make way for our far from homey quarters." We discovered one switch controlled all the lights and the cretonne-covered screen beyond the sitting area discretely hid the bathroom door.

Two girls arrived together. Eileen Welch came from Boston; her accent told us that. Natalie McCrystal informed us she was an army brat, daughter of a colonel. She bragged army regulations did not faze her. The last arrival arranged eight framed pictures of men on her bureau, before she introduced herself. Tossing back her mane of dark hair she proclaimed, "My name is Ann Paradise. These are my current boyfriends." Marie gave me a sly smile. The name seemed to fit.

At the evening meeting, Lieutenant Childress told us what would be expected of us. "You're going to work harder than you've ever worked before. The army doesn't settle for second-rate performances. Remember, I'll be with you every step of the way. I won't ask anything of which you are not capable, but I expect you to live up to your full potential."

Back in our room, Marie fumed. "One day off a week! How can we live with that? We can't even talk to the dozens of convalescent enlisted men strolling the grounds? Why not? We're still civilians and deserve to make our own decisions."

Emma reminded her of Lieutenant Childress' clear explanation. We were potential officers. Therefore, we could not fraternize with enlisted men. As time went on, those words, "Potential Officers," haunted our every move. We lived in Limbo, civilians abiding by army rules but lacking army rank.

The next morning we learned another facet of army life — forms, dozens of forms, always filled out in triplicate. After lunch, Lieutenant Childress took us on tour. She told us the area, equal to twelve city blocks, was referred to as "the campus."

Marie studied the map in her hand. "How the heck will we find our way around this maze of buildings spreading out like an octopus? Good thing they're connected by corridors." Hidden behind the main hospital, the thirty-bed wards, chapel, Post Exchange, barbershop, and other buildings gave the one hundred ten acres the complexity of a small city.

Lieutenant Childress herded us down the long block from the nurses' quarters past colorful gardens and rare flowering shrubs. We stood in awe before the imposing façade of Walter Reed Army Hospital.

Staff cars and limousines stopped on the circular drive before a fountain, where water cascaded down to a bed of orange zinnias. Thirty broad marble steps lead up to the imposing entrance. Opposite the drive, a manicured lawn sloped to a sunken garden and bandstand. Sunlight reflected from the paned windows of the greenhouses.

Betty Barnes, born in a small Ohio farming community, exclaimed, " If you add the three thousand patients here to those at the convalescent center in Maryland, you have more people than live in my home town."

The next morning, feeling stiff and formal in a starched white uniform with a white starched cap sailing above my head, I strode along the sidewalk. My first day at work! I paid little attention to the group of soldiers in prison garb sweeping the curb.

"Halt." The stern command made me freeze. An MP carrying a rifle blocked my way. "Ma'am, don't you have sense enough to know you never walk between a prisoner and his guard? Never do that again." He stepped aside. Embarrassed, I hurried on thinking; He called me "Ma'am."

For the next six months I would answer to the title "student dietitian." Although I was still a civilian, my life in the military had begun.

My First Assignment

According to the apprentice dietitians, one step up from our class of students, I had drawn a tough assignment on Ward 4 for my first weeks at Walter Reed Army Hospital. In the four-floor officers' wing, the men and their dependents rated private rooms. They had a reputation for being nitpickers. An apprentice had warned me, "You'll find officers demand more attention than enlisted men."

As I interviewed new arrivals to the medical ward — officers, sometimes their wives, and occasionally their children — they appeared courteous and appreciative. Sick, depressed, and far from home, they willingly volunteered information I needed for my questionnaire. They talked of their families and their hopes to return to civilian life.

My first priority of the day was making rounds. I handed each patient a menu. "Sir, here's something to brighten your day. Choose what you would like to eat. I may have to make modifications to comply with the doctor's diet order." I tried to tempt jaded appetites. "We serve tasty meals. Much better than the chow you ate in the field."

Although the remark prompted skeptical looks, I felt safe making that claim. Walter Reed took pride in serving the best food available. It was my responsibility to maintain that high standard by inspecting each tray before it left the ward kitchen.

From polished silverware to food temperature, every detail had to be checked. Hot foods, served on covered heated plates, must remain hot. Cold foods, kept in the refrigerator until the last moment, must remain chilled in spite of the humidity. Most important of all — coffee and tea, served in silver pots, must be steaming. In every tall glass of iced tea, there must be plenty of ice and a slice of lemon.

Generals never complained, but the wives of second lieutenants did. In the midst of a hectic meal service, one patient demanded to see me at once. "I am the wife of Lieutenant Sadonick. How could you send me such a pathetic slice of lemon for my tea?"

I stood by her bed and tried to hide my irritation. "Sometimes, we do not receive the supplies we ordered. No lemons came in today's shipment. To stretch the few we had on hand, we cut the slices thin. I'll send you another slice." Reminding myself that potential officers did not talk back to second lieutenant's wives, I hurried from her room.

Three weeks later, my assignment on Ward 4 complete, I stood before Lieutenant Childress dreading my first evaluation. Her first words sounded ominous. "As you know, you have been graded on twenty-two personal qualifications. The report is now on file with Captain Dautrich, chief dietitian."

She continued. "All are important. I look particularly at food standards, supervising ability, judgment, leadership, poise, voice, physical fitness, appearance and progress." Helpless in the face of that litany, I nodded. "For your first assignment you have done satisfactory work. I must warn you, from now on grading will get tougher."

What a relief! No black mark against my name.

Reluctant to leave my ward of friendly officers, I moved on to the office to write menus, army style. Many rules had to be considered when planning meals for a week. I stared at a large sheet of paper marked off in twenty-one squares. Down the side I printed Breakfast Lunch Dinner and across the top the days of the week. It took many hours to find a food to fill every slot.

Sometimes, I planned more dishes than the ovens could accommodate; sometimes, too much work for the cooks; sometimes, forgot to check color, texture, and flavor. Lieutenant Evans, my supervisor, glanced over my shoulder. "Never list the same item twice in one week. For example, you must come up with a different fruit juice each morning for breakfast."

Although we served mashed potatoes every day for patients on soft diets, the word "mashed" could appear only once in seven days. A list of alternative names became my best friend. Some creative person had come up with a dozen substitutes, such as snowflake, whipped, duchess.

Not one of my mistakes escaped the eagle eye of Lieutenant Evans. I stared in dismay at the sheets she handed back to me. Red marks questioned many of my choices. "What's wrong with Wednesday dinner?" I asked.

"Did you check the inventory? You should have known beef for pot roast will not be available until next month." I sighed and made no comment. Glancing at my watch, I was relieved to see I must rush to class to take an exam on the digestive system.

I could not concentrate on the test questions. My mind kept returning to menu writing. What meat was available instead of pot roast? Had I used turkey? I thought not. Maybe that would do. Picking up my pen, I wrote a definition of peristalsis.

Fatigue began to take a toll on the basement gang in Delano Hall. Even our glamour girl, Ann Paradise, regretted she had accepted a date for Saturday night. Of course, her alarm clock always went off at 5:00 a.m. She wanted to be first in the bathroom to put on her make-up. The rest of us preferred fifteen extra minutes of sleep.

Menu writing behind me, I reported to my next assignment, an enlisted men's ward. Dashing to work at 6:00 a.m. each day, the early morning chill jolted me out of my lethargy. Thirty patients waited for breakfast in one large room, the beds lined up in rows by the windows.

After supervising the tray service, I hurried through long corridors to meet my classmates for breakfast at eight-thirty. We ate in a long airless room with one window, tucked behind the staff dining room. The quick meal was followed by three more hours on the ward with the patients. After serving lunch on the ward, I rushed back to the dining room for a snack before class 1:00 p.m., sharp.

If class ended before 4:00 p.m., those of us assigned to the wards snatched a few minutes in the fresh air. We needed a boost before returning to our patients to serve supper. At our evening meal, we longed to linger, but some conscientious soul always reminded the class we'd better head for the library.

One rule, over which Lieutenant Childress had no control, made us furious. Only officers were allowed to sit in the reference room of the library. Potential officers had to stand. We studied until words began to blur and feet burned. I was among the first to give up and return to quarters to fall in bed.

The shrill jangle of Ann's alarm awoke me. I gave her ten minutes, before I stumbled into the bathroom. Catching a glimpse of my weary body in the mirror, I wondered what mark I'd receive on the next physical evaluation.

Seven weeks at Walter Reed had melted five pounds off my skinny frame.

Dr. Walter Reed

October 1944 brought a change in my training at Walter Reed. To meet a requirement for membership in the American Dietetic Association, each student had to spend three weeks at Children's Hospital, a city-run facility independent of Walter

Reed, to study childhood nutrition. Lieutenant Childress told my roommate Marie and me to catch a city bus for the half hour trip.

At 5:30 a.m. we shivered at the bus stop, our backs to Rock Creek Park. Every rustle in the bushes made Marie jump. "Marie, did you expect to be colder in Washington than in Vermont?" Before she could answer, approaching headlights made us move closer together. A sleek black car glided to a stop.

Out stepped a uniformed chauffeur. "Voud ya lika ride? My boss goin' to Russian Embassy."

"We're going to Children's Hospital. Is that on your way?"

"Ya. Hop in." We sank into the spacious back seat, grateful for the warmth blasting from the heater. Our host, weighted down by gold braid, sat next to the driver. He turned and said something to us in Russian.

Marie whispered, "Isn't this a stroke of luck? Lieutenant Childress should see us now!" We wished the drive through dark deserted streets could have lasted longer. As we left the warm limousine at the deserted entrance to Children's Hospital, we regretted neither of us knew how to say "thank you" to our benefactor in his language.

Our indoctrination into high standards set by the army had not prepared us for the appalling conditions in the dietary department of this city-run hospital. Due to a polio epidemic raging throughout the city, cumbersome machines, known as "iron lungs" crowded the rooms and the halls. The sons and daughters of foreign diplomats and government leaders lay immobilized, only their heads visible outside the tubular steel contraptions.

After our first day in the basement kitchen on the floor below those incarcerated children, Marie mused, "Has even one parent ventured down here? I guess not. If anyone had seen this mess, the resulting scandal would hit the headlines."

The porter gave us our first hint about conditions in the storeroom. We were about to take inventory when he advised, "Ladies, always kick the door 'fore yuh go in. Dat warns the rats yuh're comin'."

Twenty-five pound boxes of cookies, some without lids stood on shelves. Spilled rice littered the floor. Employees changed clothes there and combed their hair before the tipsy mirror propped against the canned goods. One colored girl reported for work with the sharp tines of an angel cake cutter protruding through her matted hair.

"Marie, we're never going to eat one bite of food prepared in this place." We settled for the same lunch every day — a banana and a carton of milk.

One dedicated, hard-working woman made light of her problems. Singing spirituals, "Pureein' Pauline" spent most of her time forcing vegetables through a strainer. When she pureed beets, we fled for cover. Our white uniforms were no match for the magenta blobs of beet juice splattering counters, walls, and Pauline.

An enormous woman, in worn down shoes, her strength amazed us. Marie nudged my arm. "Look she's ready to flatten that can." After emptying a #10 can, the largest size, containing ten cups, Pauline cut out the bottom. She stuck out her stomach, pressed the can with both hands, and flattened it against her belly. A stream of green string bean juice joined the rainbow colors of beets and carrots already decorating her midsection.

On lunch break, we carried our bananas and milk to a small park across the street. Maple trees showered red leaves on our bench, and crisp clean October air filled our lungs. I mused, "The only positive thing we've seen being done for the children is Sister Kenny's method of massaging the limbs of polio victims. Many of the patients are showing improvement. I wonder why her method is so controversial."

Late in the afternoon, tired, discouraged, and outraged over the unsanitary conditions we'd seen, we waited for the bus. The ride back took twice as long in the afternoon traffic. We dozed through innumerable stops all the way to Delano Hall.

The next morning a chill drizzle hid the bus stop sign from view. Where were our Russian friends when we needed them? No bus came in sight, but a small sedan stopped at the curb. A man, the age of our fathers, wearing glasses and a felt hat rolled down the window.

"Pardon me. Would you mind telling me what you girls are doing out here in the dark at 5:30 a.m.? This is a dangerous place for you to be."

We explained we were on our way to work. He questioned the sanity of a supervisor who would put us at such risk. "I drive this way every morning. From now on, you wait for me. Do not ride with anyone else. I'll stop every day." He never failed us. Throughout the year, he delivered student dietitians to Children's Hospital.

In November, a letter to the family expressed my despair. "Sometimes I get so discouraged. There is always more work to do. By the end of the day I am exhausted, worn out by the call-downs for endless mistakes I make. I cannot relax."

Eileen Welch, one of my roommates, expressed the feelings of all the class. "We look forward to getting away, then when we go anywhere, we're so tired we want to get back and fall into bed." Lieutenant Childress had assured us she would not ask more of us than we were capable of doing. We were beginning to doubt her words.

On the way to my next assignment, in the officers' mess, I paused in the lounge to study the large oil portrait of Dr. Walter Reed. His steady eyes and faint smile gave no indication of the difficulties he'd encountered. I'd read in high school about his heroic experiment to find the cause of yellow fever.

In 1870 when he became a doctor, patients regarded a full beard as a sign of wisdom, dignity, and bedside manner. Dr. Reed managed to raise a moustache but not a beard. He wrote his sweetheart, "It is a remarkable fact that a doctor's success during the first decade depends more on his beard than his brains."

Finding no acceptable work in private practice, he became an army surgeon. On his small but reliable army income, he married his Emilie. In 1900, he recruited a group of enlisted men to join him in a risky venture. They volunteered to be bitten by mosquitoes, which caused them to develop yellow fever. By identifying mosquitoes as the carrier of the disease, he saved millions of lives over much of the globe.

Dr. Reed's discovery made possible the construction of the Panama Canal. Yellow fever had defeated French attempts to complete the project. Two years after his break-through discovery, Dr. Reed neglected an appendicitis attack to carry on his research. The delay in treatment caused his death, at the age of fifty-two.

Saying, "Good Morning" to his portrait six days a week reminded me of his grit and determination. Resolved to succeed, I looked to Dr. Walter Reed for inspiration.

A Break in Routine

By November, I needed a change from the long hours of work and study. The life of a student dietitian was getting me down. Determined to flee Washington for a day, I called Mary Kirschner, my college roommate, and told her I'd like to spend the night at her home in York. As soon as I was off-duty at 6:00 p.m., I rushed to Union Station. I arrived two minutes late! The train to York, Pennsylvania was disappearing down the track.

I stumbled into a phone booth and called Mary. "Perhaps this visit is not a good idea. The next train won't leave for an hour. You'd have to meet me at ten-thirty."

"Don't give up now," Mary urged. "Take a nap until train time." Not in Union Station, I thought, but dozing on the train did take the edge off my fatigue. Mary met me, grabbed my bag, and gave me a wink. "Welcome home, kiddo." I took a deep breath and relaxed.

A comfortable chair! For the first time in three months, I stretched out in a comfortable chair. Mary's family peppered me with questions. I steered the conversation to funny stories about the GIs and the celebrities I'd met. During my twenty-four hours away from Walter Reed, I wanted to forget the pain, death, and tragedy I witnessed every day.

"Mrs. Roosevelt visits her boys one afternoon a week, whenever she's in town." I began. "She towers over most people. Her small felt hat is always visible as she leans over to chat with those shorter than she. Her high-pitched distinctive voice comes as a surprise." I described how her escort struggled to keep pace, as she strode briskly through the corridors from ward to ward wearing sensible oxfords and a tweed suit.

"Hollywood starlets receive whistles and shouts of approval. Mrs. Roosevelt receives love and admiration for her compassion and understanding." I told Mrs. Kirschner I had watched the first lady jot down the name and hometown of a boy lying in traction. He knew his mother would receive a call from the president's wife before the day ended. He was one of many on her list after each visit.

Doodle, Mary's fifteen year-old sister, asked, "Do you see many movie stars?" Her eyes sparkled at my reply. "Oh, yes. Movie stars, stage stars, singers, big bands, everyone comes to entertain the patients at Walter Reed." I didn't tell her I often found myself too tired or too bogged down with assignments to attend the performances.

"Did you see a movie star this week?"

"I met Alan Ladd, a leading man from Hollywood. Would you believe he is so short rumor has it he stands on a box to look in the eyes of Rita Hayworth? I also caught a glimpse of Gene Autry buckling on his gun belt for an appearance on the ward."

Mary's mother asked who impressed me most. That was an easy question to answer. "Wounded soldiers are the true heroes." I described two officers, husband and wife, who had ended up in different Japanese prison camps. Both went blind from malnutrition. Each presumed the other dead, until they were reunited at Walter Reed where they were receiving treatment. Their sight continued to improve thanks to vitamins and healthful food.

Vitamins brought to mind a letter from Mother. She had suggested I ask the doctor to prescribe vitamins to boost my energy level. I let her know in no uncertain terms that, armed with my new expertise in nutrition, I was the one responsible for maintaining the patients' vitamin levels through balanced diets.

I yawned and admitted to Mrs. Kirschner my problem was lack of sleep. Six hours a night was not enough for me. She suggested Mary and I go to bed. We did but not with the intention of sleeping. We talked until 2:00 a.m. Mary's disillusionment with teaching fourth grade came as no surprise to me. She lacked the patience to work with children.

I was relieved Mrs. Kirschner did not get me up early to help with the laundry, as she had in the past. She fed us a hearty breakfast before sending us off on a shopping spree. Stores in York displayed more merchandise in my price range than those in Washington.

Mary insisted I try on a cherry-red wool dress. It was perfect and kept alive my tradition of a new red outfit for Christmas. This day, my only chance to shop for Christmas presents, I chose gifts for the family with a Pennsylvania Dutch motif. Notepaper and coasters were unique and inexpensive with clever sayings, such as "We grow too soon old und too late shmart."

In the afternoon, we paid the obligatory call on Uncle Pete, Aunt Mary, and Aunt Florence. Uncle Pete came right to the point, "Found a husband yet?"

I laughed, "Not one person in my class has managed that." No one in New England would have asked such a personal question but I knew Mary's family well enough to expect the third degree.

Aroused from a nap by the aroma of roasting pork, I joined Mary's mother in the kitchen. She had shopped at the farmers' market for farm-fresh vegetables, good cheese, and large cuts of meat. She asked me to open the jar on the table. I told her a meal at her house wouldn't be complete without pickled beets and eggs. "You introduced me to this side dish. The only red beet eggs I've ever eaten are the ones you've canned."

At a table set with crystal goblets and Haviland china, we ate our way through a meal of seven sweets and seven sours made famous by Pennsylvania Dutch cooks. We downed large slabs of apple pie topped with ice cream, before the family rushed me to the evening train.

Twenty-four hours away from Walter Reed improved my outlook. I returned to our six-bed room in Delano Hall with spirit renewed. In the hospital, preparations for Thanksgiving put added pressure on the cooks in the kitchens and those of us working on the wards. Serving a holiday dinner on a ward presented many problems.

I stared at the menu — Thanksgiving Cocktail, Consommé Julienne, Cheese Crackers, Roast Turkey, Chestnut Gravy, Mashed Potatoes, Green Peas, Spiced Peach Salad, Hot Rolls and Butter, Cranberry Sauce, Pumpkin Pie a la Mode, Mints, Nuts, and Coffee. How were we going to find space for all that food on a patient's tray?

It took me all morning to come up with a plan. The KPs liked the diagram I drew to illustrate where to position the juice glass, large plate, small plates, nut cup, saucer, and cup. They needed good directions because they'd see little of me — I had to cover four wards.

The resentful tray carriers complained the extra dishes made the trays too heavy. I ran from ward to ward begging for cooperation. "Private, please. Put the crackers on the bread and butter plate, not on top of the pumpkin pie."

Many patients appreciated the colorful trays loaded with food. One eighteen-year old from Mississippi exclaimed, "This's almost as good as the possum I used ter git at home."

Another grabbed a turkey leg. "This sure beats the rations in the trenches. Next year 'll be better'n this. I'll be eatin' turkey with Ma and Pa."

Others lay ill and unresponsive, too depressed to care about Thanksgiving, too sick to eat a turkey dinner. My heart went out to them. I wondered about their mothers back home who could only imagine what their sons were going through.

The day had been such a busy one I had had no time to miss my family. Thankful to go to bed early, I drifted off to sleep wondering how Mother, Dad, and the boys had spent the day. I supposed Uncle Ed still told holiday diners to sit two inches from the table and eat until they touched. Of course not! Not in wartime!

We could splurge for the soldiers, but for civilians, one serving would have to suffice, even on Thanksgiving.

Christmas Leave

By the time the holidays approached, we students had grown accustomed to the routine at Walter Reed Hospital. One of my roommates, Eileen, studied the calendar on the door, "Only twenty days until January 1, 1945. Then we'll be one-third of the way to our goal of becoming second lieutenants."

Lieutenant Childress had told us she was trying to arrange for anyone living nearby to have two days off at Christmas. The thought of leaving after work on Christmas Eve to spend Sunday and Monday in Connecticut equaled the best present Santa had ever given me. Mother and Dad would be in Florida, but I could still have a New England Christmas, maybe a white one, and see Sam and Betty.

"Marie, I'll be so lucky if I get that leave. I'm the only person close enough to home to consider Lieutenant Childress' offer. Who knows where we'll be next year?"

Plans for a field trip made me wait a little longer for a decision. The class was told to be ready at 9:00 a.m. for a visit to a meat packing plant in Baltimore. "Let's sleep in," suggested Marie. That idea appealed to everyone in our dorm room. We skipped breakfast for the luxury of an extra hour and a half in bed.

On the bus, a stern lecture from Lieutenant Childress did not make us repent. For ten miles she berated us. "I'm ashamed of you. As nutritionists, you know the importance of proper eating habits to maintain good health. You needed a substantial breakfast to get you through this day."

The back streets of Baltimore led to an industrial area, where the pungent odor of cattle pens foretold our arrival at the Eskay Meat Packing Plant. When we gagged at the disagreeable smell, our Ohio farm girl, Betty Barnes, laughed. "If you think this is bad, you don't want to live on a farm." Worse was yet to come. We stepped through the door of the meat packing plant into chaos.

The screech of animals, noisy machinery, moving conveyor belts, flashing knives, and blood turned our stomachs. Blood everywhere. For the steers, the end came quickly with a cut in the jugular vein to end their misery. Amid the bedlam stood a skinny man wearing a skullcap. His feet planted firmly on the slippery floor, knee-high boots splattered with blood, he made a sign over each dying animal.

"He's the rabbi giving his blessing," yelled the guide.

We were relieved to move on. After the carcasses had been skinned, skillful butchers cut the meat into wholesale cuts. In a quieter room, we peered into huge vats filled with sausage meat and spices. When the meat was forced into casing, the casings writhed like snakes and continued to squirm until tied into inert links.

The next statement of our cheerful guide unsettled our nerves. "We do our best to meet high sanitary standards, but rats are a problem. In spite of our precautions, now and then, one gets chopped up in the sausage meat."

At lunch in the company dining room, Marie stared at her plate of potato salad and cold cuts. "Did the fellow mean what he said about the rats?"

"Of course not. He just wanted to scare a bunch of girls." I hoped I sounded convincing, but from that day on neither of us ordered bologna or salami sandwiches.

A week later, when I received a summons to Lieutenant Childress' office, I wondered whether I had made another mistake. She looked up from the papers on her desk with a smile. "Miss Morrison, you are granted leave for Sunday, December 25 and Monday, December 26." That was the news I needed to make the day brighter.

I had been shaken by my experiences on a ward where the patients had no hope of recovery — twenty-four young men all diagnosed with Hodgkin's disease or leukemia, illnesses for which there was no known cure. They had marched off to war prepared to face the hazards of battle, not to end their lives like this with a fatal disease.

Some refused to eat, others, hoping to build up their strength, tried to choke down the food. One doctor believed a concoction of folic acid, yeast, and milk might help. The patients showed no improvement. If they could have had their way, they would have tied the doctor down and forced him to drink the vile mixture.

"Cocktail time, boys." As I handed out glasses of the repulsive brown liquid, my attempts to sound light-hearted fell flat. On the chart where I recorded daily food consumption, there were few check marks opposite folic acid drink.

When a patient was moved to one of the two private rooms opposite the ward kitchen, he knew his name had appeared on the critical list. I often stepped across the hall to give a word of comfort to the lonely occupant. Early one morning a worried mother waited for me by her son's door.

"I want you to know how much your words have meant to John. I'm afraid he's worse today. Please come see him for a moment."

I held the young victim's unresponsive hand and whispered to his mother, "He 's been so brave, never complained." After I left, the door remained closed.

I had no time to check on John before rushing off to lunch followed by class. Due to a shortage of classroom space in the crowded hospital, our class met in the morgue. We hated sitting on the damp cold stone benches and hated the thought of what went on there.

As I walked by a series of jars lined up on a shelf, the name printed in block letters leapt out at me, "Norwood, John." John was gone? The autopsy already performed? I sat in stunned disbelief and heard not a word of the lecture.

My next assignment had taken me to Ward 33, such a long walk from the main entrance that the men called it "no man's land." Those patients felt free to ignore rules and regulations — inspection teams never showed up there. Many of the fellows lay in traction, impatient and bored, waiting for their bones to heal.

Late one night "unidentified persons" snuck several bottles of whiskey onto the ward. A wild melee followed. Everyone got drunk. In spite of heavy plaster casts, patients ran races in the long corridor. Some tipsy revelers removed weights from their buddies in traction and got them up to join the fun. Frantic nurses called for help. Emergency teams of doctors spent hours resetting bones.

The commanding officer immediately issued strict orders. "The incident on Ward 33 will not be mentioned or discussed." We knew why. If Drew Pearson, the leading columnist in Washington, got wind of that scandal, the repercussions would be earthshaking. To avoid publicity, the culprits remained unidentified. Drew Pearson made no mention of the debacle.

When time came to leave that ward, I made the rounds to say goodbye. "I expect you to treat my replacement, Miss Hayes, just as well as you've treated me. She's a special friend of mine." The patients wanted me to stay. How I wished I could. They had made me laugh every day.

Walking back to quarters from the library, I confessed to Ann Paradise, our beauty queen, that the ward doctor had asked me for a date. She stared at me in disbelief. "You had a chance to date a doctor and you turned him down?"

"Well, yes, I did. Going to watch an autopsy did not strike me as a relaxing way to spend my day off." I did not tell her why I never wanted to enter the morgue again.

When large boxes of Christmas menus arrived from the printer, I began counting the hours until my two-day leave. The menu cover depicted the main building on a snowy evening. Cheerful light glowed in each window of the four stories with window shades drawn to mid sash in perfect alignment. The twinkling lights on a stately evergreen reflected on the snow and glowing lamps highlighted the fountain.

Inside the card, red printing described Christmas dinner from shrimp cocktail to rum ice cream, holiday fruitcake, and coffee. On the opposite page, the Commanding General extended cordial Christmas greetings to all personnel and patients.

He assured all personnel "we had fulfilled our duties with credit." I wondered how the patients felt about that bit of propaganda. I suspected many of them in far-flung wards had never seen the romanticized entrance depicted on the menu cover.

On Christmas Eve, my roommates shared my excitement. "I wish I could take all of you with me." If I had been working on a ward, I'd have felt guilty, but my current assignment, checking in supplies for Mess II in a dreary basement, left me free to go. Before leaving, I placed gifts for my roommates under our tiny Christmas tree.

Loaded down with a shopping bag of Christmas gifts, as well as an overnight bag, I pulled Mother's fur coat tight against the damp night air. When Mother knew she would be spending the winter in Florida, she insisted I take her coat. She must have had an evening like this one in mind.

"Merry Christmas," I sang out to the cabdriver. "I'd like to go to Union Station."

War Time Travel

The cab driver shook his head. "Lady, looks lik' you're goin' tah have a rough trip. Can't get no closer to the station in this traffic jam. Want to change yur mind?"

"Oh no. Nothing's going to stop me from catching the train to New York." I handed him a generous tip and plunged into the crowd. Only on New Year's Eve in Times Square had I been trapped in such a mob. Those revelers had been rowdy but happy, these desperate travelers pushed, shoved, and fought.

I did not know, until I read the paper the next day, many doors to Union Station had been locked to keep out the overflow crowd. To clear the concourse, travelers were let through some gates before trains arrived. Those people were in danger of being swept onto the tracks. Extra cops had rushed on duty and First Aid workers revived those knocked down by the surge of people.

Hundreds with reservations missed their trains. After the crowds dissipated, cleaning crews picked up almost a ton of coats, luggage, and pocketbooks. A few children, swept away from their parents in the melee, wound up in different states and had to be rescued by Travelers Aid.

Unaware of the dangerous situation, I pushed and prodded my way toward the closed iron grillwork leading to the tracks. Departure time came and went. No one moved. As I stood with my arms pinned to my sides, my fingers grew numb from the weight of the overnight bag in my hand. The restless throng pressed harder, until someone started to sing "Silent Night." As if by magic, the gate flew open.

Like a champagne cork released from a bottle, I was propelled down the platform by the momentum of the crowd behind me. Even with a head start, dozens of people dashed past me knocking down those in their way. I set my sights on the nearest entrance to the train. With one foot on the bottom step, I grasped the icy vertical handle with my right hand. My left hand clutched the overnight bag and the bag of gifts.

"All aboard," in two minutes every car had filled. Those of us clinging to the steps fought for a toehold. The train gave a jerk. Afraid I'd be swept off the step and crushed under the wheels, I tightened my grasp. A strong hand covered mine, "I've got you. Don't worry. I won't let you fall. Someone grab her bag."

A burly sergeant, his place above me on the car platform secured by his bulk, bent down and grabbed both my wrists. I found myself air borne over many heads into his arms.

My hero reeked of beer and needed a shave. Even when shuffling feet moved to make room for mine, he was in no hurry to put me down. As the train gained speed, the sailor who had retrieved my bags passed them on. Biting cold wind enveloped our huddled group.

Long before the train stopped in North Philadelphia, I had given up my struggle to escape from the sergeant's arms. His tight embrace protected me from the bitter chill. At the station, a few passengers pushed past us to get off. My protector seized the opportunity to force me through the door into the steamy crowded car.

"Jeez, I need a beer." Like a football player charging down field, he lunged down the packed aisle leaving me behind. I never saw him again, but I did have a chance to thank my next benefactor. A man seated on the aisle next to where I stood, said, "Would you like to trade places? I'm getting off in Trenton." Grateful to be off my feet, I dozed all the way to the final stop, Pennsylvania Station.

On the cab ride cross-town to Grand Central Station, the eerie hushed silence of the blacked-out streets could not dampen my elation. My excitement didn't wane when I missed the midnight train to Connecticut by five minutes. I called my brother Sam to tell him not to wait up for me. Santa's sleigh had left without me. My arrival would be on Christmas morning instead of Christmas Eve.

The past six hours had been spent with too many people; now I sat alone in the cavernous waiting room of Grand Central. Determined to stay awake, I settled down on a hard wooden bench under a dim light. The echo of approaching footsteps seemed ominous until I glimpsed the blue uniform of a policeman. The stern man towered over me, a club in his right hand.

"What're you doing here at this hour?"

"Merry Christmas. I came from Washington, missed the last train to Connecticut. I can't get out of here until the 6:00 a.m. train."

His weary eyes softened. "Not a good start to your holiday, is it, Miss? Stay alert and hold tight to your purse. I'll check on you every hour. Merry Christmas." He kept his promise and surprised me with a donut before his shift ended.

I stared at the huge wreath high above my head on the wall. Memories of prewar Christmases crowded my thoughts. I began a letter to Mother and Dad, far away in Florida. I wrote the night away. That letter did not survive, but my father's response did.

> Dearest Carol,
>
> During the years you have been away, you have written us many beautiful letters, but it seems to me your letter written Christmas Eve is just about the nicest ever. Mother and I will always be so glad that we are a family who get a real thrill out of Christmas and like to tell the world what a grand time we think it is. We had a lovely day but we too had a big lump in our hearts for the daughter and son who could not be here. But we surely will have many more Christmases together.

Only a handful of passengers rode the first train of the morning. The pale pink of a clear dawn highlighted the bare branches of the trees. When the train chugged to a stop at the Stamford Station, two people stood on the platform looking like a Norman Rockwell Christmas card — my brother Sam, a red muffler round his neck, and his fiancée Betty, in a matching red cap.

"Merry Christmas," they shouted. "You're just in time for breakfast."

"Merry Christmas," I called back. "Isn't this a beautiful Christmas Day?"

The Ultimatum

In January 1945, Lieutenant Childress issued an ultimatum to the class of student dietitians. "If you plan to continue in this program, you must sign a sworn statement agreeing to accept a commission as a second lieutenant in the army in September. This is your last chance to change your minds."

"I wonder whether I really want to go on," grumbled Marie. "After our experience on the field trip with that stupid captain, I'm not sure I want to put up with his kind of abuse." None of us would ever forget that day. We had witnessed how the army's policy to obey orders at all times could destroy an innocent man.

The veterinary officer, a Captain, had taken us in a cumbersome army bus to the Department of Agriculture to attend a lecture on meat cutting. At the front of the tall stone building, three graceful arches led to the courtyard entrance.

The bus bumped over the curb and halted on the drive leading through the arch. The Captain, a small, fussy man, who annoyed us with his self-importance, raised his high-pitched voice. "Corporal, why have you stopped? Proceed to the door."

"I can't move forward, Sir. There is no way to avoid hitting that car." We gazed down on a bright-red convertible. Must be a big shot to have a car like that in wartime and leave it double-parked in the archway, I thought.

The Captain's voice rose higher. "He's illegally parked. Drive on."

"But, Sir," The driver had no chance to finish his sentence.

"Corporal, I said, drive on. That's an order."

We cringed as the bus inched slowly forward. Crunch! After the sickening sound of metal tearing metal, the bus lurched to a stop. We stared in horror at the crumpled side of the beautiful red convertible.

"Off the bus, girls. Now."

Silently, we filed passed the dejected driver, aware he probably faced disgrace and the end of his army career. Seated in the auditorium, we heard not one word of the lecture. A different bus with a different driver took us back to Walter Reed. We never forgave the Captain for destroying that corporal's future.

The next day brought another blow. Emma took Marie and me aside to tell us she'd decided to leave the program. Her boyfriend had asked her to marry him and convinced her "the duration of the war plus six months" was too long to wait. I was shocked that Emma had come to that decision. We had agreed to those terms before we came to Walter Reed. She, Marie, and I had shared good experiences and difficult ones during the months as students. Now she was deserting us. How could Marie and I go on to become apprentice dietitians without Emma?

We tried to hide our disappointment and make our final field trip a special day. Lieutenant Childress had saved the best for last — a tour of the kitchens at The Pentagon. As the class waited to be issued security badges at the entrance, excitement ran high. Not even the president could be escorted through restricted areas without a badge. High-ranking officers and government officials hurried past. Everyone was on the run.

The long trek through a maze of corridors to the kitchens made us realize the vast size of the place made people hurry. We stared at long lines of sparkling new equipment. I nudged Marie's arm. "Can you believe this? Imagine serving thirty-five thousand meals a day! Bet we never work in a place this modern."

As final exams approached, I spent my day off in the library. The vitamin analysis of menus for one week ate up many hours. I finished writing two case histories, one with an uncooperative patient. Next came the review of dozens of diseases, sanitation rules, purchasing principals and protocol. It amazed me that I had covered so much material in six months and gained practical experience along the way.

Just as Lieutenant Childress had promised the first day, she had been fair and she had forced us to extend ourselves further than we thought possible. Now came our reward — final exams much easier than we anticipated. Lieutenant Childress told us we deserved that break. In the future, the good grades would look impressive in our records.

She realized how hard we'd studied, particularly those last three weeks. "I want you to know how proud I am of each one of you. You've been an outstanding class and I expect great things from you."

We hated to leave our basement quarters and find our own housing off base. For the first time, we realized how much we'd miss Lieutenant Childress. Like a mother hen, she had guided us through the strict discipline and long hours at Walter Reed. Her support and understanding had kept us motivated.

Before we left Washington for a week's vacation, one assignment remained — a group photograph of the class. Lieutenant Childress' last order surprised us. "Get out the yard stick, needles and thread, girls." We had to shorten or lengthen our uniforms until skirts were exactly thirteen inches from the floor.

Mary Schroeder, the shortest, found her skirt just below the knee. Tall Myra had to rip out the hem to lengthen her skirt to match Mary's. Her remark made us laugh. "I haven't worn a skirt this long since the government decreed short skirts to save material. I feel like a tablecloth."

The class had to admit the straight hemline of sixteen starched white uniforms made an impressive picture. Our glum expressions indicated the emotion we felt over the departure of six of our classmates. Two had followed Emma's lead to leave the program and three were being transferred to other hospitals. We'd miss their companionship.

Only ten of us remained to become apprentice dietitians. We would carry on for the next six months at Walter Reed Hospital.

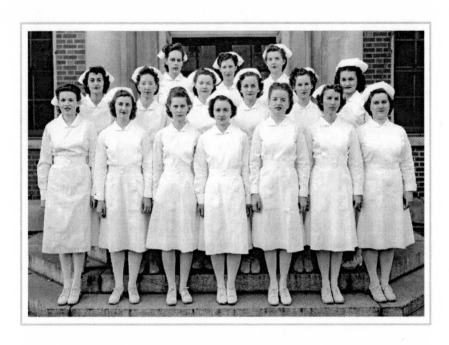

Student dietitians at Walter Reed 1945.

Victory and VIPs 1945

Vacation at last. In February 1945, my six month course as a student dietitian at Walter Reed complete, I boarded the *Silver Meteor* to Florida. Eager to see Mother and Dad at the orange grove, I didn't mind the rising temperature in the non air-conditioned coach, not after the damp chill back in Washington.

The train sped through the Technicolor landscape of Florida to Miami. I spotted Mother and Dad waiting for me in the shade of the station. Florida tans gave them a healthy glow compared to my winter pallor. After kisses and many hugs, we walked down the platform, all of us talking at once.

A worried tone crept into Mother's voice, "Dear, you're so thin."

"Well, I've lost fifteen pounds since you saw me in September."

"Let's remedy that." Dad chuckled, a twinkle in his eye. "How about an ice cream soda?"

On my first visit for Christmas 1943, I had doubted the small house under the palm trees would ever feel like home. I had missed the scenes of my childhood in Connecticut. The grove and the simple way of life there had grown in my affection during the past summer, when Dad and I had spent a month measuring the depth of the new wells.

Now, my first glimpse of Bonita Grove convinced me this was where the family should be. The swaying coconut palms towering over the little house, the orderly rows of orange trees, the brilliant magenta bougainvillea, and the heavy perfume of many plants I could not identify, filled me with awe for such beauty.

I asked Mother whether Elizabeth, the weekly laundress, still washed clothes in the huge black kettle in the back yard. She nodded. "Elizabeth says there's a rattlesnake near the packing house. She smells goat and goat means rattlesnake."

"That won't help me," I mused. "I don't know the smell of goat."

Mother flung open the door to her gift shop in the end of the packing shed facing the road. Her artistic hand and love of color had transformed a dusty storage area into a charming shop.

"I'm so proud of what we've accomplished here. In spite of the gas shortage, I've had a trickle of customers. Every little bit helps."

Bright blue cupboards lined the walls, each decorated with one large blossom of poinsettia, bougainvillea, hibiscus, or orange. When the shop closed for the summer, items displayed on the tables could be stored in the cabinets. We laughed about the day in August we'd spent in New York looking for bargains. I picked up a plate we'd found in Greenwich Village — the price now double what we'd paid for it.

"I almost had a famous visitor," Mother said. "A tall, distinguished English gentleman bought an antique cane. I heard him say Winston would be sorry he decided to nap rather than visit the shop." She showed me the newspaper describing Winston Churchill's weekend in Coral Gables.

Dad joined us on the screened porch to linger over chicken salad and chilled glasses of iced tea with lemon plucked from a tree by the door. The sun, a flaming disk in the sky, hesitated, then dropped behind the orange grove, plunging our world into darkness. Night arrived without benefit of twilight in Florida.

My long trip on the overnight sit-up train caught up with me. I sighed, "It's time for bed. We'll have plenty of time to talk tomorrow."

"I must warn you about Oscar," Mother cautioned. "Oscar is a large spider who lives in your room. He's one of our best companions. He eats bugs, many, many bugs. I couldn't get along without Oscar. Please don't kill him."

I had forgotten how relaxing a room to one's self could be. I stretched out on the bed with its cool white sheets. When I reached for the lamp switch, something overhead caught my eye. I jumped from the bed. "Dad, Dad, there's a creature on the ceiling. It looks like a miniature lobster."

"That's a scorpion. Glad it didn't bite you. One got me when I reached in to light the water heater. The pain was excruciating." He removed the little creature with the poisonous stinger in its tail by turning on the Electrolux and sucking it into the hose.

Spiders? Scorpions? How would I ever get to sleep? The next thing I knew, the bright light of the rising sun flooded the room with warm sticky heat.

Mother and Dad said they were postponing all work the few days of my visit. Dad suggested a drive to Key West. He thought I might like to get behind the wheel.

"I'm too tired for a long drive. I'd be happy to spend the day right here. Perhaps, we could call on the Robinsons."

Carl and Helen Robinson owned an avocado grove. Carl had practiced medicine in Vermont, until a radium burn on his thumb forced him to retire. When Dad and I had stayed at our grove in July, Carl had come to my aid in an emergency.

I had tried to open a can of soup with a rusty can opener and sliced a generous piece off the top of my thumb. Dad rushed me to the Robinson's kitchen. After Doc Robinson treated my wound, he queried, "How about a game of bridge?" Long after the finger recovered, we continued to play cards through the hot summer afternoons.

Now I had something to tell the Robinsons. One of my assignments at Walter Reed had forced me out of bed at 4:00 a.m. to accompany the mess sergeant to the wholesale fruit and vegetable market. Long lists of requisitions in hand, we made our way down the bright aisles past towering displays of produce.

Sergeant Smith explained the army bought only top grade and we must move quickly to find the best selection. Suddenly, I grabbed the sergeant's arm. "Stop. Stop. You have to buy some of those avocados."

I gazed up at a tower of boxes. Each label pictured a shady avocado tree above the words, "Doc Robinson's Grove, Homestead, Florida." Sergeant Smith looked dubious. "We don't have much call for avocados."

"Sergeant, I saw those avocados growing last summer. I walked under the shade of those trees with Doctor Robinson. We could serve avocados in the officers mess." The following week, a new item appeared on the officers' menu — Avocado Grapefruit Salad.

"Doc, I bragged to anyone who'd listen that the avocados came from your grove, the grapefruit from Dad's. Now, let's have a game of bridge for old time's sake."

Vacation slipped away. The long train trip back to Washington gave me time to think about the next phase of my dietetic training at Walter Reed. My new assignment would be ten weeks at the Convalescent Center in Forest Glen, Maryland. After that stint, I'd return to the main hospital but would be responsible for my own living arrangements.

I wondered what surprises lay ahead, now that I had earned the title Apprentice Dietitian.

Accepting Responsibility

Had sunny warm Florida been a dream? I had expected to return to a spring morning in Washington D.C., not icy stinging sleet on the first day of March. My planned shopping trip would have to wait.

I hurried back to Walter Reed to meet glamour girl Ann Paradise, a classmate with the same assignment as mine. We lugged our suitcases aboard the shuttle bus to the Convalescent Section, four miles away in Forest Glen, Maryland. "Even though you're an apprentice dietitian instead of a student, you look just the same," joked Ann.

"That won't last long. I've been thinking how much we'll miss Lieutenant Childress. She checked everything we did and kept us on course. Now the responsibility is ours alone."

Ann rolled her eyes. "I'll worry about that later. Just look at this place." We stared in amazement at an Italian villa, the main building of the Convalescent Center. Tucked into the hilly wooded grounds stood buildings in many styles and shapes. A Scottish castle, Dutch windmill, Swiss chalet, Southern-colonial mansion, and pagoda looked like sets for operettas.

Formerly, National Park Seminary for Girls, the students had chosen the architectural styles for their sorority houses. For the past fifty years, each graduating class had presented the school with a gift of statuary. Gargoyles, goddesses, and benches, all solid stone, appeared in unexpected places scattered through the woods.

Our home for the next ten weeks would be in the rambling building called the "Villa." Life-size statues of Roman goddesses lined the walkway, vaguely reminiscent of something Italian. What a change from our Delano Hall room for six.

"Ann, can you believe this suite?" We stared at the artistic wallpaper, wall to wall carpeting, twin beds, separate bureaus and desks, and two closets plus a tile bath, connecting our room to Jo and Dot's.

Ann smiled. "This is heaven. Now I'll have a whole bureau top for pictures of my boyfriends." She had already learned that all the patients ate in a mess hall — no wards, no trays. Now that we were free of medical lectures and class assignments, she looked forward to many dates with the recuperating officers.

We found our new boss, Lieutenant Buckman, less demanding than Lieutenant Childress had been. Lieutenant Buckman treated us like staff members, rather than inexperienced apprentices.

After our day of indoctrination, she suggested, "Lets go to the band concert in the former ballroom. I want to show you some of the beauty still evident from the days when this was an exclusive girls' school."

Three tiers of balconies circled the parquet floor. On the papered walls, nymphs dressed in filmy white danced across fields of daisies against a soft blue background.

Overhead, hundreds of prisms reflected the dazzling light of a row of chandeliers. Only girls from wealthy families would have felt comfortable in those surroundings.

Sitting in a balcony box reserved for staff members, we gazed down on hundreds of soldiers in maroon gym suits, the uniform for patients. They clapped and cheered with an exuberance we had not heard from the seriously ill soldiers at Walter Reed.

Back at the Villa, a piercing train whistle shattered the quiet night. Ann jumped up and parted the curtains. A flash of light hit the walls. With a loud clatter, a Baltimore and Ohio engine headed for the window, then veered down the track. Ann shook her fist at the window. "How often are we going to hear that?"

"Three trains an hour," Dot called from the other room. "We're only a stone's throw from the tracks." That first night we jumped every time a train passed, but we soon learned to ignore the noise.

My work hours for my first three-week assignment, 6:30 a.m. to 3:30 p.m., left time for a nap in the afternoon. After I'd taken inventory of everything in the storeroom and calculated the cost of each item, I needed the break.

Writing two sets of weekly menus, the one for enlisted men on a more limited budget than the one for officers, took great concentration. However, duplicating the name of an item twice in one week no longer presented a problem. I knew by heart every name for mashed potatoes. Due to plenty of exercise, the patients had good appetites and seldom complained about the food.

Supervising service in the officers' mess added variety to the day. A silver coffee pot and a silver vase of fresh flowers on each table added elegance to the dining room. No wonder some of those fellows were in no hurry to go home. One lieutenant took a bite of apple pie a la mode.

"Miss, a year ago I lay wounded in a foxhole. Didn't expect to live. Never imagined I'd end up livin' like this."

I laughed. "None of us did. Make the most of it while it lasts."

On the days I worked in the enlisted men's mess, I detested my job. Above the steam table a banner, printed in red on butcher's paper, proclaimed, "If your eyes are bigger than your stomach, SQUINT." Clipboard in hand, I stood by the garbage can where each GI dumped uneaten food before placing his tray on the conveyor belt.

On a list, I checked off the uneaten items and asked, "Was the meat tough? Beets not your favorite vegetable?" My poll lasted a week and, although I heard plenty of comments, not a printable one came my way. After the garbage had been weighed in the basement, I used that figure to calculate the amount of waste per capita per day.

Highlight of the day for patients and staff was an evening performance in the ballroom. Seats filled early for an appearance by Roy Rogers and Trigger. When Roy Rogers, resplendent in fringed jacket and white cowboy hat, burst into the ballroom on Trigger's back, the crescendo of cheers rising to the rafters was deafening. Only those of us seated in the balcony knew how close man and horse came to disaster.

Our vantage point placed us at eye level with a crystal chandelier. Lieutenant Buckman drew our attention to the slim chain leading to the ceiling. "That looks like a flimsy line to hold all that leaded glass. Hope someone has inspected it."

Trigger, wearing felt shoes to protect the parquet floor, pranced onto the stage. Whistles, claps, shouts, and stamping feet vibrated to the chandelier, setting up a lively chatter among the glass prisms. As Roy Rogers waved his hat, Trigger reared on his hind legs to strike their most famous pose.

The arc of the swaying chandelier grew wider. Behind us someone moaned, "It's going to crash." Unaware of the danger,

Trigger trotted off stage. Roy Rogers joined Dale Evans, perched on a fence on the sideline, to sing cowboy songs. When the performance ended, the chandelier still swung in decreasing arcs.

Ann let out a sigh of relief. "I'm so glad Trigger is safe." My concern extended to Dale Evans and Roy Rogers.

Our complaints about the antiquated wiring brought results. The following week, a strong cable replaced the slender chain.

Too Good To Last

My next assignment in the spring of 1945, at the Convalescent Section of Walter Reed, involved special diets. Doctors and dietitians emphasized the importance of good nutrition and the proper diet for every individual. In spite of encouraging patients to follow the prescribed regimen, I often questioned the results.

What good did it do to weigh every gram of food for a diabetic, when he refused to eat half of the items on his tray? Why explain a low calorie diet to a patient too heavy to walk on artificial limbs, if he sat in the PX drinking beer every night? I once caught a patient on an ulcer diet hiding under a bed with a forbidden piece of cherry pie.

My one day off was Sunday, a chance to get away from hospital routine. In February, I had written my brother Sam, an ensign in the navy stationed in Philadelphia, and suggested we meet on Palm Sunday at the end of March. His reply came six weeks later. He gave me only two-days notice, stating he and Betty, his fiancée, would meet me at the station in Philadelphia on Saturday night.

I arrived on time at 7:15 p.m. No sign of Sam and Betty. Betty's train from Connecticut had arrived hours before mine. Tired and hungry, I sank down on a hard bench. I had worked a long day, spent an hour and half getting to Union Station from Maryland, and ridden in a dirty coach to Philadelphia. Where were they?

One hour passed, then fifteen minutes more. My irritation melted when, hand in hand, the lovebirds strolled into view enveloped in a cloud of romance. Sam looked surprised, "How long have you been here?"

"Since seventeen-fifteen, the exact time we agreed to meet."

Betty bit her lip, "I'm sorry. We didn't see you." She looked up into Sam's eyes. "I was so hungry Sam took me to dinner." The closest I came to a meal was a coke and a Milky Way candy bar — Sam's treat before he sent us off in a cab to our hotel.

Betty and I kicked off our shoes and settled down to talk. I was tempted to say, "I hope my brother treats you better than he does me." But when Betty mentioned wedding plans, I forgot my miffed feelings.

"Do you know for certain you can get away for June fourteenth? I am really counting on you to be maid-of-honor. I can't get married without you in the wedding party and it's too late to change the date."

Betty would not understand the army's disregard for personal plans. I had applied in January for the time off in June. Two days was the most I could hope for — I was entitled to only one day a week. The chief dietitian had told me she'd grant me the time, provided no one on staff got sick. If that happened, I'd have to work. She'd make her decision the week before the wedding.

Betty brushed aside my concern. "We'll just have to take the chance."

The next morning, Palm Sunday, I watched the bride-to-be dissolve in tears. The belt for her new dress was not in her suitcase. She had spent hours making a silk dress, a delicate print of violets on a cream background, and now the belt was missing. I assured her Sam would never notice. She said her day was ruined.

On our way through the lobby to meet Sam, we passed a florist shop. "Betty, how about a ribbon?" The shopkeeper tied a purple velvet streamer around her slim waist and presented her with a gardenia. Betty glowed.

Ensign Morrison led us mile after mile, hour after hour, through the Philadelphia Navy Yard. "That is so interesting." Betty's glowing appreciation of dry docks encouraged Sam to describe every bolt and nut. I longed to exchange my heels for flats, even considered dropping out of sight. Sam and Betty would not have noticed and I could have avoided the return to Maryland late at night.

The following Saturday evening found me on the train to York, Pennsylvania to spend Easter with Mary, my college roommate. Mary and her mother met me at the station.

"My, you're thin," Mary's mother observed. "You need a good meal." She whisked us off to the Yorktowne Hotel for pot roast, a far cry from Sam's coke and candy bar of the previous week.

Easter breakfast brought a surprise — cream puffs. The tug-of-war between Mary's parents over church, Presbyterian Church versus Lutheran, ended as usual. Mary's Mother won. I walked down the aisle of the Lutheran Church wearing the purple orchid corsage Dave had sent Mary. In spite of Mary's lack of interest, Dave still pursued her. She wore yellow roses and purple iris from my cousin, Ted.

During the day, Mary's Uncle Pete showed up at the house three times. On each occasion he gave me a hearty kiss exclaiming, "Any friend of my niece's is as good as a niece of mine." Suspicious of his motives, I tried to dampen his enthusiasm. In my book, he remained just "old Uncle Pete."

The following Saturday, I didn't feel like boarding another train and had to force myself to catch an early express to New York to meet Betty. Going on to Bridgeport, Connecticut, for a fitting of my gown, gave us time to go over the wedding invitation list.

At D.M. Reads' Department Store, the bridal consultant took us to her office. She smiled at Betty. When she spoke to me, she looked down at her hands. "I must apologize for the long trip you've made. The yellow bridesmaid dresses are ready, but no blue chiffon has become available for your gown."

Betty and I sat in stunned silence. I had come all the way from Silver Spring, Maryland for nothing. The consultant assured Betty she would find the correct shade of blue chiffon in time for the wedding.

The uneasy woman turned to me. "Let me take your measurements. As soon as the dress is finished, I'll send it to you in Washington." After she put away her tape measure, she showed us the completed yellow chiffon bridesmaids' dresses.

Betty and I headed for the elevator. "Just my luck," I moaned. "Not only do I have to worry about getting time off for your wedding, now I have nothing to wear."

Victory In Europe

During the spring of 1945, rumors flooded the jammed hotel lobbies and crowded restaurants of Washington, D.C. The decline of the president's health, the probable collapse of Germany, and the gravity of conditions in the Pacific gave a sense of urgency and excitement to the city. April twelfth brought darkness and despair. President Roosevelt was dead.

His death in Warm Springs, Georgia came as no surprise to Washingtonians. Before his election to a fourth presidential term in November, members of Congress had seen a gravely ill man. "Off the record," they spoke of him in hushed tones.

People throughout the United States and the world reacted to the shocking news with profound grief and alarm. Even the dishwasher on KP had an opinion. "How can we win the war without 'im? Victory in Europe seemed so close, but Truman don't know nothin'." My return to Walter Reed from my assignment at the Convalescent Section in Forest Glen, Maryland had come at a propitious time in history.

My classmate Marie and I, delighted to be on the same schedule for the next six weeks, hunted for a rent within walking distance of the hospital. We stood in a dismal room in an unattractive yellow brick apartment building a block from Walter Reed.

Mrs. Hazelette, the landlady, dusted the bureau with her hand. "If you decide to stay, you can use the twin beds near the window" An overgrown tree blocked the view and any possibility of a breeze. "My daughter Donna, likes the bed against the back wall and I plan to sleep on a cot on the porch."

"Marie, we're lucky to find a room in this tight housing market. I'm not keen on sharing sleeping space with a sixteen-year old but we have no choice." After Mrs. Hazelette moved her possessions to the crowded porch amid a jungle of plants, we unpacked our suitcases in the stuffy bedroom.

"The bathroom's so small we'll have to keep our towels and toothbrushes in the bedroom," Marie complained. An open transom high on the bathroom wall provided the only ventilation in an area the size of a closet. Bathrooms on five floors shared the same airshaft. We learned to ignore the sounds of unseen neighbors brushing their teeth and flushing the john.

Our search for a room and the new assignments at work did not blot out our interest in details about the president's death. Eager to witness the early evening departure of the funeral cortege from the White House to Hyde Park, we changed from uniforms to cotton dresses and ran to catch a bus.

Marie's brown eyes sparkled. "This is history in the making. Aren't we lucky to be the only apprentices on the early shift?" On Pennsylvania Avenue, we elbowed our way into the crowd of mourners. At our vantage point in Lafayette Park, opposite the White House, we were surrounded by a surge of people who overflowed the lawns and trampled the flowerbeds. Agile climbers scrambled into the branches of the trees.

Across the street, the White House glowed in soft, yellow light. Like a stage setting, it served as a backdrop for the flag-draped coffin resting on a caisson beneath the portico. The horses, flanks shining, and brasses gleaming, stood motionless waiting for the order to escort the body of the Commander-in-Chief to Union Station.

The solemn strains of hymns played by the Marine Band, floated over the heads of the crowd and rose to those partially hidden above amid the tender fresh green leaves. "Forward. March." As the funeral procession moved slowly down the drive, the heartfelt sobs and grief-stricken bewailing of the crowd melded into one single cry. That caterwaul of despair drowned out the strains of "Abide with Me."

Marie whispered, "This must be the most moving expression of public grief since the death of Abraham Lincoln." Our attention was centered on the proud and solitary riderless horse, when the solemnity of the moment was shattered.

From high in a treetop, a deep voice rumbled, "Hey, dietitian! What's for breakfast?"

Marie and I froze. While mourners searched for the source of the disturbance, we took advantage of the confusion and pushed our way toward the edge of the crowd. Hoping no one had realized the soldier directed his remarks at us, we beat a hasty retreat down Pennsylvania Avenue.

The weeks at the Convalescent Center in Forest Glen had flown by. I hated to leave the patients and staff to return to the main hospital. Living arrangements in the Villa had been so comfortable and the entertainments in the ballroom better than Broadway. Most of all I'd enjoyed the landscape and the woods, still awash in a spring display of bright azaleas and delicate cherry blossoms.

Unlike the Japanese cherry trees in Washington, no Marines had to protect those in Maryland. In the city, as long as the fragile blossoms graced the trees around the tidal basin, Marines stood guard twenty-four hours a day. Anti-Japanese sentiment threatened anything connected with Japan.

Before returning to duty at Walter Reed, a group of officers had taken three of us dietitians to Castle Inn for farewell cokes. When writing home, I did not mention the cokes had been laced with rum. Our escorts, a colonel, a captain, and a lieutenant, regaled us with their adventures the previous night.

The colonel spoke first. "We were among the lucky ones invited to dinner at the home of Evelyn Walsh McLean." One of the wealthiest women in Washington and its leading hostess, she invited sixty service people every week for a sumptuous meal.

"You should see that place," chimed in the captain. "Elaborate table service, huge flower arrangements, and champagne flowing like water." He described the grand dame seated at the head of the mile-long table presiding over dinner. The Hope diamond sparkled on her gown. "It looked like a rock, but that wasn't enough for her. She wore several other jewels as well."

The lieutenant broke in. "When we sat down to dinner, I worried I'd pick up the wrong fork, or something. I felt uneasy until Mrs. McLean shouted toward the kitchen."

She had rapped on her glass and cried out, "God dammit! Where are those mashed potatoes? If you don't hurry, I'm coming out after them!" The lieutenant said he'd concluded Washington society lived in luxury but talked like everyone else.

On my rounds of the kitchen to say "Goodbye," I had stopped to talk to Private Kowalski, the young Polish pot washer with the deep blue eyes. I told him I'd tried many times to get him transferred to a less boring job, but the response was always the same.

"You're so reliable and do such a good job you're considered irreplaceable."

He put down the bristled scrub brush. "Thanks for trying. Two years in the army and all I've done is wash pots. This damned war better end soon."

Back at Walter Reed, I thought of private Kowalski on May 7, 1945, the day part of his wish came true. Germany surrendered.

The hospital patients did not participate in the jubilation exhibited by civilians on the streets. The shattered lives of many of the wounded could not be rebuilt. Their war would never end. They were relieved Germany had surrendered, a step toward victory, but their thoughts centered on their buddies engaged in fierce battles in the Pacific.

When General Marietta, Commanding Officer at Walter Reed, spoke at a ceremony to commemorate the historic day, I represented the Dietetic Department. Of all the dietitians, I happened to be least busy.

Several patients were given the honor of speaking. They talked about the war with Japan, not the defeat of Germany. General Marietta gave the usual speech praising the actions of soldiers and staff. He emphasized our work load would increase. The end of hostilities in Europe would free up ships to carry hundreds of wounded men back to hospitals in the states.

I skipped the refreshments and hurried back to work. For the hospital staff, the war ground on.

Coping with A VIP

After the cherry blossoms faded, the high humidity and enervating heat of summer hit Washington. Every morning I awoke sweaty and tired. At 6:00 a.m., when I hurried from Mrs. Hazelette's to my new assignment, my starched poplin uniform dissolved into a soggy mass of wrinkles.

On Ward 8, hazy sunshine flooded the spotless white-tile kitchen. Like soldiers on parade, trays stood on racks stacked five across and five down, ready for inspection. Water for poached eggs simmered in a large skillet on the two-burner gas stove. Private Williston, the angry depressed soldier, who ran the kitchen on Ward 8, began each day with the same complaint.

"Where are those damn girls? Can't you make them come on time?"

"I try. But you know the carefree attitude of southerners to work. It's not just these colored girls who disregard the clock." None of my pleas or threats changed the unreliability of the three civilian workers. Beulah May, Florine, and Annie usually arrived about the time the food cart bumped down the hall.

The hot food arrived, in a steam-heated cart, from the main kitchen in the subbasement four floors below. On ward 8, an officer's ward, patients selected their food from several choices on the menu. I modified requests to meet special diet requirements. This resulted in dozens of containers, labeled fat-free, salt-free, minced, pureed, etc.

Although they took a haphazard approach to their work, there was no time to reprimand the tardy girls. They placed the cold foods on the tray; Williston prepared eggs and dished up the hot items. In a final check, I could spot a missing spoon or sloppy plate. Once I discovered a cockroach peering over a slice of melon on a colonel's tray.

Cockroaches! No matter how clean the kitchen, cockroaches thrived in the moist, steamy conditions of the south. The bane of every housekeeper and cook, I would have had a hard time explaining that to a colonel.

I tried to speed up the pace in the kitchen. "Let's hurry and serve as many trays as possible before George comes for General Pershing's breakfast."

General Pershing, Commanding General in World War I, over eighty and frail, lived in a penthouse on the top floor. Three times a day, George, his corpsman, came to pick up the General's tray. His meals took precedence over all others. Tray service was suspended while I poached General Pershing's eggs — two poached eggs, seven days a week.

"George, does the General know you can't poach a bad egg? Is that why he orders them poached?" George shrugged.

Even the army could not guarantee the freshness of eggs in wartime. Sometimes, I tried a dozen before finding two that did not disintegrate in the water. What a relief to slip two perfect poached eggs onto wheat toast, add a metal cover to keep the food hot, and send George on his way.

Williston, the three girls, and I doubled our efforts to finish tray service. Often, before we could serve the last patient, George reappeared at the door. "I'm sorry. The General dozed off. He's forgotten he already ate breakfast. He's demanding his eggs." One morning, after I poached eggs for the third time, eggshells littered the table. Williston, always worrying about inspections, hastened to clean up the mess.

Inspection day brought added tensions for Private Williston. The three civilian colored girls, who set up trays and carried them to the patients, reacted with sullen indifference to his criticism. To prepare for the 10:00 a.m. inspection, Williston had begun work at 4:00 a.m. and griped all morning.

"You said to take it as a good sign when General Pershing ate only one breakfast. It didn't help one damn bit. Those blasted inspectors drove me nuts. Do you know what they did?" They had brought a ladder. The captain had climbed up and dusted the light bulb with his white glove. With a smirk at Williston, he held up his hand to display a greasy smudge.

Williston trembled with rage. "I knew he'd run those damned white gloves over the gas stove, but I missed a perfect grade because of one lousy light bulb."

I had watched him soak the grilles from the stove in ammonia and I had prodded the girls to swab the corners in the refrigerator. Not a drop of water had marred the waxed tile floor. Not a streak had spoiled the shine on the windows. Only one "lousy light bulb" stood between Williston and perfection.

Lunch service got off to a bad start. After being blasted by Williston, the girls were in no mood to cooperate. As I called off the items to go on each plate, Williston muttered to himself and paid little attention. I grew exasperated.

"Wait a minute. That plate calls for fat free fish, not salt free chicken."

Williston slammed the fish on the plate. "That does it. I can't take anymore, even from you." He hurled the plate toward my head.

I must have ducked. As the plate sailed by my ear, I felt a whoosh of air. The girls watched in stunned silence. The heavy piece of crockery smashed against the wall, falling in a dozen pieces. Mackerel, mashed potatoes, and peas clung in gobs to the gleaming tile.

Shaken, I took a deep breath. "Beulah May, you go to the kitchen for another piece of fish. Williston, let's get these trays out before George comes for General Pershing's lunch. You can clean this mess up later." Our usual routine took over. None of us ever mentioned the incident.

Miss Pershing and Fifi

I never had time to eat breakfast. Coffee cup in hand, I'd hasten to my office for the daily conference with Miss May Pershing. The General's sister arrived promptly at ten to plan lunch and dinner for herself and her brother. An imposing figure, white hair piled high, ramrod straight back, she dictated orders as though she had negotiated the victory in World War I.

Her first words foretold trouble. "Miss Morrison, must I tell you again? The red-topped sugar shaker goes on my tray for lunch, black on the General's. For dinner mine is black, his red." I sighed. I knew that after I had inspected the tray, someone would switch the sugar shakers just for spite.

I looked forward to Tuesdays, when the meeting with the General's sister took less time than usual. On that day, General Pershing's son Warren came for lunch. The menu never varied, always steak and ice cream. Miss Pershing almost smiled at me. "Major Pershing will be here. We'll have the usual."

Her smile changed to a frown. "Now about dinner. Why can't you people get the correct color sugar shaker on each tray?"

Major Pershing, not only had to follow in the footsteps of a famous father, he had to live with tragedy, which struck his family when he was five. His father was in Texas on August 27, 1915. His mother had entertained in the family home at the Presidio in San Francisco. After she retired, devastating fire swept through the house.

Coals smoldering on the grate in the living room had tumbled onto the floor. The polished wood surface, highly waxed to meet army standards, burst into flames. Within seconds, the wooden structure became an inferno. Mrs. Pershing, trying to protect her three daughters, encircled them with her arms.

She perished along with Helen, eight, Anne, seven, and Mary, six. Firemen rescued Warren from a second story roof, his life saved by the maid.

General Pershing, in El Paso preparing a new home for his family, was handed a telegram by an orderly. "Go on. Read it," ordered the General. In a faltering voice, the orderly informed him of the death of his wife and their three beloved daughters.

I wondered how Major Pershing, after losing his mother, had coped through the years with the imperious manner of his aunt. She intimidated me. A week later Miss Pershing voiced new complaints.

"Miss Morrison, I can't understand why the General has to put up with such unappetizing food."

I tried to give a positive response. "Miss Pershing, we go to great lengths to prepare tasty, healthful meals for you and General Pershing. What is wrong?"

She threw back her shoulders and glared at me. "This is intolerable. The 'tow-ma-tow' juice is much too dark, the bouillon much too pale."

I bit my lip trying to think of something diplomatic to say. I considered, "We'll try another brand." Nothing was going to suit her. Why waste my time?

When George, the corpsman, came for the trays, I called him aside. "George, what am I going to do? Miss Pershing insists the 'tow-ma-tow' juice is much too dark, the bouillon much too pale."

"I wouldn't worry about the tomato juice," he laughed. We both knew the General detested tomatoes in any form. "Take it from me, all the staff is feeling the heat." Miss Pershing had suggested the afternoon visits of the General's friend, Fifi, left him exhausted.

George picked up a tray. "The General's so mad at Miss Pershing he hasn't spoken to her in three days. That's made her furious. She's taking it out on all of us."

During World War I, General Pershing had closed the brothels within five miles of every American base in France. At the same time, the French government furnished him with elaborate quarters in Paris plus female companionship. When the war ended, Fifi came with him to the United States.

Only those of us in close contact with General Pershing seemed aware of her existence. Fifi resided at the Shoreham Hotel, a short drive from Walter Reed Hospital and convenient for her afternoon visits with General Pershing.

After lunch, Miss Pershing left in a staff car for her apartment. Fifteen minutes later, a limousine glided to a stop at the side entrance to the hospital. With the dramatic flair of a movie star, Fifi emerged, the personification of a Paris fashion plate circa 1918. Wearing a large picture hat and a flowered silk gown, which swirled gracefully to her ankles above pointed-toed shoes, she ducked into the elevator.

Two hours later, she left with as little fanfare as she had arrived. Ten minutes after her departure, Miss Pershing returned in the staff car. Due to precise planning by General Pershing's aides, the two never met face-to-face.

George had confided, "No matter how good the General's mood before Fifi leaves, he's depressed afterwards. No wonder he eats so many eggs for breakfast. He seldom enjoys his dinner. Hates the sight of that tomato juice."

A Study in Contrasts

For some unfathomable reason, the State Department handled General Pershing's guests. One call from a State Department official prompted me to phone Captain Dautrich, the Chief Dietitian.

"Captain Dautrich, I have a problem. The State Department just informed me General Pershing will have twelve guests for breakfast tomorrow. Does this call for linen napkins?"

"Absolutely. You'd better go the butcher shop for twelve strips of bacon. I'll send a requisition."

I explained we had only a dozen napkins. It took five each day, one for General Pershing's breakfast, two for lunch and dinner with Miss Pershing. Another five were in the laundry."

"I'll take care of that. You'll have the napkins this afternoon." I wondered where she'd find them. Shelves in linen departments had been empty for months. Three hours later, a large box arrived from Woodward and Lothrop, one of Washington's leading department stores.

In the gray box, individually wrapped in tissue with a gold seal, lay twelve large damask napkins worthy of a banquet. Apparently, wartime shortages had not enticed anyone to pay the exorbitant price for the last remaining dozen linen napkins in Washington. Not until the army had to cope with guests of General Pershing.

Next morning I arrived at work an hour early to polish thirteen silver-plated coffee pots. That task crossed off my list, I hurried to the subbasement. The butcher handed me a package — the twelve precious strips of bacon, one for each guest of the General.

The first breakfast trays on Ward 8 went out early to make room for the twelve extra trays with the polished coffee pots and those elegant napkins. The breakfast hour came and went. No call from the penthouse. No word from George. At 10:00 a.m., the apologetic corpsman appeared at the door.

"All we need is two pots of coffee." He stared at the row of trays set up for the guests. "Guess no one told the visitors breakfast was included in their chat with General Pershing," he mumbled.

Never again did I have to worry about linen napkins. I had twelve damask beauties locked away in the bottom drawer of my filing cabinet.

A few days later, I had more on my mind than guests for breakfast. The war in Europe over, General Eisenhower had made his triumphant return home. He basked in the adulation of a populace eager to honor their Commander-in-Chief. Protocol demanded he pay a call on President Truman at the White House and a visit to General Pershing in whose footsteps he had followed.

A directive had gone out to every department in the hospital. "General Eisenhower will arrive tomorrow morning at 1100. He will proceed from the main entrance to Ward 8 for a meeting with General Pershing. All personnel are encouraged to give him a warm welcome."

Patients and staff jammed the halls to catch a glimpse of General Eisenhower. Amid shouts and cheers, his aides cleared a path and hurried the smiling hero along. He had retained his boyish grin in spite of the responsibilities he had shouldered throughout the war.

During the early days of the war, the Washington papers had often reported the visits by U.S. Army chief-of-staff, General George C. Marshall, to General Pershing. After reminiscing about World War I, the two men would discuss the progress of the war in Europe and the problems in the Pacific. In recent months, those meetings had seldom taken place. At eighty-two, General Pershing could no longer grasp the complicated details of World War II.

Miss Pershing wanted her brother to appear at his best. She had insisted he rehearse for two days the remarks she hoped he would make to General Eisenhower. George, the General's corpsman, doubted the repetition would help. "These days the General is more aware of his war, World War I, than World War II."

When George came for the General's supper trays, I asked him how the General had responded to General Eisenhower's visit. He shook his head. "At Miss Pershing's insistence, we coached him again on what to say. The old fellow did his best."

Dressed in striped pajamas, General Pershing had tried to sit erect in bed. After returning General Eisenhower's brisk salute, his attention seemed to waver.

"General I want to congratulate you on winning, on winning, on, on ..." His words melted away. Miss Pershing took over and finished his sentence. General Eisenhower eased the situation by praising General Pershing for his leadership in World War I.

Two days later, another directive went out to department heads. "Tomorrow, Friday, General George S. Patton will follow his visit to President Truman at the White House with a meeting with General Pershing at 1100. General Patton has ordered all corridors be cleared of non-essential persons. Duty personnel are required to ignore his presence."

The visit from the most controversial general of World War II would include a reunion with his son-in-law, Colonel Waters, who occupied the room next to the ward kitchen. He had arrived at Walter Reed gaunt and undernourished from a German prison camp. American forces had rescued him during the Battle of the Bulge, the costly campaign waged by his father-in-law.

I had grown fond of Mrs. Patton, the general's gracious supportive wife, who spent many hours with Colonel Waters. She often tapped on the kitchen door, a glass bowl in her hand. "I hope this won't be too much trouble. I've made wine jelly for the Colonel. Could you keep it in the refrigerator until lunchtime? Thank you so much."

After the door closed, I'd threaten those irresponsible girls working in the kitchen. "Don't you dare sample this jelly. You hear me? Not even one tiny taste." Mrs. Patton had no idea I needed an MP to guard the colonel's dessert. Lacking that, I'd become protector of the delectable wine jelly.

The imminent arrival of General Patton made me reiterate the orders of the day to the kitchen help. "General Patton wants all personnel to stay out of sight during his visits to General Pershing and Colonel Waters. Thought you'd like to know what's going on, when you hear the commotion next door. Don't forget. Keep the kitchen door closed."

My warning aroused the curiosity of the three girls. That led to their downfall. When they heard talking in the hall, Beulah May opened the door a crack. Her action brought dire results.

General George S. Patton

Tension ran high on Ward 8 that June morning in 1944. Staff members were on guard, having been alerted to the impending arrival of General Patton to see his son-in-law Colonel Waters. General Patton's order that the halls be clear of onlookers had left the corridors deserted.

With more immediate problems on my mind, I hurried down the hall toward my office. As I passed Colonel Waters' room, the door opened a little. A small blond boy, the colonel's son, pointed his finger at me. "Bang, bang. I gotcha." The four gleaming stars on the army cap tilted toward his ear spoke louder than words. Grandpa Patton had arrived.

Clutching my head as though I'd been shot, I staggered down the hall followed by a child's laughter. He got off one more shot in my direction before a gruff voice inside the room issued a sharp command, "Shut that door."

"What happened to you?" The nurse, with whom I shared an office, looked at me in surprise. I smoothed my hair and straightened my cap. "General Patton isn't the only member of the family who likes warfare. I got wiped out in a gunfight with his four-year-old grandson." Before I could explain, the heavy tread of boots made us jump to our feet.

General Patton strode into the room surrounded by an aura of static electricity. Ignoring the nurse in her striped seersucker army uniform, he confronted me in my starched white apprentice outfit. Perhaps, my cap reminded him of nurses of an earlier day. "I want to see General Means," he barked.

"I'm sorry sir, I am the dietitian. Lieutenant Barlow can help you."

He pivoted on his heel to face her. "God dammit, I want to see General Means, now."

Color rose in her cheeks. "He has just come from surgery, Sir. No one is allowed in the recovery room without permission."

"Well, by God, get it," he thundered. She jumped when he struck the corner of the desk with his riding crop. With trembling hand, she called the Chief Surgeon. General Patton paced the small office from wall to wall like a caged lion.

The deep voice of the surgeon came over the phone in measured tones audible across the room. "General Patton has my permission to see General Means for exactly five minutes. I am notifying the recovery room he's on his way."

Lieutenant Barlow gave General Patton a snappy salute. Without a word to either of us, he strode from the room. She collapsed at her desk. "Did I do the right thing?"

She repeated her question. "Oh, did I do the right thing? He scared me when he struck the desk with his riding crop." She had had no choice. She could not disobey the surgeon's orders, not even for General Patton.

I grinned. "Wonder whether he'd have shot you, if he'd been wearing his ivory handled revolvers?" The Washington Post had reported that authorities on protocol deemed it inappropriate for General Patton to wear the revolvers for the first stop on the day's itinerary — his call on President Truman at the White House.

Steps, two at a time, pounding up the stairs next to the office caught us by surprise. Lieutenant Barlow turned pale. "Is he coming back?" Before I could reply, a breathless colonel burst into the room.

He approached her desk. "Did you call me about General Patton?"

In a wavering voice she replied, "Yes Sir."

He smiled. "Let me shake your hand. You did a very brave thing. I congratulate you." The Chief of Surgery knew it took guts to cross General Patton.

A glance at my watch sent me scurrying to the ward kitchen. The food cart for lunch would arrive any minute. Inside the kitchen door, I faced catastrophe. Annie and Florine huddled over Beulah May. She sat on the floor crying and wringing her hands.

Florine looked up at me, the whites of her eyes enormous, as though she'd seen a ghost. I turned to Williston. "What's going on here? What happened?"

Private Williston tossed his head, waving a slotted spoon in the direction of the sobbing girls, "Ask them."

I put my hand on the distraught girl's shoulder. "Beulah May, what happened? Pull yourself together. We have to serve lunch." She tried to stifle her sobs. She said she heard noise in the hall and she wanted a peek. She opened the door just a bitty bit.

"Dat genral he look so mean. He hit the door, hard, with a stick in his han. Then he shouts at me." Her words almost lost in her tears, she gulped, "He yell at me, 'What the hell you think I am? A damn exhibition?'"

"I'm sorry Beulah May, but I warned you not to open that door. Now drink this glass of water and come help us serve lunch." The rest of us turned our attention to filling plates, but not Beulah May. When George came for the Pershing trays, he stared at the crumpled heap on the floor. I offered no explanation for the tearful girl cowering in the corner.

Unable to find a way to comfort Beulah May, I left for my afternoon break. She still lay on the floor, her face to the wall. I never saw her again. She fled without stopping to pick up her paycheck. She had my sympathy, but finding another job would not be easy.

Many a person, stronger than Beulah May, including me, had quaked at the sight of General Patton. Nurses, who had served under him overseas, told me they hid when he came through field hospitals on inspection. Although used to profanity, they cringed at his language and they could not tolerate his insults to the patients.

Williston, Florine, and Annie struggled to cover Beulah May's share of the workload. No replacement materialized to take her place.

General Patton had cost me the most reliable of my three employees.

Sam and Betty's Wedding

Sam and Betty's wedding day, June 16, 1945, was only two weeks away. As I waited for the chief dietitian's approval of my two-day leave, my anxiety grew. I began to doubt I would be maid-of-honor at the marriage of my brother and my dearest friend. "If no staff member is sick next week, I'll grant you the time off," Captain Dautrich had said. I prayed no one would go on sick call.

The unavailability of blue chiffon for my gown had seemed a bad omen. Betty relieved my mind about the dress. True to her promise, the bridal consultant had found the material, but not in time to mail the gown to Washington. I would have to go to Bridgeport for a fitting the day before the wedding.

I worked thirteen days straight to accumulate time for a two-day leave. Five days before the deadline, Captain Dautrich granted her permission. My classmates marked the day with a party. On Thursday evening, I sneaked away from Ward 8 an hour early and grabbed a cab to the airport. Wedding plans paled in comparison to the experience ahead — my first plane ride.

The plane picked up speed on the runway and I held my breath. The whine of the propellers intensified and, until the ground dropped away, the vibration set up quivers in my stomach. As the plane pierced the fluffy white clouds and rose into a pink sky, I reveled in my bird's eye view of the sunset. My spirits soared higher than the clouds.

Beneath me in the deepening dusk, pinpricks of light multiplied turning the scene into fairyland. On the approach to LaGuardia Field, a dip of the wing revealed the Statue of Liberty, a miniature far below outlined by the rising moon. The first person in my family to travel by air, I had fallen in love with flying.

In spite of my new interest in plane travel, my loyalty to the New York, New Haven and Hartford Railroad did not waver. On the ride from Grand Central Station to South Norwalk,

Connecticut, the old train car, which reeked of dusty plush, stale air, smoke, and newsprint, seemed like an old friend.

Eager to be the first one off the train, I jumped to my feet before the conductor called, "Souuuth Norwalk." I rushed to the door where hot sticky humid air hit me in the face, a reminder that Connecticut sometimes felt like Washington.

"Sam, Betty over here." They had been too engrossed in each other to notice me. Sam grabbed my suitcase. Betty stumbled over her words in her eagerness to fill me in on details for the festivities ahead.

"You're sleeping at my house. It'll be a short night. You have to be at D.M. Read's in Bridgeport at 9:00 a.m." The seamstress, who had worked overtime to finish my dress, would be there to make any last minute adjustments.

In the fitting room, I stared in the mirror and wanted to cry. The lovely blue material reflected the color of my eyes, but the dress hung on my skinny frame like a limp rag. "You've lost a lot of weight since I measured you six weeks ago." The seamstress talked through pins protruding from her mouth.

"Now don't you worry, Dearie. I'll rip the dress apart, cut off an inch all the way round. You'll look beautiful tomorrow."

"But there is so little time and I can't come back again."

"Of course not. I'll put all my girls to work on it right now. The dress will be delivered to your house in the morning. You just relax." She assured me there would be no extra charge for the service. "We always do our part to make a wedding day special."

The hours melted away in a blur of activity. When I saw my eighteen-year-old brother Sherman, I paraphrased his last letter to me, which began, "Old Girl, can you believe our shy, easily embarrassed brother is getting married?" We shook with guilty laughter. So often in the past, we had teased Sam just to see him blush.

Late in the evening, after the rehearsal had ended, Betty, her mother, and I gathered in the kitchen. Although we realized this might be the last time our threesome would chat over coffee cups, no one mentioned the changes ahead. Betty seemed reluctant to break the spell.

I gave Betty a hug, "Well Miss Urban, it is midnight. We'd better get to bed. In case you don't remember, tomorrow you'll be Mrs. Morrison." For a moment, apprehension showed in her tired eyes.

Then she smiled. "Sam says your parents never told you how to behave when you went out in the evening, as my father always did. They gave you only one bit of advice, 'Remember your name is Morrison.' Tomorrow I'll officially become a Morrison. Hope I can live up to the name."

"You'll do fine. You'll also be my sister. The sister I've longed for and never had."

Not a breath of air stirred the curtains in my small bedroom. I fell into a fitful sleep until the whine of a mosquito disturbed the silent night. At the first hint of daylight, I crept down the stairs and tiptoed out the back door. As I passed the rose arbor and the colorful gardens, the manicured grass felt cool under my bare feet. Birds in the trees kept up a lively chatter proclaiming Betty's wedding day.

I sat on a log by the Norwalk River, watching the mist rise from the gently moving stream. The day before, my college roommate, Mary, had exclaimed, "You call this a river? I anticipated something as wide as the Susquehanna."

The thoughts I tried so hard to suppress overwhelmed me. Three years and two weeks had passed since Betty's brother, Ernie, had been killed in an army plane crash. Ernie and I had often double-dated with Sam and Betty before Ernie enlisted in the army in 1941. After that summer, we'd had few opportunities to be together.

Seeing Sam and Betty's happiness made my feelings of loss and loneliness hard to bear. I missed Ernie desperately and felt crushed by the pain and suffering I dealt with every day at Walter Reed, a constant reminder of his death and so many others.

The splash of a fish in the river brought me back to reality. I rose to my feet telling myself, "You must not think that way today."

After lunch, Betty and I, trying to ignore the oppressive heat, sat on her bed in our slips. Betty pushed back her damp hair. "When I needed someone to calm me down this morning, no one had time for the bride." She said she felt Aunt Irene and her crew cared more about groom's cake, wedding cake, pastry, and punch than her jitters.

"It upset me that you and Mother were both away at the beauty shop when I needed you."

I felt my hair. "I might as well have stayed here with you. A lot of good it did me to sit under a dryer. This humidity is turning my hair to frizz." As I slipped Betty's wedding gown over her head, her reflection appeared in the full-length mirror. She gave me a dazzling smile and pirouetted like a dainty ballerina.

In the back of the church, I waited for the two bridesmaids in soft yellow to proceed ahead of me down the aisle. For a second, the packed pews changed to people in dark clothes instead of pastel frocks. Ernie's flag-draped coffin stood before the minister. Blinking, I swept that image from my mind.

I remembered the minister's advice at the rehearsal to walk in a straight line by keeping my eye on the seam in the carpet. Instead, I gazed at Sam standing by the altar, stiff and handsome in his white uniform. He peered over my shoulder to catch a glimpse of his bride.

The first notes of the "Wedding March" swelled to a crescendo. Yellow daisies in my bouquet cascaded down the swirling skirt of my blue gown, now a perfect fit. Head held high, I began my majestic slow march down the aisle.

At the reception in the garden at Betty's home, guests in the receiving line tried to stay in the shade. Betty's father acknowledged compliments about his lovely daughter with a smile, but his chest swelled with pride whenever the guests mentioned his award-winning roses. A professional gardener, he had spent the morning watering the flowerbeds to insure perfection on his daughter's wedding day.

Although the roses did not wilt, the lengthening shadows did little to counteract the stifling heat for the guests. Sherman touched my shoulder. "Anything I could do for you, Sis?"

"How about bringing me a gin and tonic? I'm about to collapse." We concluded Betty's outgoing Hungarian relatives were breaking down the New England reserve of our Morrison aunts and uncles. Perhaps, the frequent trips of the men to the bar in the cool basement led to the convivial conversations of those seated under the trees.

Mother, wearing a pink lace dress and picture hat, stood by the rose arbor unaware of the artistic picture she made. I overheard Dad whisper to her, "I might be prejudiced, but to me you outshine the bride." She gave him a radiant smile.

Sherman threaded his way in our direction past groups of chatting guests. He held a tall glass, dripping beads of moisture. Before he could hand it to me, Mother spoke over my shoulder.

"Sherman Morrison, what are you doing with that drink in your hand? Get rid of it right now." Sherman shrugged his shoulder toward me, turned, and retreated down the garden path.

The afternoon passed much too quickly. Misty eyed, I watched the bride and groom run through a hail of rice to Aunt Hannah's borrowed car. Tin cans tied to the bumper made a din long after the newlyweds disappeared from sight.

I turned to Dad. "I, too, must go. Can't miss that plane to Washington."

His eyes glistened. "I have a surprise for you. I'm going to take the train with you to New York."

Unaware of other passengers in the crowded car, we relived the highlights of the past forty-eight hours. As the train approached Grand Central Station, the mixed emotions of the long day caught up with me. My head dropped on Dad's shoulder and I sobbed.

He told me he understood in his next letter. He mentioned the wonderful wedding, so beautiful in every way and over so quickly. He said it did his heart good to go to New York with me and know I was returning to Washington by plane.

"I just loved you Saturday night with all my heart, 'Little Honem.'" That had been his pet name for me when I was a baby. He continued, "I guess everyone has a little breakdown some time or other. Somehow, on reaching important milestones in our family life, there is always a tug on the heartstrings."

He wrote that when Sam, Sherman, and I were small children, he doubted there was ever a Christmas night he did not have a lump in his throat when he went to bed.

His words brought fresh tears. The future looked so uncertain to me.

The home where we had shared those memorable Christmases had been sold. Sam and Betty would soon establish a home of their own, but Mother and Dad faced a struggle to make the orange grove profitable. Sherman added to everyone's worries by announcing he wanted to become an aerial gunner. I felt unsure and alone facing two years in the army.

Inevitable changes were rapidly altering our lives. We would need the strong family ties uniting us to meet the challenges ahead.

Summer In Washington

The morning after the wedding, I stumbled through the breakfast routine on Ward 8 in a state of euphoria. Lack of sleep for three nights wasn't going to get me down. When I bragged to George, General Pershing's corpsman, that I felt fine, he shook his head, an indication he didn't believe me.

As I poached the General's eggs, the slotted spoon seemed to chase the congealing egg whites round and round the bubbling water in the skillet. I had cracked only two eggs but thought I saw a dozen. Before I could capture one elusive slippery yolk, I felt my knees buckle. Like a rag doll, my limp body sagged to the tile floor. The slow descent spared me injury but wounded my pride.

George bent down to fan my face with the General's linen napkin. Williston stopped serving trays to hold a glass of water to my lips. After they helped me back on my feet, I stumbled off to sick call.

The doctor pulled down my eyelids. "Have you had trouble keeping down food?" he asked. Before I could respond, he gave his diagnosis. "Food poisoning." He sent me off duty with orders to rest, drink tea, and eat dry toast. I wondered why he had chosen food poisoning when I had not mentioned nausea. Even I knew the symptoms for exhaustion differed from those for food poisoning.

I didn't argue. He had given me the excuse I needed to catch up on sleep. Mrs. Hazelette, my landlady, fed me milk toast before she tucked me into bed. The following year another wrong diagnosis by an inept army doctor would have life-threatening consequences.

Two days later, renewed and full of energy, I returned to work, not on Ward 8, but to my new assignment in Mess I. Writing requisitions with a mess sergeant seemed easy compared to dealing with Miss Pershing. Our paths never crossed again. She proved to be my toughest assignment during the year at Walter Reed.

Freed from the late hours on Ward 8, I joined my friends on the long summer evenings. Marie and I preferred the humidity outdoors to the hotbox at Mrs. Hazelette's. On the Fourth of July, our day off, we tried to escape the heat by following the example set by President Lincoln.

Abraham and Mary Lincoln had spent their summers in a rambling white shingle house on the grounds of the Old Soldiers Home. Only three miles from the White House, higher elevation, green lawns, and groves of trees offered a respite from the soggy nights along the Potomac River.

We sat on the grass in front of the Lincoln home waiting for the fireworks. As darkness fell, the first skyrocket shot into the hazy air. Boom! White light filled the sky, revealing a row of limp American flags outlining the porch of President Lincoln's residence.

Marie grabbed my arm. "This gives me goose bumps. Fireworks after all the years of blackout! I'd forgotten how intense the light could be. Just being here makes us part of history. I think I see Old Abe rocking on the porch."

In August, the pace picked up for apprentice dietitians. I called my brother Sam and his new wife in Philadelphia with distressing news. "I can't visit you on Wednesday, which breaks my heart. I have to take my army physical — on my day off. It isn't fair when I have only one day off each week."

My brother, now a seasoned Navy man, laughed, "Welcome to military life. You'll learn in the military no one cares about your day off, except you." He warned me the physical would be tough.

As a gruff army colonel checked me over, inch-by-inch, inside and out, Sam's words saved me from panic. The doctor ignored my punctured eardrums and skinny frame. He nodded approval over my normal blood pressure.

The following day, August 6, brought the biggest, blackest headlines since the end of fighting in Europe — ATOMIC BOMB DROPPED ON HIROSHIMA.

The stunned country, which had never heard of an atom bomb, reacted with disbelief and alarm. Two days later, after a second bomb flattened Nagasaki, the horror began to sink in. The United States had killed thousands of civilians in a matter of seconds on a scale beyond comprehension.

Our patients, who had served in the Pacific, expressed no guilt over the civilians killed or left horribly injured. To them any means of destroying the enemy and concluding the war was justified. They did not have long to wait for the end. On August 14, Japan surrendered.

Every city, town, village, and hamlet in the United States, erupted in wild celebrations. Marie and I considered joining the crowds headed for downtown Washington. Curious to see what was going on in the neighborhood, we walked to the corner of 16th Street. Hundreds of impatient people shouted, pushed, and screamed in an attempt to board overloaded buses.

After I recounted the rowdy New Year's Eve scene I'd once witnessed in Times Square, Marie agreed it might not be safe in the city. We turned back and slipped into the chapel on the grounds at Walter Reed.

Sun shining through the stained glass windows suffused the hushed silence in tones of blue and rose. The somber notes of the organ drowned out the murmured prayers for peace. Gradually, the music became brighter and louder until the joyful sound soared to the rafters high above. Victory had come at last on this day, which would go down in history as VJ Day.

Some of the hospital wards remained quiet. Those men with broken bodies and minds faced only pain, hospitalization, and loneliness. The new optimism of the outside world held little promise for them. On other wards, recuperating soldiers went wild. They shouted, whistled, danced in the halls, and lined up to call home.

Sadness lay heavy in my heart. Ernie had been killed so long ago, in 1942. The Brooklyn boys Mary and I had dated on campus had been part of a battalion wiped out in Italy, and I had just heard that John Zimmerman from Danbury had been promoted to captain before losing his life when his plane was shot down over Germany. At least the killing was over, but too late for so many.

The end of the war left our class of apprentice dietitians confused and uncertain about our future in the military. Twelve million Americans in uniform were eager to leave the service and return home. In fourteen days, we would be commissioned second lieutenants and don our uniforms for the first time. We wondered whether we could expect any changes in our commitment to serve.

"Absolutely not," snapped Captain Dautrich. "You are needed more than ever to relieve personnel who have served for years. Now that the war is over, instead of serving for the duration plus six months, you face two years in the army. You will be sworn into the army on the first of September, two weeks from today."

Final Days At Walter Reed

During the year at Walter Reed Army Hospital, there had been no time to think of fashionable clothes. Now, in August 1945, my classmates and I set out on a shopping spree, but not to Woodward and Lothrop, Washington's luxurious department store. We headed for the Army Supply Store.

Glamorous Anne Paradise turned away from the long rack of khaki uniforms. "I don't think I can survive two years in khaki and olive drab. How can we boost the boys' morale if we can't wear evening gowns?" No one had an answer to her question.

I tried to pull the laces tighter on the sensible B width brown oxfords. My narrow feet required quadruple A. The corporal handing out boxes of shoes had only one solution—wear extra socks. I wondered how many pairs it would take.

When my turn came to stand before the mirror in a khaki uniform, the transformation amazed me. I looked taller and confident — ready to face the challenges ahead. The tailor marked with chalk the necessary adjustments for a perfect fit. "Lieutenant, your uniform will be ready on Monday." He was the first person to address me with my new rank — we had not yet been sworn in.

Monday evening, Marie and I spread a jumble of uniforms and insignia on the bed. Marie grabbed the ruler from her notebook "I know the gold bar has to be one inch from the shoulder seam. Does the U.S. go on the lapel above or below the caduceus?"

Our classmate, Mary Schroeder, who had come back to Mrs. Hazelette's with us, draped a tie around her neck. "Who knows how to tie this thing?"

"I do," I laughed. "Guess you don't have any brothers." She replied, "Men on the farm seldom wear ties, only to a wedding or a funeral." I told her I'd show her after I pressed a dress to wear to the garden party at the Chinese Embassy.

"La-di-dah! You're going to a garden party at the Chinese Embassy?" Marie's brown eyes glowed with excitement. "Do you have a date with that Chinese fellow you met at your aunt's? You took such offense the night I teased you about going out with a Chinese laundry man."

Her insensitive remark had bothered me. I still resented it. "No," I replied evenly, "but I suppose I might see him."

Mary looked confused. I said, "Mary, I don't think you heard me say a friend of my Mother's, Edith Wilson, whom I call Aunt Edith, is social secretary to the Chinese ambassador. She's invited me to go to an embassy party." I passed around the invitation to the reception, which honored General Shang Shen, Chief of the Chinese military mission. He was returning to China.

Uniforms and insignia forgotten, Mary and Marie turned their attention to my two summer dresses. "You'll have to wear the white flower print on blue," Marie decided. "That one looks cooler and matches the blue ribbon on your straw hat. Hope your gloves are clean. Want to borrow my silk purse?"

The next afternoon I hurried off duty to shower and dress before passing inspection by my friends. Marie had taken care of the details. "Your lipstick, hanky, money, gloves, and invitation are in your bag. Hope you snag a colonel." She suggested I drink a Manhattan for her and assured me she'd wait up to hear about the evening.

My confidence wilted on the hour ride by crowded streetcar and bus to Aunt Edith's. I had no idea how to act at an embassy party. Aunt Edith assured me I'd have no problem. "Strict rules of etiquette take care of everything. I hope you don't mind going on the bus. It will be much quicker that way. We're going to a beautiful estate called Twin Oaks."

We left the bus to take a shortcut up a hill through a vacant lot. "No one except the caterer will see our undignified arrival," Aunt Edith explained. "This is the quickest way for me to get to work." Climbing the hill, we giggled at the incongruous sight we made in our party frocks and summer hats on a dusty path lined with weeds.

We paused by the caterer's tent to push back our damp hair, powder our shiny noses and don white gloves. I pulled a burr off Aunt Edith's skirt before she stepped briskly around the corner.

As we took our places at the end of the line, I gasped at the beauty of the wide expanse of lush green lawn and the blazing colors of the gardens. An endless procession of limousines slowly climbed the long paved drive. I asked why some of the chauffeurs left their cars and disappeared inside the embassy.

Aunt Edith straightened her hat. "They're dropping off calling cards of those unable to attend. One corner of the card is turned down to indicate the invited guest sends regrets. I'm glad we'll soon be inside out of the heat."

Following the slow-moving line we ascended the marble steps into the cool great hall. I recognized some of the generals, admirals, and diplomats from their pictures in the newspapers. Aunt Edith placed her calling card, with my name added to it, in an enormous porcelain fish bowl decorated with koi and lily pads.

Both Ambassador and Mrs. Wei held up the line to speak a few personal words to Aunt Edith, a treasured member of their staff. Mrs. Wei, charming and vivacious, wore a white Chinese gown, brocaded with delicate flowers. A binding of black around the standing collar and down the front of the straight dress contrasted with a tiny edging of green, which matched her jade earrings.

After shaking the hand of the last person in line, we stepped onto the vine-covered veranda and gazed across the huge expanse of brilliant green grass clipped smooth as velvet. Strolling in the lengthening shadows, Chinese ladies in gowns of glowing silk stood out like jewels among military uniforms and the formal clothes of diplomats.

Few people stopped at the tea table to chat with friends of Mrs. Wei, who served fragrant tea in fragile porcelain cups. Most guests headed for the cocktail tables weighed down with glasses for every type of drink — Manhattan, martini, old fashioned, gin and tonic, highball, and wine. Waiters in colorful silk jackets handed the libations to the guests.

On opposite sides of the lawn under the spreading trees stood buffet tables laden with ham, turkey, beaten biscuits, and many delicacies. Knives flashing, the waiters carved thin slivers of meat and deftly slid them on the tiny biscuits. The guests sipped their drinks and nibbled the dainty morsels while strolling across the lawn.

Aunt Edith whispered, "Isn't this funny? Everyone is so hungry for a taste of meat in these days of rationing they cross back and forth from table to table meeting the same people."

Someone jostled my arm. A cold liquid splashed down my leg. "Excuse me, a bit crowded here." I glanced down at the dark stain from a spilled drink spreading across my white shoe. I heard the familiar voice again. "I really am sorry about that."

I looked up and found myself staring into the smiling face of Lieutenant Commander Douglas Fairbanks, Jr. The only movie star I'd seen all evening had just spilled his cocktail on my foot.

Lieutenant Commander Fairbanks ignored the buffet feast. He crossed the lawn from one cocktail table to the other, growing less steady with each trip. In a loud voice, he argued with a slim woman in black. "Just one more. Damn it. Just one more." Face flushed, cap askew, he swayed on his feet. An aide grasped him by the elbow and escorted him out of sight.

Mr. Lee, the young attaché in the embassy, whom I'd met at Aunt Edith's, bowed from the waist. "Pardon me. I have completed my duties. Would you care to see inside the embassy?"

We stepped into a serene room decorated with priceless treasures from China. The silence took us a world away from the hundreds of people milling about outside on the lawn. The subtle scent of incense filled the air. It would have taken days to absorb the beauty of the teak furniture, silk walls, porcelains, ivories, and jades.

I concentrated on Mr. Lee's words. "Only personal guests of Ambassador and Mrs. Wei ever see this room. When Madame Chiang Kai-Shek visits, she likes to sit here looking out at the garden."

I noticed her autographed photo on the grand piano, along with those of President Roosevelt, Mrs. Roosevelt, Prime Minister Churchill, General Eisenhower, and many other dignitaries, all in matching silver frames.

Aunt Edith appeared at the door. "The party is breaking up. It's time for us to make our escape." I thanked Mr. Lee and reluctantly said goodbye. Aunt Edith led me through a dark hallway, past waiters carrying trays of empty glasses. While honored guests waited under the front portico for their limousines, we left by way of the kitchen door.

Plunging down the hill on the uneven path, we removed our gloves and hats. As we waited for the bus, an angry red sun sank behind the trees. Sleek limousines from the embassy party swept past. I laughed. "Bet none of those people recognize us, even though a few minutes ago we were sharing refreshments."

After a cold glass of iced tea at Aunt Edith's, I made the long trek by bus and streetcar back to Walter Reed. Tired and bedraggled, I found my room jammed with friends. Marie had rounded up the crowd to hear about the embassy party.

She shrieked with delight. "Douglas Fairbanks spilled his drink on your shoe? He really did? He talked to you? Even Ann, with her dozens of dates, hasn't snagged a movie star."

I didn't mention to Marie that I was more impressed by the quiet moments with polite Mr. Lee in Ambassador Wei's drawing room.

Class of '45

The year at Walter Reed Army Medical Center ended as it had begun—filling out forms and trying to absorb dozens of new rules and regulations. On August 31, 1945 we ten apprentice dietitians, shed our old status for a new one. No longer students or apprentices, we had achieved the same army rank as our former instructors. For the first time, we ate dinner, not in the stuffy students' back room, but with the staff in their dining room.

"Lieutenant Morrison, welcome to the Army." Lieutenant Childress' words took me by surprise. She was the first officer to address me as Lieutenant. Some time, during that busy day, I'd raised my right hand and been sworn into the army. I had also been awarded a pin making me a member of the American Dietetic Association.

At a farewell dinner, the instructors welcomed us as partners. No longer serious and remote, Lieutenant Evans cracked jokes. Captain Dautrich, chief dietitian, congratulated each of us by name before turning the program over to Lieutenant Childress.

"When I spoke to you for the first time, I assured you I would not ask more than you were capable of doing." We laughed when she said there must have been times we doubted that. She emphasized that part of her job had been to make us tough and resilient. She had watched us grow, learn, and become responsible women.

She presented each of us with a rose. "Graduates of the Dietetic Intern Program at Walter Reed Army Medical Center, class of 1945, you have successfully completed the most rigorous training offered by the army. Whatever duties you are called on to perform, you are prepared to meet the challenge. I salute you."

Her next words made Marie and me cringe. "Lieutenants, I turn the program over to you." Busy with important matters, we had resented our assignment to provide the entertainment. Not until that morning had we come up with an idea.

I handed Marie the box of crepe paper rosettes we had made for awards. She called on Lieutenant Childress. "Our first award goes to you for putting up with us. You molded a group of scared, immature college girls into women proud to don the army uniform." Marie's voice grew unsteady. "Lieutenant Childress, we'll miss you. We could not have made it without you."

Our next award went, in absentia, to Marion Dow, one of three transferred to another hospital after the first six months. We could never forget the trouble she had brought on herself and a soldier on sentry duty parading in front of Walter Reed. When he passed behind the broad marble steps, Marion shoved a bite of her dessert in his mouth.

As he emerged on the other side, he could not take his hand off the rifle to remove the crumbs of chocolate cake around his mouth. The hapless soldier found himself face to face with an enraged colonel. Marion earned her award by talking her way out of that situation. Probably, the private had landed in the guardhouse.

Marie smiled at Myra. "Now, on a lighter note. Myra, you win our award for being a glamour girl both day and night. While the rest of us retired in cotton nightgowns, you matched the stars of Hollywood in your pale blue, baby doll pajamas."

Marie turned to Mary Schroeder from Illinois. "Mary, we recognize you for your high-pitched shriek at your first glimpse of a crustacean in that fancy restaurant. Your scream startled diners at nearby tables. They feared they were under air attack." Marie described how the waiter had heard this westerner say she'd never seen a lobster. He had brought a live one on a huge aluminum tray for her inspection.

The next award went to Eileen Welch. She had proved at the Eskay Meat Packing Company in Baltimore that 'wearin of the green' meant more than one's outfit. After witnessing the slaughter of the animals, none of us had relished cold cuts for lunch in the company dining room, least of all Eileen. Her green face had matched her green sweater.

I wondered what Marie would say about me. "Carol, we recognize you for your ability to maintain order in the Ward 8 kitchen while poaching General Pershing's eggs again and again."

After Marie handed out her last award, she smiled at the staff dietitians. She noted they had to go on duty early, not on vacation like us. It was time to conclude the program. I jumped to my feet. "Marie, before we go, you've earned the gold star."

The audience laughed over Marie's humiliating experience with an over-worked obstetrician. After delivering babies all through the night, he asked Marie to bring a breakfast tray to his room as soon as possible. He thought he'd have time to eat before the next delivery.

In her haste, Marie tripped in the doorway. The tray flew from her hands. She crashed to the floor spewing coffee and juice in all directions. The doctor surveyed the mess, as she lay sprawled in a jumble of eggs, toast, and jam. He stepped over her prostrate body and hurried to the delivery room. Marie had the presence of mind to call out through her dripping hair, "Sir, when you return your eggs will be ready."

Our light-hearted spoof ended the evening on a high note. After the party broke up, for the last time our class walked through the lobby past the portrait of Dr. Walter Reed. We paused at the top of the broad marble steps, linked arms and skipped down to the sidewalk. Eager to pack for vacation, we raced away in the sultry night air without a backward glance toward Walter Reed Army Hospital.

The class of 1945 had been granted one month's leave. We were ordered to report on October 1 to Fort Sam Houston, San Antonio, Texas.

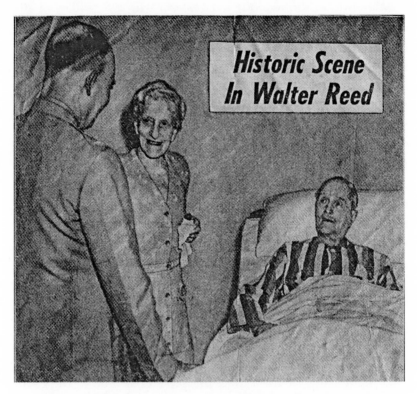

General Eisenhower meets with Miss Pershing and
General Pershing at Walter Reed Hospital in 1945.

The New York Daily Mirror printed this photograph on
Wednesday, July 21, 1948 after General Pershing's death.

Part III. Army Life

Part III. Army Life

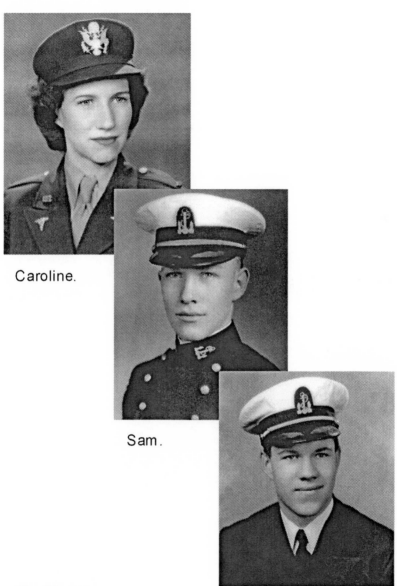

Caroline.

Sam.

The Morrison
siblings in uniform.

Sherman.

Basic Survival Skills 1945

After the long year at Walter Reed Army Medical Center, vacation in September 1945 did not live up to my expectations.

On the day of my arrival at Pennsylvania Station in New York, Mother, happy and excited, ran down the platform to greet me. After nine months apart, she rambled on without stopping for breath. "Dad longed to come but he's anxious to finish the job in Amherst, Massachusetts. We're eager to return to Florida. He'll come to Bethel to see you this weekend. Aunt Hannah is delighted you'll be staying with her."

Stay with Aunt Hannah? I was going to stay with Aunt Hannah? A wave of homesickness for my childhood home, sold the previous year, brought tears to my eyes. The reality of my situation hit me hard — I no longer had a room to call my own.

Mother gave my hand a squeeze. "I'm sorry, dear. I'm keeping house for Father. There's no room there for you there, unless you sleep in the sitting room."

I agreed I couldn't rest with Grandpa's antique clocks chiming at all hours. Mother said, "We'll be only a block apart and we can spend lots of time together."

As the train from New York clicked along the humming rails toward Bethel, I studied the familiar countryside. I had missed the indestructible stone walls. Even though our home was gone, those sturdy boundary lines built by early settlers remained. To me, they stood for strength and endurance. Those were qualities I needed to cultivate.

Mother's account of family and friends went on and on. When I asked whether she missed our home in Danbury, she laughed. "When you children were growing up, I loved our home but it has served its purpose. Now Dad and I are happy with our new life at the orange grove in Florida."

The train slowed to a stop in Bethel, the town where Mother, Dad, Sam, and I had been born. Only half a dozen people followed us down the steps to the platform. The deserted station dozed in the lengthening shadows of the hazy September afternoon.

Mother and I took turns carrying my heavy bag one block up Greenwood Avenue. Dad had been born in the tall, Gothic house at 219 Greenwood. His sister Hannah still resided there. His sister Margaret, and her husband, Arthur, shared Hannah's home when not in Florida.

Mother unlocked the double door with a skeleton key. "Hannah is working at the library until nine tonight. She said you should not to wait up for her. She'll see you at breakfast."

Mother glanced at her watch. "I must hurry to get Father's supper. We eat at five-thirty sharp. Come on up when you are ready." Leaving me to unpack, she disappeared up the hill toward 248 Greenwood Avenue, the modest cottage where she had been born. Grandpa lived there with his dog, Skippy.

Left alone, I set my bag next to the imposing hall tree. As long as I could remember, the same hats had hung on the brass hooks. In the high-ceiling parlor, glossy dark woodwork and drawn green shades at long windows cast gloom over the quiet room. To protect rugs and drapes from the sun, the shades were seldom raised. Only the lonely tick of the clock broke the silence.

I felt smothered, needed fresh air. Unpacking would have to wait. As I approached Grandpa's house, my spirits rose. His dog, Skippy, wagged his tail and licked my hand as though he remembered me. Rounding the corner of the house to the back door, I caught a glimpse of Grandpa coming out of his pumpkin-colored barn, a tin pan of fresh eggs in his hand.

He set the pan on the ground, wiped his hands on his pants before seizing my hand in his firm grip. "Glad to see you Carol. Good thing it's suppertime. You must need a meal. You're skinny as the coon dog I used to have."

I towered over my grandfather, who never weighed more than one hundred and eighteen pounds. He may have been lacking in stature but he felt no reticence about expressing his opinions. To me, he seemed one of a vanishing breed of men — a true Connecticut Yankee. A hatter by trade, he never owned an automobile or a horse.

I remembered him telling me, "All a man needs is two good feet. Mine have taken me far. You learn a lot walking ten to twelve miles a day. It's gol darn unhealthy fer people to rush around like chickens with their heads cut off."

Our conversation brought us to the house where he and Grandma had lived for fifty-four years until her death the previous year. The small, cozy, low-ceiling rooms brought back memories of happy hours spent with my grandmother.

Mother served supper on time, just as her mother had always done. After Grandpa washed his hands and face at the kitchen sink, we sat down to our evening meal.

"Gosh Hazel, I hope you've made plenty of pie. Carol looks like she needs some food that'll stick to her ribs."

After supper, I offered to help with the dishes but Grandpa wouldn't hear of it. Mother washed the plates and silverware in the battered metal dishpan. She placed them in the dish drainer, which stood in the sink next to the dishpan. Grandpa carried a teakettle of boiling water from the coal range across the kitchen and poured it over the dishes. The routine had not changed since Mother learned to help when a small child.

I said goodnight and strolled back to Aunt Hannah's. I lugged my suitcase up the stairs, being careful not to scrape the wallpaper at the sharp bend half way up. In the back bedroom, an iron bed, covered with a pristine white counterpane, stood waiting for me. I folded the spread and sat down with a jolt. Aunt Margaret's orthopedic mattress felt as unforgiving as a rock.

After a restless night, I arose early. I held on tight to the rail going down the steep dark back stairs to the drab gray kitchen. An orange stood on the enamel top of the gas range warming over the pilot light. In the dining room, the most cheerful room in the house, sunshine poured through the long narrow windows.

Aunt Hannah rose from the table to give me a kiss. "I hope you slept well. The chill will soon be off your orange. We'll start with the prunes."

This fussy prim gray-haired lady bore little resemblance to the fun loving Aunt Hannah of my childhood. The one who had given me the newest books to read, brought me an antique locket from London, and introduced me to summer theatre.

Three prunes sat in a puddle of juice in a white sauce dish before me. "I don't care for any, thank you."

"Oh, you must eat them. They are good for you." I bit my tongue, felt tempted to say that I had majored in nutrition in college and had written hundreds of special diets in the past year. She probably needed to eat prunes. I did not.

Instead of speaking out, I picked up my silver spoon and ate the prunes. The training of my childhood would not let me rebel. "Do as you are told. Always show respect for your elders."

That vacation, I longed to see one person my age, someone to whom I could relate. Surrounded by older members of the family, I felt isolated and alone. Thoughts about the uncertain life in the army stayed uppermost in my mind.

I began counting the days until I could escape to Texas.

Texas, Here We Come

In late September, a hint of fall color crept over the Connecticut hillsides. When the brilliance of fiery maples and golden birches reached the valley, the time had come to leave Bethel for basic training in the army. Every colorful tree seemed to shout, "Don't Go. There's nothing to equal this beauty in far-off Texas."

After climbing the steep stairs to Aunt Hannah's attic to pack away my civilian clothes in the wardrobe trunk, I was tempted by the letters and photos stored in the bottom drawer. I shook my head —this was no time to get nostalgic about the past. Wham! I slammed the lid shut.

As I draped a sheet over the top of the trunk, I wondered how long I would have to call this space "Home." Four square-feet under the eaves, the only place in the world I had to store my few possessions.

That evening Marie Lanou arrived from Vermont. Before leaving Walter Reed, we had made plans to travel together to basic training. Seeing her for the first time in her trim uniform revived my spirits. She made our future sound exciting.

"Did I get a lot of attention on the train! Before we buckle down to 'Yes Sir' and 'Yes Ma'am,' we're in for lots of fun — three days and two nights on the train to San Antonio." She admitted she still felt like a fool trying to salute. After I donned my uniform, we walked around town intending to practice our technique.

We found no service men on the streets in Bethel. Saluting each other sent us into spasms of laughter. One hour of training in military procedure, given by Lieutenant Childress before we left Walter Reed, seemed woefully inadequate to get us to Texas.

Striding along Main Street side by side, we gained confidence in our new role as lieutenants in uniform. When our hair sagged in the afternoon humidity, we wondered how we could keep the stray locks one inch above our collars. "I know that's the rule," Marie complained, "but I refuse to cut my hair any shorter."

The following evening, our last night of vacation, Mother and Dad took us to the Spinning Wheel Inn in Redding for dinner. Just as Marie had predicted, our first public appearance as women in uniform brought us lots of attention. After we'd finished the chicken potpie, the waitress served large slices of apple pie topped with cheddar cheese.

She smiled. "The apple pie comes compliments of the Inn. Dessert for military personnel is always free."

Back in Bethel, Mother insisted we stop at Grandpa's "for just a minute" to say goodbye. As Marie and Grandpa traded stories, the hour grew late. Grandpa's words left us laughing. I wished I had written down some of his tales, now it was too late for that. I might not see him again — he was almost eighty!

From his rocking chair, he directed his remarks to Marie. "I want to tell you 'bout an old feller here in town named Mike Todd. He had lots of money but hated to part with even one cent." Grandpa recounted how a 'widder lady' down Redding way got her eye on Mike Todd and snagged him. They got married in Redding and planned to spend the night at a hotel in Danbury, twelve miles away.

Grandpa rocked slowly. "Well, old man Todd, he put his new wife on the train. Told her to get off in Danbury and wait for'im. Then he took off his shoes and walked the twelve miles to save shoe leather and train fare. He was the tightest gol dern feller I ever knew."

Marie reciprocated with a story about her brother. Studying for the priesthood, he was helping the parish priest in Atlantic City where her family spent the summer. Her father, tall and dignified, walked past the church on his way home from the office and decided to stop for confession.

After he had talked for some time, the voice on the other side of the grille said, "That's enough, Pop. Tell Mom I'll be late for supper." Mr. Lanou's fury over the audacity of his son in hearing his own father's confession, forced Marie's brother to stay out of sight for days.

The visit ended with everyone laughing.

Early the next morning, Mother and Dad waited on the chilly platform to see Marie and me off on the train to New York. There seemed to be so much I wanted to say but could not. The shrill whistle of the engine rounding the bend warned us time had come for a final hug and kiss. Clutching the official government envelopes containing our orders, Marie and I scrambled aboard the train.

Once in New York, our concerns over saluting faded fast. We became experts in a matter of minutes. Service men, most of them veterans on their way home to civilian life, jammed the streets. Every enlisted man we passed grinned at us before giving us a snappy salute. They recognized a couple of greenhorns when they saw them. We returned salutes until our right arms ached.

As soon as we entered our train compartment, Marie kicked off her shoes. "Thank goodness, we don't have to make this long trip in coach. Take off your tie. Let's get comfortable. After we pass Philadelphia, we'll head to the diner for lunch."

What an obstacle course that turned out to be. We fought our way through crowded coaches, where many passengers without seats stood in the aisles. Trying to appear nonchalant, we ignored the whistles and catcalls of soldiers, sailors, and marines.

"Halt." A burly sergeant MP stuck out his nightstick to block our path. "Lieutenants, I must inform you, you're out of uniform." We checked each other over and saw nothing amiss. The sergeant smirked, "Your neckties do not match your skirts."

As I issued my first order, I tried to keep my voice from trembling. "Sergeant, our uniforms were purchased at the leading army supplier in Washington, D.C. They are in compliance with the dress code. Now let us pass."

"Yes Ma'am." I didn't have the nerve to tell him to wipe that sneer off his face.

Marie charged ahead toward the diner. "Thank goodness, rank takes precedence over inexperience. At least, it saved us this time. Bet that old bully has been in the army twenty years."

Lurching down the aisle on the swaying train to the diner remained an ordeal. The harder we tried to ignore the remarks of the enlisted men, the more they taunted us. "They're too skinny." "Oh, you beautiful doll. Want a drink?" The fun and excitement we had anticipated did not materialize. Our lack of knowledge about proper procedure kept us holed up in our compartment.

Sixty hours after leaving New York, the train pulled into San Antonio, long after the sun had set. The mission-style station charmed us. Until that moment, only in the movies had we seen men in Stetson hats and boots and Mexican women in ruffled blouses and colorful skirts.

The hot breeze that sapped the last of my waning energy did not keep Marie from singing "Deep in the Heart of Texas."

Fort Sam Houston

Fort Sam Houston, San Antonio, Texas. On the cab ride to the base, Marie and I were too exhausted to pay much attention to the surroundings. The sentry's instructions to the cab driver led us past row after row of identical two-story army barracks. We felt lost until we spotted our friend, Mary, standing in a doorway.

"Where have you been?" she called. "You're the last ones to arrive. You're stuck with the worst beds." The rest of her news did little to reassure us. Women had never been quartered in that part of the camp before. There weren't even window shades.

We climbed steep stairs and faced two long rows of cots covered with khaki blankets stamped US in large letters. The beds at the end of the line had been left for us, numbers twenty-nine and thirty.

Back at the entry stood our footlockers. As we wrestled the heavy chests up the stairs, Marie complained, "This is a heck of a job to do in heels. What I need is a shower and bed."

Squeals of laughter filled the room. "What's so funny? Why're you laughing at us?"

Vi a large bossy woman with a deep voice explained. "Jane, one of the first to arrive, thought she'd beat us to the shower. Was she ever sorry!" Vi insisted San Antonio hadn't heard such screams since the Alamo. "You know why? Cockroaches.

Hundreds of cockroaches. They're true Texans. Baby ones measure two inches long."

At 6:00 a.m., all thirty of us stepped into the so-called shower to shampoo our hair. In the long narrow room, a pipe near the ceiling with punched holes every six inches dumped water, either ice cold or boiling hot, directly on top of our heads. Privacy and modesty forgotten, together we fought the cockroach invasion.

That first night in the barracks, Vi had more advice. "Get your name on the sign-up sheet to do your ironing. The ironing board's busy from morning 'til night."

Before she could continue, someone shouted, "Turn out the damn lights so we can undress. The dimwit who put us here had better get window shades in this place tomorrow."

Even a lumpy mattress could not keep me awake. Sometime after midnight, loud laughter, cursing, and breaking glass interrupted my dreams. What was happening? Vi jumped up from her cot muttering, "Those damn drunks." She raised the screen and leaned out the window. In a husky voice she yelled, "Shut up you bastards. Don't you know it's 2:00 a.m.?" I had never before heard a woman use that kind of language.

"My God, there're women in there." Bam! A heavy object hit the front door. Our first night in the army and we were under siege by our own men. The din grew louder. "Scatter," hissed a low voice. "Here come the MPs." Aware that Vi's salty language and go-to-hell attitude needed no help from me, I drifted back to sleep.

When the chief dietitian heard our complaints, she took action. By noon, window shades had been installed and a sentry had been posted in front of the barracks. For the next six weeks, a guard remained on duty day and night.

We questioned whether the program for basic training had kept pace with the change in conditions. Since fighting had ceased with the surrender of Japan in August, why should we be trained for battle conditions? We saw no reason to crawl on our stomachs under barbed wire with bullets screaming over our heads. The chief dietitian told us we had no choice — only the High Command had the authority to alter the rules.

The first week a drill instructor took control of our lives. He made no effort to conceal his contempt for a bunch of women whom he must bully into marching form. He showed us no mercy.

"Forward march," he shouted. "About face." As we practiced the same maneuvers again and again, our make-up melted and our hair grew limp. When we bumped into each other, we snickered. In language we did not care to hear him repeat, he informed us such behavior would not be tolerated.

By Friday, he had turned us into a cohesive unit. To our surprise, we marched in a review without disgracing our tough drillmaster.

After surviving those scorching hot mornings in the sun, we looked forward to afternoon assignments in the hospital. In contrast to the old brick buildings at Walter Reed, tall, gleaming Brooke General Hospital appeared modern and efficient.

Marie straightened her seersucker cap. "I wouldn't mind being stationed here."

"Great thought, but there's not a chance," I replied. "Only those with pull get assigned to a post as popular as this one." Not many army posts could equal the social life available to officers there. The lush green polo field attested to that. We decided to relax and enjoy the few weeks we expected to be at Fort Sam Houston.

Much to our relief, training for battle conditions was cancelled and we had extra time to explore San Antonio. Our classmates from Walter Reed staged a reunion at a Mexican restaurant. After a month apart, we chatted and giggled without the restraints we had felt under Lieutenant Childress' supervision.

I liked the informality of the untidy eatery — the intense bright blue windowsills, bouquets of huge crepe paper flowers on bare tables, and the lively music of strolling musicians. Most of us had never tasted margaritas or Mexican food. Anne, most sophisticated among us, urged us to try the margaritas.

"Don't drink too fast," she advised. "This is strong stuff."

Mary hesitated before taking a sip. "Salt on the rim of the glass? That's strange." We laughed remembering Mary's reaction of disgust at the sight of her first lobster.

She did not looked reassured by Anne's words. "The salt cuts the flavor of the cactus juice. You'll like the food. Much of it's made from corn. That's something you know about in Illinois."

On Saturday, I had a visitor. My cousin Ted, a corporal in the Air Force, stationed at nearby Foster Field, traveled by bus to San Antonio to see me. After my last class ended at noon, I hastened to town to meet him. He looked lean and fit, thinner than I remembered him.

"Ted, this seems too good to be true. Both of us stationed here two thousand miles from home. We're so lucky to have this day together."

Our lunch surprised me as much as the Mexican combination of ground beef, refried beans, and cheese in a tortilla had done. Sizzling steaks served Texas style, not on plates but platters. The size of the portions astounded me. "I can never eat that much beef," I protested.

Ted grinned. "Wait 'til you taste it."

We lingered over coffee. I looked down at my platter surprised to fine it empty. "Ted, you were right. If Texans call this lunch, what is dinner like?"

Ted grinned. "I knew you needed a good meal. Can't beat Texas beef." He grew nostalgic. "Just think. Our parents have never been west of the Mississippi and here we are in Texas. Any amount of marching is worth it to spend a weekend here with you."

Catching up on family news, we wandered along the walk by the river. Few in carefree Texas bothered to salute when off the base. However, many enlisted men, seeing me with a corporal, forced me to return their salutes. Although relatives could be together regardless of rank, a group of GIs followed us shouting, "Verboten. Verboten."

We retreated to the Saint Anthony Hotel for dinner. Ted studied the menu. "Let's have lobster for old times' sake. Remember how we used to pick out live lobsters from the pen of sea water at Captain Allen's Clam House at Compo Beach?" Much to our dismay, the lobsters arrived smothered in Mexican hot sauce.

The next day, tired of saluting, I came up with a plan to escape the soldiers' attention. "Ted, let's rent a car. My treat. Now that I'm finally making money, I'll blow my first paycheck on a day in the country." Ted chose a convertible, a red one.

Driving through posh neighborhoods, we admired enormous houses with towering white columns, endless green lawns, stables, horses, and more horses. Only in movies had we seen such places. "Let's head for the open road." Ted suggested. "You haven't seen the expanse of this land, so different from hilly Connecticut."

We headed for Hondo forty miles away. Flying along the gleaming highway in the shiny convertible, wind rushing through my hair, I felt free as the bird circling overhead. Ted poured out his unhappiness over the treatment he'd received from my college roommate, Mary Kirschner. Said she'd broken his heart.

"Last week she sent me a 'Dear John' letter. Guess I never really had a chance with her but I kept hoping. Now I'll have to find a new girl, someone less fickle than Mary."

His words gave me a guilty conscience. Although I had known of Ted's feelings, I had rooted for Dave to win Mary's affection. Her ambition would have overwhelmed Ted. Moreover, he could not have stood up to the opposition expressed by both mothers — his as well as Mary's.

I changed the subject. "Those must be the celebrated long horn cattle. This land seems to go on forever and the sky is huge. Oh, Ted. I wish we could drive farther but we must turn back.

The car has to be returned by six." Before parting, we made plans to get together again on Ted's next leave.

Next morning reality wiped out all thought of those two carefree days. I climbed into the back of a truck headed for a tent in the broiling hot desert.

The next five days would be spent working under field conditions at Cook and Bakers' School.

Cook and Bakers' School

In mid October, the heat of summer still gripped Fort Sam Houston. Our group of dietitians, trying to adjust to basic training, filed off the bus and stared in dismay at the desolate desert. "This is crazy," murmured someone behind me. "Why make us take training at Cook and Bakers' School under field conditions when the fighting is over?"

As we marched into a huge stifling tent, hot rays of the sun made our starched seersucker uniforms stick to our backs. A blast of heat rose from the coal ranges in the still air and hung like a cloud under the heavy canvas. A scowling mess sergeant called us to attention.

"I don't like this any better'n yah'll do. My assignment is to teach yah'll to bake and cook. By damn that's what I'm goin' ta do. Latrine is out back. Watch out fer snakes. Drink plenty o' water. First person to pass out flunks."

He ordered us to open our field manuals to the list of equipment. "Today we'll learn what yah'll have ta' work with under field conditions. If you're lucky, you'll be far enough behind the lines to have a black beauty lik' this one." He cast an admiring glance at the imposing black cook stove.

The next day he introduced us to dehydrated foods. "Lieutenant Morrison explain the use o' powdered eggs and how to make 'em."

Thank goodness, I knew the answer. "Under certain conditions," I quoted the manual, "it is more expedient to furnish dried whole eggs than fresh eggs to the Army cook. This product represents the solid portion of the egg with only shell and water removed."

He ordered me to continue. "One hundred pounds of liquid eggs without the shell consists of twenty-six to twenty-seven pounds of egg solids and seventy-three to seventy-five pounds of water. Dried eggs should be reconstituted with cold water. Hot water will ruin the eggs. They should not stand more than thirty minutes."

The hours passed slowly. We made our way through dried milk, dried onions, dried cabbage and carrots, dried apples, and dried prunes. Through the long afternoon, we purified water before reconstituting dozens of samples. Each item had to be graded as to color, texture, and flavor.

Marie blew on a lock of hair, which had escaped from her hairnet. "I thought those onions would make me sick. Hope tomorrow's less boring. At least we'll be combining all this stuff in recipes."

Thursday morning found us in high spirits. A light breeze stirred the air outside the tent. Inside we stood behind long tables covered in white butcher paper. Following the mess sergeant's orders, we lined up equipment to make cakes. Confident of our reconstituting abilities, we added water to the dry ingredients.

Intent on stirring the contents in large stainless steel bowls with long handled metal spoons, we did not notice visitors standing at the entrance to the tent. "Tenshun." The gruff command of the mess sergeant startled us. With a loud clatter, a dozen spoons hit the table.

An inspecting general, followed by his staff, ordered us to proceed. We were lucky the inspection took place before we baked the batter. The finished cakes rated low on our survey sheets. The mess sergeant showed his displeasure over the dropped spoons.

"Yah'll acted like scared rabbits."

On Friday, after serving a meal of cooked dehydrated foods, we graduated from Cook and Bakers' School with certificates to prove our proficiency.

During four weeks in Texas, we had mastered army protocol, drilling, hospital procedures, and cooking in a tent. We had grown accustomed to the living arrangements — thirty women officers in an army barracks with an armed guard to protect us. Now we were ready to leave that security for our first assignments. Day after day, we waited for orders to move out.

Two by two, people, like the animals in Noah's ark, people left until only ten of us remained. Ordered to report to the chief dietitian, I eagerly anticipated my new assignment. I was baffled when she did not mention my future post.

"Lieutenant, do you know how to paint?" She answered her own question. "I'm sure you do." She pushed a can of black paint and a brush across her desk. "Go to the third room on the right. Paint faces on the pumpkins you find in there. They're decorations for the officers' Halloween party."

Sitting alone in the quiet room surrounded by a hundred pumpkins, I smoldered. More scowling faces than happy ones came to life under my brush. I wondered why I had to carry out this task all by myself. It would have been fun if someone shared the work with me. It would have been even better if I'd been invited to the party.

Three days later, I received my orders. "Report for duty within five days to Battey General Hospital, Rome, Georgia." I griped to my few remaining friends in typical army style. "What kind of a place would be named Battey? Where the heck is Rome, Georgia? Why do I have to travel alone when the others have gone with a partner?"

At a farewell dinner in our favorite Mexican restaurant, even a second margarita could not lift my spirits. Marie and Mary had orders to head for California. I wished Mary were going to Rome, Georgia and I to San Francisco with Marie. From our first day of training at Walter Reed, Marie and I had shared good times and bad. Now I faced a lonely trip without my best friend to a hospital named Battey in far-off Georgia.

I wondered whether Marie and I would cross paths in the future. Although we corresponded for the next sixty years, we never again met face to face.

Rome, Georgia

Disconsolate at the thought of traveling alone from San Antonio, Texas to Rome, Georgia, "wherever that might be," I anticipated a dull trip to my first army assignment. Contrary to my expectations, the next two days brought good companionship, good food, and fun.

The porter in the Pullman car led me to my compartment. An air force captain sat at a tiny table, which filled the space between two facing seats. Tall and lean, his tousled brown hair seemed at odds with his tailored uniform. He pushed aside his papers to give me a cordial smile. "I'm Captain Warren on my way to Virginia. Where're you going?"

"I'm Lieutenant Morrison on my way to Rome, Georgia. Did you ever hear of that town?"

"It's about two hours out of Atlanta. Kind of an out-of-the-way place." At the sight of the shiny gold band on his left hand, I relaxed. I wouldn't have to worry about his intentions. Only a man devoted to his wife wore his wedding ring.

By the time we reached the front of the line waiting for a table in the dining car, we had scrapped the formality of rank in favor of Bob and Carol. I enjoyed the luxury of starched table linen, fresh flowers, and a flavorful steak served with an endless supply of fresh, hot biscuits. In spite of Bob's company, I could not keep from yawning. He grabbed the check. "You've had a long day. The porter must have the berths made up by now. Let's turn in."

I did not hear my traveling companion climb the ladder to the upper berth. Grateful that my ticket specified the lower one, I had already fallen asleep. Unaware when the train crossed the

Mississippi during the night, I opened my eyes to bright sunshine in bayou country.

As the train drew into New Orleans, Bob pointed out landmarks he recognized. "This is an exciting city. Since our train for Atlanta doesn't leave until evening, how would you like Bob's guided tour of New Orleans?" I was amazed at my good fortune. Marie had predicted army travel could be fun. Bob's invitation proved her point.

Before we could investigate the city, we needed reservations for the sleeper on the next leg of our journey. Apparently, the army had expected us to sit up the second night. Even Bob's persuasive voice could not cut through the red tape quickly. I watched in awe as he threatened, cajoled, and, eventually, came up with reservations for a compartment on the overbooked train to Atlanta.

He put the tickets in his pocket. "Let's grab a cab and head for the best Shrimp Creole in New Orleans. It's a little out-of-the way place far from the tourist crowd."

On the half dozen tables in the restaurant, red check tablecloths echoed the informality of candle wax dripping down the sides of wine bottles. Bob warned me to take small bites until I got used to the hot intensity of New Orleans cooking.

He was right. The first taste of Shrimp Creole seared my throat. A large sip of coffee to put out the fire gave me a jolt. The strong bitter coffee, stronger than any I had ever drank, took me by surprise. Bob laughed. "It's chicory added to the coffee beans, goes well with the fiery food," he explained.

We lingered until candle wax cascaded down the buildup on the wine bottle onto the tablecloth. The other mid-day diners had long since departed. We left the restaurant to stroll through the French Quarter. I tried to absorb new sights and sounds — the delicate iron-grille balconies, street musicians playing on the sidewalk, and jazz pouring out of dark mysterious bars, all surrounded by the aroma of jasmine, pralines, coffee, and frying fish.

As we rushed back to the station, the orange-red October sun disappeared behind the palm trees. After so many new experiences packed into in a few hours, the cool calm of the compartment brought a welcome chance to relax.

Bob spread out graph paper on the small table between us. "How could I be so lucky as to meet a dietitian, someone who knows about kitchens? I want to surprise my wife with plans to remodel ours."

We changed traffic patterns, lowered the height of counters, moved a wall to make space for a breakfast nook. By midnight, we could think of no more improvements.

Sleep proved elusive the second night in the lower berth — so many impressions to absorb from one day, so many uncertainties to face on the morrow, and so many cups of New Orleans coffee.

Morning found us in Atlanta. While Bob went to the hotel barbershop for a shave, I sat in the lobby and wrote a hurried letter to Mother and Dad. I mentioned Captain Bob Warren but did not disclose he had a wife. Thought it fun to leave them guessing about our relationship.

We dallied over breakfast and spent an hour browsing on Peachtree Street. Bob's train left before mine. "Thanks, Bob, for making this trip so much fun. I shall never forget my introduction to Shrimp Creole and coffee laced with chicory. Without your help, I might have wandered around Georgia for days trying to find my way to Rome."

"Enjoyed your company. I'll tell my wife how you helped improve the plans. Once in a while unexpected good company comes along, even in the army. We have to make the most of each day. Good luck." He waved and disappeared in the crowd.

Two hours later, I boarded a dirty coach with few passengers. The train lumbered along past tar paper shacks and tumble down houses. Black children wearing tattered clothes, or none, played in the grassless, red clay yards. It seemed doubtful they would ever escape the poverty of that worn-out land.

The view outside the window changed and I enjoyed passing through groves of trees. How I had missed trees in the wide-open spaces of Texas. WELCOME TO ROME, GEORGIA — that sign on the outskirts of town brought me back to concerns about Battey General Hospital.

The train jolted to a halt. I straightened my tie and smoothed my wrinkled skirt before stepping onto the platform. A private gave me a sluggish salute. "Lieutenant Morrison? The car's over yonder in the shade. If yah give me yore claim checks, I'll git yore bags."

My spirits soared. I had not expected to be met by a staff car. The driver took off in a cloud of red dust. He turned his head to say over his shoulder, "Battey General Hospital ain't much. Don't know why they sent yah here, Lieutenant. The hospital goin' ta' close by the end of the month."

Battey General Hospital

After the driver's warning that Battey General Hospital would soon close, I did not expect the warm welcome I received. The informality of the staff made it seem more like family than the army. The chief dietitian, a chatty captain, walked me to my room along a corridor lined with pots of African violets.

"I'm sorry to tell you the rumor you heard is true. This hospital is being phased out. Patients are already being transferred to other facilities. While you're here, your assignment will be to write special diets and supervise in the kitchen." She told me I would be entitled to a half day off one week, one and one half days off the next.

The following morning at 6:30 a.m., Lieutenant Winfield, in charge of the kitchen, took me on a tour. "This is a great place to work, with one exception — the commanding officer is a tough, old grouch. Oh, oh, here he comes. He inspects this department every morning." She sighed before giving the colonel a smart salute. "Good morning, Sir."

Waving his limp hand toward his cap in return, the gray-haired, overfed officer glared at her. "By god, I'll decide for myself when the day's good and when it's not."

As he strode out of sight, Lieutenant Winfield whispered, "Now you've met the menace. Relax. He won't cross our paths again until tomorrow."

One of six dietitians, I enjoyed the casual approach of the staff to their jobs. Lieutenant Childress at Walter Reed, with her insistence on strict military standards, would never have condoned leaving work to stroll to the post office, nor would she have allowed breaks mid-morning and mid-afternoon to drink cokes.

Much of my energy went into making a cook out of Elroy. A backwoods Georgian, tall and gaunt, shoulders hunched, arms dangling helplessly at his sides, he moved at only one speed — slow, really slow. Lieutenant Winfield advised me to ignore him. "He's good at chopping vegetables, not much else." Curious about his lack of motivation, I asked him whether he had always lived in the area.

He looked at me with pale, watery blue eyes. His Adams apple rose and fell in his throat. "Wal Lootenant, Ah was borned in the mountains. Ma' pappy moved us down here when Ah turned five. Only made it in school ta third grade." No wonder he has trouble following a recipe, I thought. He can't read.

Next time we worked the morning shift, I handed him a card. On it I had printed in large letters the list of ingredients for Chicken and Noodle Casserole. I read the words to him, made him repeat them.

"Now line up all the things we talked about on the table. Count to make sure you have them all." I discovered he could count to ten. "I'll tell you how much of each item to use."

When the dish came out of the oven, fragrant and bubbly, Elroy stared at it in amazement. "Lootenant, I made that? I made that all by myself?"

"You did Elroy. You're going to be a good cook." By the end of the week, he had mastered cream sauce and chocolate pudding. His locomotion had progressed from really slow to just plain slow.

On Saturday, my afternoon off for the week, I explored Rome, Georgia. It proved to be a hopeless place to shop. I could not find even one Christmas gift. A week later, with a whole day at my disposal, I endured a bumpy bus ride to Chattanooga, Tennessee. There I discovered a real city with Christmas decorations on the streets to put me in a holiday mood.

When I dropped a quarter in the red kettle of the Salvation Army lassie, she responded with a nod of thanks and renewed enthusiasm for ringing her bell. Only a few pennies and dimes lay in the bottom of the large pot. Laden with packages, I caught the bus back to Rome. As I slipped off my shoes to rest my tired feet, I laughed. Were the hillbilly ways of Georgia already rubbing off on me?

The slow-paced life at Battey General Hospital ended too soon. The chief dietitian called me to her office. "Lieutenant Morrison. I can give you a choice of new posts — Kennedy General in Memphis, Tennessee or Letterman in San Francisco." It took me only seconds to make my decision.

"Ma'am, I'd prefer Kennedy." Dot Barnard, my classmate from Walter Reed, was in Memphis. San Francisco seemed a million miles away from the family. Following my snap decision, I went back to work to announce the following day would be my last.

In the morning, Elroy stood waiting by the door to my office. He shook my hand. "Lootenant, ah told my wife las' night, she shore is lucky she found me first. She wouldn't have stood a chance, if I'd set eyes on y'all 'fore I met her."

The stubble on his chin quivered. I looked into his pale eyes. "Elroy that is the nicest compliment I ever had. Just keep studying those word lists we made. You're going to be a good cook." We shook hands again before he shuffled down the hall.

At lunch, Lieutenant Winfield came up with a bright idea. "Why don't you ask for a delay en route? If you leave tonight you could spend a couple of days with your family in Florida."

"Can I do that? I've been in the army too short a time to know all the ropes."

"Give it a try. Call Kennedy General and ask for the adjutant. I'll help you." Much to my amazement, I was granted three days delay en route. While Lieutenant Winfield checked train schedules, I rushed off to sign papers, pick up my orders, and pack.

I glanced around my room one last time to check for anything I might have overlooked. After a hasty supper, the staff dietitians treated me to a taxi ride to the station. In the three weeks I had known them, they had become good friends. Now it was time to say goodbye. It seemed to me I was always saying goodbye.

As the train pulled away from the station, the moon rose over the Georgia pines. I dozed, dreamily planning the reunion with Mother and Dad less than twenty-four hours away in Miami, Florida. A sudden thought made me sit bolt upright.

My nylons! What a disaster! Every pair of nylons I owned, except the ones on my legs, hung freshly laundered on the towel rack behind the door in my room at Battey. In those days of rationing the loss of four pairs of nylons was a catastrophe.

I consoled myself thinking of the bonanza they would be to the maid who cleaned the room.

Memphis, Tennessee

A three-day leave with Mother and Dad in Homestead, Florida had seemed such a good idea. After a long sleepless night on the sit-up train from Atlanta to Jacksonville, Florida, I regretted my impulsiveness. During a long layover there, I dozed on a hard wooden bench. To my chagrin, I slept through the departure of the noon train to Miami.

"Miami. Track Nine." Late in the evening, that blaring announcement jolted me to my feet. Grateful for a reclining seat on the modern streamliner, I fell asleep before the train left the station. A new world greeted me in the morning — green grass, swaying palm trees, pastel buildings, and magenta bougainvillea.

After the red soil and scraggly pines of Georgia, Florida appeared to be a fanciful dream. As the train glided to a stop in Miami, I spied Mother and Dad before they saw me. They were intent on scanning the sea of uniforms hurrying past them.

"Here comes our lieutenant." Dad gave me a comforting hug.

Mother kissed me and then stepped back. "Let me look at you. I had no idea you would be so stunning in your uniform. Welcome home. Carol, we're going to make this the best vacation you've ever had."

That promise left me short on sleep but long on memories. On the first day, dazzling sunshine bounced off the brilliant sea surrounding the Florida Keys. After we drove half way to Key West, Dad, sensing my fatigue, suggested we turn back. Later, I regretted that I never saw Ernest Hemmingway's town.

The next morning my parents and I took off to see a Florida craze — animal jungles. We visited The Parrot Jungle, where hundreds of brilliant birds perched in the trees and flew overhead.

I preferred The Monkey Jungle, perhaps because of the slogan: "Where The Humans Are Caged And The Monkeys Run Wild." We walked inside a chicken wire enclosure, while over our heads the monkeys chattered, swooped, and hung from tree limbs by their tails. Our grove lay only a few miles away, and occasionally, an escaped monkey on a spree scampered among our orange trees.

A leisurely lunch at the Tap-a-Wingo Restaurant featured a specialty of Florida cooking — key lime pie. I described the meal in New Orleans to Mother and Dad, and bragged my travels were introducing me to the best of southern cooking, as well as the worst.

On my last morning, we shopped at the Sears skyscraper in Miami. Sears and Roebuck, familiar throughout the United States for the mail order business generated by their catalogue and drab stores in small towns, had startled the retail world. The windows in this gleaming building featured stylish, colorful clothes. The ground floor displayed a wonderland of costume jewelry, raffia purses, and floppy hats.

I hated to leave the vacation atmosphere of Miami for the long trip to Memphis. By the time I reached Tennessee, I had made up my mind to never travel hundreds of miles out of my way again for three days of pleasure. Perhaps, if I had arrived in Memphis by daylight instead of darkness, I would have felt less forlorn.

When I spotted Dorothy Barnard waiting for me, my spirits rose. After returning her salute, I laughed and grabbed her arm. "Dot, when you were assigned to Kennedy General, I never expected I'd be joining you." I told her I had chosen Kennedy over Letterman in San Francisco because I would be working with her. I wanted to be with a friend, someone to help me learn the ropes.

On the taxi ride from city streets to a residential area, Dot's comments convinced me I'd made the right choice. "The fourteen dietitians on staff have lots of fun. We live in the nurses' quarters. Although much newer, Kennedy General reminds me of Walter Reed."

The hospital had opened in January 1943 and in three years had become one of the largest army hospitals in the country. The patient population had peaked in June at six thousand. Now in December, the census had returned to the usual number of forty-five hundred.

I asked Dot about her job. "I'm working with paraplegics, spinal cord injury patients. Many of them will never walk again. A few are paralyzed from the neck down. Great group of guys. It's considered such a tough assignment no one is expected work there for more than three months."

The taxi pulled up in front of a large, two story brick building. Dot led me through a spacious lounge furnished with polished mahogany furniture and upholstered chairs and sofas. On the second floor, she opened a door. "Here's your new home, not fancy but comfortable. You share the bath with Naomi, a nurse on the other side. I'll come for you at 6:00 a.m. and take you to breakfast."

Next morning I reported for duty to Captain Smith, the soft-spoken, unassuming chief dietitian. She introduced me to Lieutenant Cubillis. "Lieutenant Cubillis will spend the week with you introducing you to all phases of the dietary department. I'll decide later where to place you."

As we walked the long corridors, Carlota Cubillis and I talked of Miami, where her Cuban family lived. She told me stories of the many months she had spent overseas. The most competent and charming dietitian I had met, I felt privileged to work with her.

By the end of the week, she bragged we had walked all eleven miles of corridors connecting the wings of the hospital. My aching feet attested to that. The following morning she was gone. Instead of being discharged as she had hoped, her orders sent her to Brazil for three months.

On Monday morning, Captain Smith ended the suspense over my assignment. "Lieutenant, you are going to work on Ward 2B, a paraplegic ward. Lieutenant Cubillis recommended you for this demanding assignment." Just as Dot had told me, Captain Smith emphasized I would be relieved after three months for a less stressful job.

Paralyzed patients were subject to severe infections. Proper nutrition played an essential role in their welfare. Captain Smith explained my responsibilities. "Every day you will receive lab slips giving plasma protein levels. The patients with the lowest numbers are at greatest risk of developing infections."

It would be up to me to keep them well nourished, even if I had to prepare special foods to appeal to their depleted appetites. Another part of my job would be to calculate nutrients consumed at every meal by each patient.

Captain Smith hesitated a moment. "One more thing. You will be assisted in the ward kitchen by three German prisoners of war."

Kennedy General Hospital

My first day on duty on Ward 2B, December 1, 1945, I wondered how I would communicate with three German prisoners of war. I spoke no German, they little English. According to international law "a prisoner must be accompanied by a guard at all times." This edict had been revoked at Kennedy General Hospital to allow well-screened prisoners to relieve the acute shortage of hospital personnel.

I stepped into the ward kitchen and faced three men dressed in coarse blue jackets and blue pants. They stood stiffly against the wall. "Good morning. I'm Lieutenant Morrison."

A tall man with thinning hair snapped to attention. He bowed from the waist. "Goot Morning. I am Otto." He pointed to the next man, "This iss Rudolph." Rudolph's face remained blank. "This iss Edmund." Edmund, a head shorter than his partner, gave me a shy smile.

Arrival of the food cart from the main kitchen saved us from further attempts at conversation. Edmund placed juice, cold cereal, and milk on each tray. Otto added hot food — eggs, toast, and coffee. I checked the tray before Rudolf carried it to the patient's bedside. Under Otto's direction, the three men worked with efficiency and speed.

As Rudolph returned the empty trays to the kitchen, I calculated food intake. The names of the patients were printed across the top of the form, the foods to be served at each meal down the left. I put a check mark by the foods eaten by each patient. Some days I had to work overtime to finish my calculations of the carbohydrate, fat, protein, vitamin, and mineral intake.

Leaving Otto in charge of the kitchen, I met patients, starting with those who had not eaten breakfast. At the end of the hall, ten enlisted men shared a ward. Other rooms for enlisted men had one to four beds. A corridor separated them from the private rooms of the officers. I hunted for the name Thibeaux on a door.

"Good morning Captain Thibeaux. I'm Lieutenant Morrison. Not hungry this morning?" As I stared at his stiff body and useless hands strapped in braces, I marveled at the friendly smile he gave me.

"Well, I'll tell you how it is. I have to be fed. That's the nurse's job. Sometimes, when the tray comes, no one's here to feed me. Can't stand cold eggs."

"I can take care of that. How do you like your eggs? I'll cook some for you and send someone to help you before the plate gets cold."

Back in the kitchen, Otto watched me fry two eggs. "Over easy." Otto repeated my words but looked confused. I made motions with the spatula to show what I had just done. "Over easy."

He grinned "Yah, yah. Over easy." I never cooked another egg. Otto had just become a great short order cook.

Not all patients wanted to cooperate. Private Jones lay with his face to the wall. "Go away. I ain't goin' ta eat this crap."

What did you have for breakfast at home?"

"Nothin'. Maybe a chaw o' snuff."

It would not be easy to reach Private Jones. Paralyzed from the waist down, he had been shot in the back by a buddy cleaning his rifle. At the time of the accident, Private Jones had been in the army three weeks. He was eighteen years old.

Activity on Ward 2B became routine until I received a communication from the commanding officer. It concerned garbage. "Lieutenant Morrison: This is to inform you Ward 2B has the highest ratio of garbage per capita of any ward in the hospital. If this situation is not remedied, you will report to me in person one week from today on December 15, 1945."

After the evening meal, Rudolph carted the garbage can to the main kitchen where he weighed and recorded the contents. Paraplegic wards always had the worst record. Bedridden patients had poor appetites and often refused to eat their food. Cupcakes and other treats, forced on the patients by good-hearted Red Cross ladies, ended up on the returned trays and contributed to the total waste.

The commanding officer's letter in hand, I pointed to the garbage can. "Too much, too much." Otto, Rudolph and Edmund stared at me. "Yah" usually meant that someone understood. This time Edmund caught on. He placed his hand near the top of the can, pretended to scoop out some of the contents. "Yah," I said. We all laughed.

The next evening, baked beans, an unpopular dish for finicky appetites, appeared on the menu. We had finished serving, when an urgent announcement crackled over the PA system — "Plumber to Ward 2B, Plumber to Ward 2B." My resourceful helpers had found a way to dispose of the hated beans — in the toilets.

Discovering new ways to beat the system became a game. Beets, the least popular vegetable, disappeared into empty saltine cracker boxes to be disposed of with waste paper. Nurses were notified nothing could be returned on trays that had not originated with the dietary department.

My next communication from the commanding officer brought astounding news. "Lieutenant Morrison, you are to be commended for the lowest ratio of food waste per capita of any ward in the hospital. Congratulations."

No one questioned how such quick results had been achieved. As long as I remained at Kennedy General Hospital, Ward 2B had one claim to fame — the lowest figures reported, week after week, for garbage disposal.

In spite of language barriers, Otto, Rudolph, Edmund, and I had become an efficient team.

Christmas On Ward 2B

Santa Claus dominated the Christmas decorations on Ward 2B — a Santa only paraplegics could think up and appreciate. Stuffed with pillows, dressed in a maroon exercise suit similar to those worn by the patients, this Santa sat in a wheelchair. A plastic tube ran down his leg to a gallon jug on the floor by his feet. Even Santa could not escape a catheter on Ward 2B.

When the staff had asked the patients to volunteer to decorate for Christmas, several men refused. Far from family and friends, trapped in deformed bodies, they found memories of previous Christmases made this one too painful to contemplate.

As I tacked sprays of artificial greens over the doors, I thought back to the long strands of princess pine I used to weave around the spindles and the banister on the stairs in our Connecticut home. I had added red bows to the greens to give the hall a festive. The fire marshal brought me out of my reverie. "Take that stuff down. You can't use that. It isn't fireproof."

"For only three days? Can't we please have decorations for three days?"

He glared at me. "I said take it down."

Seeing my dismay, the patients came to my rescue. "We'll help, Lieutenant. We'll fix up a Santa Claus. You find some treated paper we can use for decorations."

I skipped my afternoon break to help redecorate. At first, only a few patients cut, pasted, and glued strips of red and green fireproof construction paper into paper chains. That childhood activity brought back memories we all had in common. Soon everyone was sharing stories of flour and water paste, paper chains, first grade, and Sunday school.

Our colorful hand-made decorations hung in graceful swags over doorways and looped across walls. Plenty of chains remained to decorate the Christmas tree and the beds in the ward. "Hey, Jonesie, your bed is next," called Jake to his ward mate.

For the first time, Jones showed interest in activities around him. The paper chains remained on his bed for a week. Our decorating efforts harking back to childhood, brought Ward 2B an award for the most creative Christmas decor in the hospital.

On Christmas morning, twelve patients, unable to go home, remained on the ward. The chief dietitian suggested we try something new — serve dinner at tables in the recreation room instead of carrying trays to the patients. That took precise planning — two stretchers and ten wheelchairs required a lot of space.

Lieutenant Beaman refused to say whether he planned to stay for dinner. When I asked him, he shrugged. "Naw. I don't think so. The food ain't fit to eat." Ignoring his remark, I went in search of a corpsman to place blocks under the table legs. The table height had to be raised to accommodate the wheelchairs.

Private Pinsky called to me from his room. "Lieutenant, want to see pictures of my niece and nephew?" I had been warned to keep my distance from him, but, preoccupied with the tables, I moved toward his bed. As I reached for the pictures, he grabbed me by my wrists in a vise-like grip. Arms forced to my sides, a strong jerk landed me full length on top of Private Pinsky.

The many hours he had spent lifting weights had given him massive strength in his upper body. He had me pinned down and I could not escape. My feet beat against the blankets. "Let me go," I hissed. "Let me go."

"I'd like to keep you forever." Only after giving me a quick kiss did he release me. He winked. "Merry Christmas, Lieutenant." As I smoothed my hair and adjusted my cap, I vowed to never again get closer than ten feet to Private Pinsky.

Back in the kitchen, the German prisoners, Otto and Rudolph, had lined up their gifts to the patients. Each poster-painted water glass depicted realistic scenes of their homeland — snowy villages, mountains, and children at play. Edmund and I carried the glasses with care to the rec room where we were setting the tables.

"I bet these paper tablecloths aren't fireproof," I muttered. "They are colorful and the fire marshal certainly won't be around on Christmas morning."

At each place, I added a paper cup of mints and nuts, place card, menu, crayon-decorated napkins sent by school children, and a pack of cigarettes. Oranges made a golden streak of light down the center of the tables. The European scenes on the water glasses stood out like jewels. Santa Claus sitting in his wheelchair, cigar in hand, seemed to nod his approval.

First to arrive, Lieutenant Beaman. "You said you weren't coming." Although making room for an extra wheelchair caused a delay, I refused to show my annoyance with the troublemaker. As Bing Crosby's rendition of "Jingle Bells" filled the air, the two stretcher patients arrived wreathed in paper chains followed by a parade of wheelchairs. The nurses and I stood by the door to wish our guests a cheery, "Merry Christmas."

"Hey, Lieutenant, the menu says cigarettes and cigars. Why don't I see any cigars?"

"I'm saving those to go with dessert. We want to take pictures for your families before the room turns blue with cigar smoke."

On my way from the kitchen with a pot of hot coffee, I met Lieutenant Beaman in the hall wheeling away from the rec room. "Told you the dinner wouldn't be fit to eat," he snarled.

"Good riddance," shouted Jonesie. "Lieutenant, he didn't eat even one bite, just stuck cigarette butts in the mashed potatoes and left. Now that stinker's gone, we can have some fun."

An hour later, leaving the men puffing cigars in the smoke-filled room, Otto, Rudolph, Edmund, and I dragged ourselves back to the kitchen to face stacks of dirty dishes. I stared at the clock.

"Oh, no! Otto, you've missed dinner. The one day of the year when you're served a good meal and you've missed your Christmas dinner." Only on Christmas was the prisoners' usual fare of beans and black bread replaced with the same dinner menu as that served to the patients.

Otto brushed aside my apologies with a wink. "It's O.K. Vee eat vell." He flung open the oven door. Food returned on patients plates filled several containers.

"Lieutenant, ve have sometink for you." With a flourish, Edmund lined up four of the decorated glasses on the counter.

Even Rudolph smiled. Otto, a towel draped over his arm, poured a murky liquid from a ginger ale bottle.

"Merry Christmas, Lieutenant." We clinked glasses. The first sip sent a shudder from my head to my toes followed by a delightful warm glow. My Christmas present had some kick to it. I wondered what was in that potent concoction. Where had they kept it hidden? Otto gave me only one clue. He had saved the orange and grapefruit rinds from breakfast to start his brew.

After he divvied up the remains in the bottle, we drank a final toast. Being careful to walk in a straight line, I left in a happy daze to join the staff for our evening dinner. The day had turned out well. For a brief time patients, prisoners, and personnel had been united in a common bond. We had overcome our animosities, our homesickness, and loneliness to make this a special Christmas day.

Later, as I opened my Christmas gifts, I realized I had forgotten to take one of the glasses Otto had decorated with such skill. By the time I returned to Ward 2B, the paint had washed away in the hot water of the dishwasher. The magic of Christmas along with the designs had disappeared.

Life returned to what was normal for Ward 2B.

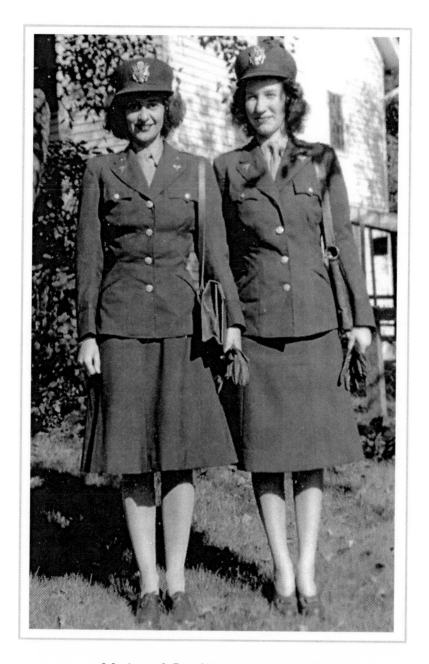

Marie and Carol in new army uniforms.

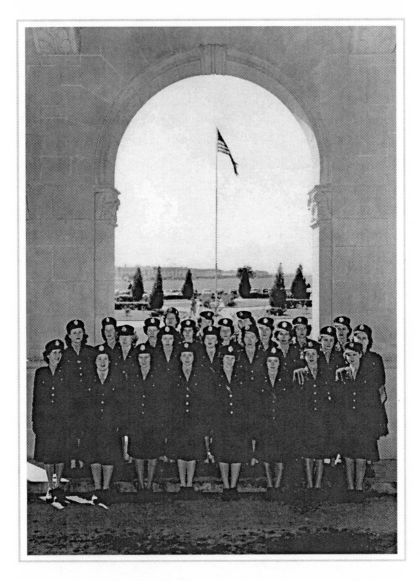

After Basic training. Fort Sam Houston 1945.

From Memphis to El Paso 1946

New Year's Eve 1945, I sat alone and forlorn in my room in the nurses' quarters. The din from the New Year's Eve party in the reception rooms below grew louder. As the old year faded away, laughter and screams were mixed with the sounds of splintering wood and breaking glass. What a way to end a year and start a new one!

On New Year's morning, those of us who had avoided the New Year's Eve party no longer regretted our lonely evening. A corpsman told me many of the officers had arrived drunk. After someone slipped an unidentified substance into the punch, many of the women passed out. It took the MPs to stop the ensuing brawl.

The next day a notice on the bulletin board made me angry. "All residents will be assessed a fine of ten dollars toward repair of furniture and rugs damaged on New Year's Eve." I protested in vain that those of us who had not attended the party should not be required to pay.

After the excitement of the holidays, the patients fell into a slump. No matter what the menu offered, they complained. However, I was unprepared for the display of dissatisfaction I faced one evening when making rounds. On the ward, every man had dumped salad, bread, butter, napkin, and bottle caps into the stew on his plate. The polite officers sent back their trays untouched.

I fumed on the long walk to the main kitchen for three-dozen eggs. I could not let the patients miss a meal, so I made egg salad sandwiches to replace the stew. One patient told me, "Stew's just a way to use up old garbage." Only in his mind did the flavorful dish made from top quality beef resemble the unsavory slop served under battle conditions.

Another group of men were appreciative of the efforts of the dietary department. I went on duty at midnight to feed a convoy of one hundred and fifty new patients arriving by airlift from Europe. Regardless of the hour, new arrivals always received a steak dinner with all the trimmings. Their astonishment over a hearty meal in the middle of the night made that a fun assignment in spite of my loss of sleep.

My offer to help my friend Dot, led to more sleepless nights. When she described her panic over an upcoming appointment with the dentist, I volunteered to go along. I could be her support and have my teeth cleaned at the same time. The dentist told her she had no problems. His serious expression told me I was not that lucky.

"You have an impacted wisdom tooth which is going to give you trouble any day. Why not make an appointment for me to extract it?"

Dot whispered, "That captain is so cute, you'd better take him up on it." He did seem capable, a more important attribute than charm in my estimation.

The following Monday, before leaving the kitchen for the dental clinic, I told Otto I would return in time to serve lunch. I managed to keep my word, although I did not anticipate returning pale and weak with a swollen face and bloody stains trailing down my uniform.

In the dental clinic, a much older man, a colonel who headed the dental department, had replaced the smiling captain. He held the x-ray to the light. "Never saw a tooth with a root that long. Must be a distorted picture."

My heart sank. I remembered Dad's experience with Stan, our dentist at home. "Longest roots I ever met up with," Stan had said. When he could not budge the tooth, he told Dad to lie on the floor. With his knee against Dad's chest, Stan found the leverage he needed to yank out the molar.

The jab of a dull needle into my jaw made me wince. The colonel gave me two more shots of Novocain before he pulled, and pulled, and pulled. The resistance of the stubborn tooth increased the ugliness of his profanity. Color rose in his face, as he gave a mighty tug on the forceps.

"God Damn." The tooth broke into dozens of pieces. "I don't have the tools to handle this. Follow me." I staggered from the chair into the hall. Half way up a flight of stairs, the colonel turned and glared down at me. "Lieutenant, I said follow me."

Holding tight to the banister, I dragged myself up the steps. He reached the end of the hall, strode into the last room, and barked at the patient in the chair "Get up." A startled private scrambled to his feet. The colonel thundered at me. "Sit down."

Within seconds a call could be heard over the PA system, "Oral surgeon to Room 10. Emergency. Oral surgeon to Room 10." A major burst into the room. "Open wide." He stared in my mouth. A flicker of disgust crossed his face. He turned to the colonel. His rage raised his voice to a high pitch. "What the hell did you think you were doing to her? I'm not sure I can get all those roots out."

While I wondered would happen if the roots could not be removed, he began to pick out the shards of tooth. The Novocain wore off and daggers of pain shot through me. I writhed in agony. Three corpsmen were summoned to pin down my thrashing arms and feet.

When the ordeal finally ended, the oral surgeon patted my shoulder. "I'm going to sew up the hole now." His words only increased my anxiety. The length of thread he measured from a spool looked a yard long. As soon as he finished his needlework, he hurried away.

Once again the patient of the colonel, I did not expect much help. "Come back in three days and I'll take out the stitches," he muttered. Before I could ask how to care for my throbbing jaw, he disappeared.

Too distraught to think clearly, I stumbled back to Ward 2B. Exhausted, I slumped to the floor. The alarmed Germans gathered round me on their knees. "Vee so sorry, so sorry." Their show of sympathy almost made up for the disdain of the cold-hearted dentist.

Back in my room, I paced the floor like a mad woman. One of my friends dropped by. "I know a fellow in the dental clinic. I'll call him." She returned with codeine and instructions to stay on my feet to avoid a dry socket. Even with the medication, the throbbing pain kept me walking from wall to wall until dawn.

Three days later, still unable to eat solid food, I returned to work. In the following weeks, constant fatigue and loss of weight dragged me down. Something else seemed wrong. I did not realize that grim experience would lead to dire consequences affecting the rest of my army career.

My three months on Ward 2B came to an end. I reported to the chief dietitian for a new assignment. Captain Smith repeated the words expressed on my first day. "No one is expected to work more than three months on a paraplegic ward. I'm aware of the long hours and mental fatigue you experience there." She glanced at a paper held in her hand. "However, I must show you this."

She unrolled a yard-long scroll. Black letters at the top proclaimed:

"Hear Ye. Hear Ye. Don't Take Lieutenant Morrison away. We need our fav'rite dietitian. Please let her stay."

Every patient on Ward 2B had drawn a stick figure in color above his name. Jonesie had added a comment. "For you I'll even eat beef stew."

Captain Smith looked concerned. "I leave the decision up to you." She hesitated, "But I'd advise you to let me transfer you."

Leave Jonesie, Captain Thibeaux, Private Pinsky! Even Lieutenant Beaman had signed the petition. I couldn't desert my boys. Tired as I was, my task was nothing compared to theirs.

I squared my shoulders, "Captain Smith, I'd prefer to stay on Ward 2B."

A Breath of Fresh Air

By February 1946, the three German prisoners of war and I had few communication problems. At night, when they were confined in a compound behind high fences topped with barbed wire, they made rapid progress studying English.

When I gave them the news they had waited so long to hear, they pounded each other on the back and reverted to speaking German. "The word is official — Kennedy General Hospital will be turned over to the Veterans' Administration on June 30. In the meantime, civilians will gradually replace army personnel. I expect to be reassigned soon."

I hesitated to give impact to my next words. "You won't have to wait much longer to go home. The first two hundred prisoners return to Germany next week."

The following Monday, Otto, my most dependable employee, said "Goodbye." I hated to lose him and feared the uncertain future he faced. During those long days in the ward kitchen, we had developed mutual trust and respect. I could always count on Otto. Under different circumstances, we would have been friends.

"Lieutenant, I don't even know if my family has survived. If I find them, where will we go? The country is in shambles. No need for professors now. How will I feed my children?"

"Otto, if you do find your family, I'm confident you'll use your ability and determination to build a new life. Could anything be worse than what you've already experienced in the war? Perhaps, you'll come back to this country. You've taken the first step by learning English."

He grabbed my hand. "You've done so much to make my life easier. Thank you. Auf Wiedersehen." We parted with tears in our eyes.

Otto's departure left the ward kitchen in disarray. The surly PW assigned to take his place annoyed the patients. "Lieutenant Beaman vants jelly," he reported. I took a paper cup of apple jelly to Lieutenant Beaman. He responded with a loud curse. "Not Jelly. Chili."

One of the new patients, a young recruit from Tennessee, called me to his bedside. He pointed to the dessert on his tray, "What's that?"

I smiled. "One of our most popular desserts — a chocolate éclair."

He pushed the plate away. "I ain't goin' ta eat no hot dog roll with frostin'." He refused to taste the glistening chocolate-coated pastry.

Every day brought new rumors, changes in routine, and more work. Aided by a new dietitian on the paraplegic service, I covered six wards. Supervising food service at so many locations kept me running from morning 'til night. Dot Barnard's reassignment to San Francisco left me dejected. Just like basic training, others left while I remained behind.

Who would have expected two middle-aged ladies in geometric printed dresses, fussy hats, and sensible shoes would lift everyone's spirits? On a day when the first buds of spring swelled on the trees, Helen Keller and her companion, Polly Thomson, paid a visit to the patients. Wherever they went, a breath of fresh air swept through the wards.

I had seen Lena Horne electrify the GIs, who attempted to jump the balcony railing to reach her on stage. I had heard claps and whistles of approval for Benny Goodman and laughter for Bob Hope. Never before, had I seen men moved to tears. The courage and faith exhibited by Helen Keller made an unforgettable impression on all of us.

Sixty-six years old, an illness had left her blind and deaf at eighteen months of age. Conversing with the patients, her guttural speech came slowly in tones she herself had never heard. Her first teacher, Anne Sullivan, had taught her to speak. Young Helen had learned the sounds one at a time by putting her fingers on Miss Sullivan's throat. With repeated practice, she learned to make each sound herself.

I found Polly Thomson as inspiring as Helen Keller. She spelled out words in Miss Keller's hand using the manual alphabet. At a play or movie, she could spell out dialogue as fast as eighty words a minute.

Since the war began, this twosome had brought encouragement to thousands in over eighty military hospitals. Bending over to touch the head of a GI with close-cropped hair, Miss Keller said, "Your hair stands up like your spirit." She kissed others, leaving them flustered by her kindly attention and her heartfelt words. "This is my way of thanking you for all you have done." Wherever the patient's hometown, she talked about that part of the country. Even the battles in Europe and the Pacific were familiar to her.

Helen Keller urged the paraplegics to accept the challenge presented by their intensive therapy. As a result of her inspiration, many men worked with renewed determination to drag useless limbs encased in heavy braces across parallel bars. Others spent extra time lifting weights to strengthen upper body muscles. Some tried again and again to master the art of guiding a spoonful of food from plate to mouth.

After Miss Keller's visit, renewed hope prevailed in the wards. My efforts to meet the patients' nutritional requirements paid off in fewer infections, better appetites, and weight gains. Officers and enlisted men gathered in the parking lot to inspect the first Ford automobile equipped with hand controls for operating the car. Seeing that vehicle gave many patients a glimpse of a future with the freedom to drive again. They began to emphasize what they could do rather than dwell on what they had lost.

Even my life got a boost. One of the dietitians living on my floor talked me into a blind date. I met a handsome, blond, attentive flight officer named Don. We danced until midnight in the Balinese Room at the Claridge Hotel, before going to Donley's for steaks at 1:00 a.m. My first evening on the town since college was an indication of how lacking my social life had been in the army.

Don stroked my hand. "Have you seen the mighty Mississippi from the air? No? I'll rent a plane on Saturday and take you up to see a sight of unbelievable beauty."

I wondered how much time we would have to get to know each other. My orders to leave Memphis might come through at any time.

Too Good to Last

My new friend, Don, kept his promise to take me up in a small plane. Flying over the Mississippi into the sunset took me into a new world. The sinking sun, a fiery ball, turned the river into a wide red ribbon slashing the darkening landscape. The small plane buzzed along like a mosquito, infinitesimal in that vast space. How shocked Mother, who feared flying, would have been to know I had put my life in the hands of a man I had known only a week. I felt no such qualms.

Approaching darkness forced Don to turn back toward the miniature airport far below. Back on the ground, he gave me a hug. "We chose a good evening. I've seen many kinds of weather up there; never saw a more dramatic sky. Very special, just like you."

Over late supper in a coffee shop, I told Don about one of my patients, Captain Thibeaux, a special guy paralyzed from the chest down. When the tray carrier placed a dinner tray over his prone body in bed, neither man noticed the plate slipped. The metal rim of the hotplate, which I had heated in the oven in my determination to serve "hot things hot," left a burned gash two inches wide.

"I felt terrible, but Captain Thibeaux treats the accident as a huge joke. He cannot feel pain and tells everyone I burned him on purpose. 'Look what Hot Dog did to me.' He insists the HD on my collar stands for hot dog, not hospital dietitian. Now all the patients call me that."

Don left for ten days on flight duty, which gave me time to catch up on sleep and letters. I agonized over my feelings about the sale of the orange grove in Florida. When Dad wrote that he and Mother had accepted an offer too good to refuse, my heart sank. Three years before, they had paid twenty-two thousand dollars for the orange and grapefruit groves. They were selling the orange grove for twenty-seven thousand dollars and expected to get five thousand for the grapefruit grove.

I reread Dad's explanation of their decision to sell. "You know, dear, we have worried about hurricanes. Two years ago, when howling wind tore along the coral wall, sparing us, but wiping out our neighbor, we realized how vulnerable we were. I think I still have some good years left in construction back in Connecticut."

I doubted that. Healthy and relaxed in Florida, it seemed a mistake for him to return to the stress of writing competitive bids and putting in ten-hour days on a construction site. He and Mother were ignoring the seriousness of his heart condition.

I was haunted by his words at the time they bought the grove. "I've been working for a mad man for years." Now, lured on by wild promises, he planned to work again for Ford Osborne, owner of Osborne-Barnes Construction Company in Danbury, Connecticut.

During my childhood, a bottle of Milk of Magnesia and a soupspoon stood on the windowsill over the kitchen sink. When preparing a bid, Dad relied on that remedy for his upset stomach. That familiar blue bottle had never showed up in the Florida house. I suspected Mother's discomfort in the muggy heat influenced their plans.

To me, it seemed a mistake to leave their enjoyable life and start over again. I tried to be diplomatic in my response but my heart was not in it. They had been so happy at Bonita Grove. I felt dejected for them and for me. Once again, there was no place we could call home.

When Don returned from ten days of flight duty, my spirits revived. We celebrated his return at a USO show in the base theatre. It turned out to be funnier than any comedy we'd seen in the movies. Most of the big name entertainers had given up performing for service men to return to their peacetime careers. A valiant group of second raters carried on.

The announcer and leading talent, formerly a baritone with the Metropolitan Opera Company, was now reduced to a monotone. His long hair disappeared beneath his collar and his acting style seemed limited to casting an amorous eye on the generous proportions of the soprano.

Unfortunately for her, the spotlight centered on the broad, black satin expanse of her mid-section, accented by a red velvet rose. Her accompanist, an anemic young man wearing glasses, bow tie and pin striped suit, looked like an overgrown child prodigy. Perched on an unstable seat, a pile of music, he played variations on Chopin in a style Chopin would not have recognized.

A violinist with a squeaky violin, an unsmiling cellist, and a motionless mezzo-soprano completed the group. The soprano stood cold and distant as a marble statue. When the baritone gazed into her eyes and crooned, "We could make believe I love you," the audience burst into laughter.

"No you couldn't," shouted a GI.

In contrast to that debacle, the following Saturday night was filled with glamour and excitement. Don took me to a dance in a southern colonial mansion turned over to the army for an Officers' Club. As we approached the expansive white house, made taller by fluted columns gleaming in the moonlight, the aroma of boxwood and gardenias filled the air.

I winked at Don. "I may be wearing a uniform but I feel like Scarlett O'Hara." Actually, I liked wearing my well-tailored uniform. It saved the hassle of worrying about an appropriate outfit.

"Rhett Butler at your service," whispered Don, sweeping me onto the ballroom floor. Never before had I danced with a partner who could lead me with such ease through the most intricate steps. I seemed to melt into Don's arms and float around the room. The dance was one to remember, a night of pure magic.

After we left the mansion, Don found a parking place under a huge, protective tree on a dark street. I suspected he still thought of himself as Rhett Butler. I lost all illusions of being Scarlett when my straight khaki skirt, in contrast to her hoops, hampered my ability to move.

Don pulled me close and nuzzled my hair. Firm fingers undid the brass buttons on my uniform. I giggled over his struggle to remove my necktie. "Are you trying to strangle me?" I murmured.

"That's hardly my intention," he replied.

In spite of his hints that I remove the inhibiting skirt, I had no intention of going that far. Suddenly, bright light lit up the interior of the car. As I cringed and tried to sink from sight, Don muttered, "Damn. What's that guy think he's doing pulling in next to us? Let's get out of here." The moment of suspense slipped away, not to be regained.

Back on base, properly attired with tie tied, buttons buttoned and hair still awry, we strolled toward quarters. Don's voice changed, no longer light and carefree. "Let's sit on the steps, I have something to tell you."

He slipped his arm around my shoulder. "This isn't going to be easy. Might as well blurt it out." The pressure of his fingers dug into my flesh. "My orders came today. I leave for Japan on Monday."

I never saw Don again.

Final Weeks At Kennedy

Soon after Don's departure for Japan, I took a flight of my own to Connecticut. My cousin Polly had, finally consented to marry navy Lieutenant Sherman Glass on May 18, 1946.

On the morning of my flight to Connecticut, I felt uneasy about a taxi ride alone to the Memphis airport at 3:00 a.m. My arrival at a low dark building near the runway did little to reassure me. A dim row of light bulbs pointed the way to a dingy room furnished with a counter, wooden chairs, and a water cooler.

I felt better, when the stewardess, smart in her tailored uniform and perky hat, stepped forward. "Welcome aboard. We expect to depart for New York on time."

She herded the straggling passengers across the dark tarmac in the sticky night air to the plane. Before I could stow my flight bag, I saw the stewardess lean over a man scrunched down in a front seat. After a long conversation she was joined by the pilot and two harried officials. Their heated discussion turned into a shouting match.

The passenger next to me grew restless. "What's going on? I need coffee." He had to wait an hour before an announcement brought action but no explanation.

"This flight is cancelled. Please collect all personal belongings and report to the terminal."

The first streaks of dawn pierced the dark sky. Tired and confused, I lugged my flight bag, coat, and purse back to the depressing boarding area in the terminal.

"Step this way." The stewardess had lost her cheerful smile. "After you've been issued a new ticket, return to the plane to the seat you occupied before. Move quickly. We're anxious to get under way." She gave no opportunity to question her instructions.

By the time the plane roared down the runway, a bright golden sun had risen over the Mississippi. Coffee at last! As the stewardess added cream and sugar, she explained the delay. A passenger, who had boarded in New Orleans with a ticket to Memphis, refused to leave the plane. He demanded he continue on to New York.

The weary stewardess sighed, "The only way to get him off the plane was cancel the flight and rebook the rest of the passengers. I never had this happen before."

At the terminal in New York, I rushed toward Mother and Dad, who stood waiting arm in arm, just as I had last seen them. We all shed a few tears of happiness. This would be a day to enjoy being together. There would be time later to talk about their decision to sell the orange grove, and the fact we were now homeless.

Mother said she had good news. "Carol, you won't have to stay with Aunt Hannah this time. You can be with us at Grandpa's. He's in the hospital for minor surgery. You can sleep in his room."

The rainy weather, which had plagued my days off in Memphis, followed me on vacation. Each gloomy day seemed to sap my waning energy. It took black coffee to keep me going. One morning my queasy stomach forced me to stay in my room. I lay in Grandpa's bed under the ornate walnut headboard wondering whether it would crash down on me. Something was wrong, but what?

On the day of Polly's wedding, the desperation in Aunt Pauline's voice made me forget my concern over my health. The mother of the bride needed help. "Carol, this rain isn't going to stop. Come as soon as you can. We have canceled plans for the reception in the yard and on the porch. Everything must be moved indoors. Only you have the know-how to make that happen."

Just as Aunt Pauline expected, my military training served me well. I assigned one team to carry small furniture upstairs and another group to push the heavy dining room table against the wall to create open space. Others followed sketched diagrams showing the placement of napkins, silverware, and plates. Before leaving for the church, I snatched the heavy punch bowl from a wobbly tea wagon in imminent danger of collapse.

Under the dripping trees before the Methodist Church, ushers stood ready with huge umbrellas to escort guests through the deluge. In spite of their efforts, many women entered the sanctuary in bedraggled damp frocks with color running from their ruined dyed shoes.

I had no such problems in my crisp new summer uniform, beige trimmed with maroon braid on the sleeves and matching maroon tie. Rain had not affected the high polish on my closed toe leather pumps. I walked down the aisle on my cousin Bob's arm, confident that I looked my best.

The reception turned into happy chaos. The guests, packed in tight as sardines in a can, sat on the stair landing and jammed the dining room, living room, and hall. Those who tried to escape to the porch were driven back to the kitchen by wind and rain.

Until time for their departure, the bride and groom ignored the weather. As they dashed down the path to their car, wet confetti stuck to their clothes in globs. Polly's gray suit developed red and blue polka dots from the clinging bits of paper. Later she laughed over her ruined suit. "That's what I get for being married on the wettest day in the wettest May on record."

After the wedding guests left, I issued orders, army style, to recruit a clean-up crew. With the house in order, only one task remained — pack my bags for my return flight to Memphis.

The trip went smoothly. On the plane, only a nagging concern about my next assignment disturbed my slumber. Relieved to be back in quarters, I stared in disbelief at the clutter in my room. Dot and Corinne had moved on leaving me a chair, footstool, lamp, plants, cokes, and, best of all, a small fortune in soap flakes.

Back on duty, I found morale on the wards had hit an all time low. Jonesie wheeled his chair around me in the hall. "Hi chicken, how's my slim little ole' dietitian? We tried to get you back on Ward 2B. Went to see the chief dietitian. She said we looked well enough fed to get along without you."

That evening the kitchen girls did not show up. Edmund, the only remaining German prisoner, helped me serve fifty patients. "Lieutenant, I go back home tomorrow. How vill you get along? I vorry about you. Vil you give me your address? Some day when things get better I write to you."

How I hoped things would get better for hard-working, serious Edmund. From the day he had told me about his background, I had felt his pain. "I only small shop keeper in Czechoslovakia. Don't know politics. Captured first by Germans, then Russians, then Americans. Maybe my wife not alive."

Edmund's request for my address put me in a difficult position. What was the penalty for corresponding with a prisoner of war? I looked in Edmund's troubled pale eyes and took the chance. On a diet slip, I printed Grandpa's address in Connecticut.

He stuffed the paper in his pocket, "Auf Wiedersehen, Lieutenant." Trying to hide his emotion, he swallowed hard and disappeared down the hall.

Two years later Edmund kept his promise. The letter came from Wiesbaden, U S Zone Germany. His words about "forbidden fruit" surprised me. I had no idea that was how the PWs described the food returned on patients' trays, the food they hid in the oven to eat later.

Dear Miss Morrison.

After I left America as PW I found new home in Wiesbaden and now I keep my promise and I send you a few lines. I hope you remember me as PW Kitchen boy of 2B. I thank you once again for all the good treatment I received from you. You was always so good to us and shut your eyes when we went on the forbidden fruit to better our Camp life. In those times we were better off than we are now as we have no ice box to go to fetch something. I expect you have seen from the Papers how life is here in Germany. As I was not allowed to enter my old country GSR I was very pleased I found friends in Wiesbaden who took my Wife and my self in. My plans to get to Canada has not come to any thing yet.

So we live here from day to day and wonder what the next time will bring. We have nearly lost all hopes of better times. We shall be very pleased to hear from you and hoping my letter will find you in the best of health.

Kindest regards

Yours sincerelly

Edmund Borek

My answers to Edmund's letter brought no reply.

A New Assignment

The takeover of Kennedy Hospital by the Veterans Administration loomed one month ahead, July 1, 1946. Each day dumped more work on the weary dietitians. Friction with our new bosses from the Veterans Administration turned the hospital into an uproar. I hated the place.

Only seven army dietitians remained. Lieutenant DeWees had transferred from our unit to become chief dietitian for the Veterans Administration. When she refused to listen to our complaints, my friends appointed me to do the unthinkable. In desperation, I went over her head to confront our commanding officer, Colonel McIvers.

"Sir, we are working harder than the PWs ever did. It is impossible to serve meals to fifty patients using broken equipment aided by one inept helper."

He made no comment but that afternoon four listless slovenly girls showed up on each ward to serve supper. We no longer lacked personnel in numbers, although four girls did not equal three PWs in terms of efficiency.

The Army blamed the Veterans for not hiring enough people. The Veterans blamed the Army for transferring personnel too soon. Civilian help got mad and quit. Lieutenant DeWees never once came to the wards to observe our problems. She did brag about "a great morale booster" for our patients. Pastel paper napkins would replace white ones.

The lieutenant in charge of ordering food in the main kitchen concentrated on plans for her wedding. When she got ahead on milk, she cancelled the milk order for three days. The milk on hand turned sour. When she cancelled the bread order, the bread turned blue with mold. Patients complained bitterly about sour milk, moldy bread, and scorched meat. I was embarrassed, and resented the inefficiency of the dietary department.

To escape our disillusionment, we dietitians accepted an invitation from Jesse, a colored cook in the main kitchen, to visit his restaurant. The taxi took us through slums worse than any we'd seen in Washington, D.C. In a neighborhood of small homes, poor but respectable, the driver stopped in front of a low unpainted building with a Coca-Cola sign tacked next to the screen door.

"You ain't going in that nigger place are yah?" We ignored his remark.

Smiling Jesse stood at the door of his modest café, eager to greet his first white guests. He led us past a row of stools and six tables in the dining room to the kitchen and urged us to sit at a table covered with butcher paper and decorated with bouquets of garden flowers in milk bottles. Heat rose from the wood stove, and soon the back of my dress stuck to the chair.

The efficient equipment in the immaculate kitchen surprised us. Jesse helped his wife cook, while their son waited on the table. "I brought y'all a coke. Here's the menu," beamed young Jesse. We sipped the refreshing ice-cold cokes, wrapped in paper napkins, and tried not to smile at his hand-printed words.

Special — Fride Chicken. Stake. Comonation salad. Peese. Ice cream. Cake. $1.00

The meal would have been a bargain at twice the price — crispy fried chicken with fluffy mashed potatoes and cream gravy, beaten biscuits, fresh peas, combination salad, homemade ice cream and cake, plus all the cold coke we could drink.

After dinner, our words of appreciation brought a glow of pride and satisfaction to the faces of Jesse, his wife, and their son.

Jesse stood tall. "Now y'all know how I like to cook. Those vet people ain't got no ideah what to do. I'll call one of my frien's with a taxi to take yah back. The white fellows won't come to this neighborhood to pick up passengers."

That delightful evening stood out in sharp contrast to the following Saturday night. All duty personnel were required to attend a farewell party for Colonel McIvers at the Officers' Club. When Lieutenant DeWees had asked me to take charge of refreshments, I refused. Regardless of her expectations, I was too exhausted to handle a party. One of my friends volunteered for the job.

She supervised the bountiful buffet table and the glasses of sparkling champagne. The food could not match that served in Jesse's hot kitchen. Many guests skipped the buffet in favor of the bar. An unlimited supply of liquor awaited them there.

Late in the evening, Colonel McIvers arose from his place of honor at the head table. The time had come for his farewell speech. He beamed at the officers assembled before him. "It's been a pleasure to work with such a good natured bunch of bastards."

A strange silence fell over the room. Even in jest, such an insulting remark was inappropriate. He mumbled a few words and sat down.

Next on the program was the colonel in charge of the Veterans Administration. He staggered to his feet, swayed back and forth a few times, and gave up his attempt to address the crowd. A nurse living on my hall topped his performance by hurling insults at her date in front of the assembled guests. The evening had turned into a fiasco. In the morning, I concluded the participants had no recollection of the previous evening, not when they bragged about the great party.

My immediate concern was an appeal by Lieutenant DeWees to the chief dietitian in Washington, D.C., requesting that the four of us without orders be left at Kennedy on detached service for a month. We dreaded another four weeks of hearing about VA policy. "In the Veterans Administration we do this, in the Veterans' Administration we do that."

Someone must have understood our predicament. Next morning we received orders from Washington to proceed to new assignments. What a blow! I was headed back to Texas.

My new post would be Beaumont General Hospital at Fort Bliss, El Paso. Worse than that, I would travel there with Peg Ward, our party girl — Peg, who had liked to hide out in the Officers' Club rather than spend time with her patients.

The thought of the trip with Peg, plus living in another hot climate wore me down. I envied my friend, Edith Roberts, who was going to Old Farms Convalescent Hospital in Avon, Connecticut. How I wished I had been sent there. I blocked out that thought and turned my attention to the sad task of saying goodbye to the patients. My experience with the incoming administration did not bode well for their future.

Peg burst into my room. "I have a great idea. Since we have five days before we report for duty, let's hitch a free plane ride with the Air Transport Command. That way we can cash in our travel vouchers. I need that chunk of free money."

She hurried off to pack. I rushed to the pay phone to call home. Short of change, I called collect. "Hello." I heard the voice of my brother Sherman.

The operator broke in. "I have a collect call from Memphis, Tennessee. Will you accept the charges?"

"Just a minute while I think about it." I waited nervously for Sherman to decide. After a long pause, he agreed. "OK. I accept. Hi, Sis, What's up? Mom and Dad aren't here. Couldn't decide whether you'd want to spend the money to talk to me when you probably want to talk to them."

"Hi, Sherman. Glad you decided I'm worth it. Tell Mother and Dad my orders came through. I leave Memphis in the morning for El Paso, Texas. I'll call them in a few days, as soon as I arrive at Beaumont General Hospital."

After a frenzied night of packing and some tearful farewells, Peg and I picked up our orders and headed for the military airport. In the waiting room, a huge chalkboard announced arrival and departure times. Officers and enlisted personnel scanned the board for destinations and the number of seats available for departing flights.

Within two hours, a plane to Austin, Texas appeared on the board. It had four seats available and was leaving in fifteen minutes.

"Where's Austin?"

Peg shrugged, "Hell, I don't know but, if it's in Texas, it has to be closer to El Paso than Memphis, Tennessee. Let's go."

We grabbed our bags and dashed across the hot concrete toward a small plane, propellers already in motion. An orderly greeted us at the door, "Welcome aboard."

We looked around us in disbelief. We had not anticipated traveling to our new assignment in such luxury.

Guests of the Colonel

When Peg and I had decided to hitch a ride in army plane from Tennessee to Texas, we had anticipated bucket seats in a cargo plane. We were unprepared for quilted leather walls, man-size upholstered chairs, a card table, and current magazines. The orderly behind the bar asked Peg for her drink order.

She shook her head. "Not yet. Who rates a plane like this?"

"Colonel Duke, Commanding Officer at Bergstrom Field in Austin. He's boarding right now." A tall colonel followed by two captains bounded into the cabin. Our crisp salutes were rewarded with his broad grin.

"Welcome Lieutenants, glad to have yah aboard. John takin' good care o' y'all? We'd be honored to have yah join us in a friendly little game of poker." Much as Peg liked the attention of officers, she had the good sense to decline the opportunity to play with pros. A few moments later poker was forgotten.

The plane lurched down the runway, struggled into the air and bucked like a rodeo horse. A terse announcement from the pilot froze us in our seats.

"Returning to the base, Sir. Hang on for a rough landing." The plane shuttered, twisted, and jerked. Peg and I gripped each other's hands. Below, the landscape looked like jagged collages of torn paper. Approaching ground level, the ashen face of the colonel emphasized the seriousness of our situation.

The plane hit the runway, bounced high in the air, bounced a second time before rolling to a stop. Peg and I, too spent to speak, huddled in our seats. Colonel Duke followed by his aides rushed out the door. Although we could not distinguish the words, we heard angry shouts, orders, and curses filtering up to our level from the ground.

The colonel stormed into the cabin, his anger still evident. "Ladies, I apologize for the fright y'all must'a felt. Some damn fool forgot to take the pin out of the tail. That was a close call. Now it's time for some serious drinkin' to calm our nerves. What'll yah ladies have?"

None of us paid attention to the smooth second take-off, nor did the men play poker. John kept our glasses full all the way to Austin. The colonel related many tall tales about Texans. I came up with a few of my own about New Englanders.

As the plane touched down on the runway in Austin, Colonel Duke apologized again for giving us a fright. "No flights go out tomorrow, Sunday. I've arranged for y'all to stay over in the nurses' quarters. Good luck with a flight on Monday." He brushed off our thanks and hastily left the plane.

Peg and I stepped through the cabin door into a blast furnace. Withering dry heat rose up to meet us. We clutched our skirts to keep them from rising like kites in the stiff hot wind. By the time we descended the steps, my face already felt parched and wrinkled.

As if by magic, a staff car appeared in front of us. "Lieutenant Morrison? Lieutenant Ward? Private Simpkins to drive you to quarters. How y'all like the heat? Typical Texas day, only one hundred eight degrees. The sun'll go down soon. Then it'll be a bit cooler."

A captain, her hair blowing across her face in the stiff breeze, welcomed us to the nurses' quarters. She said she hoped our room was ready.

"Colonel Duke didn't give us much warning that he was bringing guests who would be staying here." Peg and I tried to hide our surprise. We had not realized we rated VIP status.

The two nurses who greeted us at the door were under that impression. One of them pushed back her straggly locks. "Wow. Have we had a struggle to clean this room for you on such short notice. Who are you anyway? Colonel Duke sent word we should go all out for you."

I laughed. "Hate to tell you after you've worked so hard. We're just a couple ordinary gals trying to get to El Paso. We hitched a ride from Memphis on the colonel's plane." I thought it prudent not to mention the near catastrophe in the air, the probable reason Colonel Duke felt responsible for our welfare.

Our new acquaintances said they'd come back to take us to the Officers' Club for dinner. We found it paid to be guests of the commanding officer. We received the best table in the room, along with iced champagne and Texas-size steaks. Lois, who had lent her sheets to make the beds, sipped her second glass of champagne.

"I'll clean your room anytime for treatment like this. How about coming back at nine for the dance?"

Peg's eyes lit up at the mention of a dance. Mine did not. Back in the room, we had our first disagreement. "Peg, I'm beat. All I want is a shower and bed. No sleep last night and this long day have done me in. You go anyway." She refused to go alone but berated me for spoiling her fun. I turned my face to the wall and fell asleep.

The next morning we both slept late. By the time we had donned our olive drab dresses, cooler than our uniforms, Peg had perfected her plan to snare dates for the afternoon. "We'll go to the Officers' Mess for lunch at twelve-thirty. At that hour we should have our pick of several hundred men."

At precisely half past twelve, I followed her into the dining room. She cut short her intended grand entrance and swore under her breath. I wanted to laugh at her discomfort. The room resounded with chatter, every word in Chinese. We had stumbled into a group of three hundred pilots in training for Chiang Kai-shek's army. Unable to communicate with them, we ate in silence at a table for two.

On Monday morning, Peg was responsible for an unpleasant incident. Without asking permission, she helped herself to food in the kitchenette. The nurses, upset to find their breakfast eggs missing, were so mad they refused to say goodbye. Before we sneaked away, I wrote a note of thanks and an apology. Controversy and Peg seemed to go together.

Back at Air Transport Command, we boarded a flight to San Antonio in a troop carrier — no special treatment on this leg of the journey. We found ourselves the only passengers in a plane, which in wartime would have been crowded with dozens of soldiers. During a rough ride, seated on a bench against the wall in a windowless cabin, we bounced around like ping pong balls.

On the ground at nearly deserted Kelly Field in San Antonio, Peg and I hunted for transportation to town. A couple of MPs offered us a ride in their jeep. "Lieutenant, I'll get you there in record time," said the driver. He kept his word by careening around corners breaking the speed limit all the way. He deposited us, dusty, windblown, and breathless, in front of the Gunter Hotel.

"Peg, let's go to the coffee shop. I ate there a couple of time during basic training." Had it been only eight months since I left San Antonio? It seemed years ago.

The MP had warned us few military planes flew to El Paso. We took his advice and booked a commercial flight on Continental Airlines at 9:00 p.m. I offered to give Peg a tour of Fort Sam Houston but she insisted a sight seeing tour of the city.

I could have told her the Alamo would be a disappointment. The dusty, poorly lit rooms with an odd assortment of furnishings not related to the battle had not changed. The entire city seemed to have lost much of its vitality. The deserted streets cried out for the thousands of the service men who had been discharged and sent home.

At 11:00 p.m., the Continental flight still sat on the runway. The plane finally took off in spite of bright flashes of light on the horizon. After the pilot skirted storms for two hours, he met one he could not avoid. During a rough ride, hail pounded on the roof. The engines glowed red hot. Jagged streaks of lightening came at us from all sides. Peg grabbed my arm.

"Do you think our luck is running out? We had our backs almost broken in a troop carrier. We survived a wild jeep ride before an endless afternoon in a stifling tour bus. Now ice is forming on the wings. This is too much for one day."

"Let's wait 'til we're back on the ground to worry about that," I replied curtly. "After all it was your idea to hitch rides to save money." When the plane dropped beneath the clouds and bounced to a stop, we slapped each other on the back. Our luck still held.

The stewardess stood by the door. "Welcome y'all to El Paso, Texas. Local time 2:00 a.m."

Peg's shoulders sagged. "That woman should be shot for being so cheerful this early in the morning."

We checked into the Hotel Cortez. I loosened my tie and kicked off my pumps. "After this twenty hour day, I've had enough traveling. I'm ready to stay put."

Peg shook her head. "Don't say that. When we cash in the travel vouchers, we'll have money to take our next leave in San Francisco."

That idea didn't appeal to me then, but would the next day when I saw the desert by daylight.

Barren Mountains

Everything seemed out of sync at 2:30 a.m. I was relieved Continental Airlines had reserved a room for us at the Hotel Cortez but Peg was not ready to settle for sleep. She grabbed the phone and berated the desk clerk. Her voice grew shrill.

"Dammit, I know it's the middle of the night. The sheets on my bed have not been changed and I expect you to get a maid up here this instant." Half asleep, I turned toward the wall. The night clerk must be glad he didn't have to meet her face to face.

By the time the hapless maid knocked on the door, Peg's fury had turned to frenzy. I felt sorry for the trembling girl. "Peg calm down. It's not her fault. Don't make a scene. Let's not get thrown out of here at this hour."

Peg gave me a look of contempt before she marched into the bathroom. Bam! The door slammed shut behind her. Go to San Francisco with her? Never! Her tirade over, Peg had no trouble falling asleep. I lay awake until dawn.

Curious to see my new home, I stood at the window watching shafts of early morning light strike the treeless mountains. Those jagged stone pinnacles appeared to be a barrier thrown up to stop Texas from spreading farther west. The vast expanse of the Texas landscape made me feel lonely.

Below, in the middle of the street, stood a dead tree trunk surrounded by a fence. Was that a memorial to one of the few trees in sight or the relic of a hanging in a bygone era? Maybe a dose of Texas justice would make my roommate change her unruly ways.

On the taxi ride to Fort Bliss, we saw little grass but plenty of cacti. Landscaping consisted of colored stones, or hard packed soil, softened by desert plants. Brilliant flowers against high walls added a Mexican touch, often emphasized by a plaster donkey cart painted bright red and yellow, or a plaster peasant figure asleep under a huge sombrero.

On our arrival at Beaumont General Hospital, the grounds came as a surprise — an oasis of green grass, shady trees, and flowers. Only the army could afford to run sprinklers every day in the dry desert air. Not only lawn sprinklers, but air conditioning in our quarters.

The chilled air made up for lack of space in the small single rooms with a communal bathroom down the hall. Though I would miss my private bath, I welcomed the Bendix washer in the basement. A warning posted on the wall sounded ominous. "Frequent dust storms clog the filters causing air conditioners to be out of order for days."

Captain Lord, Beaumont's chief dietitian, made a good first impression compared to Lt. DeWees, my last boss.

"Lieutenant Morrison, welcome. Take today off to get settled. Tomorrow, after completing the paper work, report for duty in Mess 2." She smiled, " You'll be happy to know Congress passed the pay increase bill."

I left Captain Lord's office walking on air. Before I worked one day, my base pay had risen from one hundred sixty to one hundred eighty dollars a month.

Sleep took priority over unpacking. After a refreshing nap, I called Mary Schroeder, my classmate from Walter Reed. She arrived on the next bus from her post at the Annex, three miles away in the desert. After a reassuring hug, she looked at me and frowned, "Carol, what's happened to you? You're so skinny."

"I have lost weight. Wish I could take a few days off to rest. The hectic pace at Kennedy took so much out of me. I couldn't eat in that heat. Ninety-five degrees in muggy Memphis felt hotter than one hundred five degrees here in dry El Paso. I'm down to a hundred and fifteen pounds." I showed her the safety pins holding up my skirt.

Mary warned, "This climate is tough at first. Drink plenty of water." She plopped down on my bed. "Carol, I'm so glad to see you. Talking about 'the good old days' at Walter Reed is like being with family. Remember last Fourth of July when you and Marie and I sat on the lawn at the Old Soldiers Home to watch the fireworks?"

"Seems years ago. What about the night we introduced you to your first lobster? You'd never seen anything like that in Illinois."

I changed the subject. "Tell me, how do you like Beaumont Hospital?"

"As long as I'm stationed at the Annex, it's great. I'd hate to be in this location under the eagle eye of Captain Lord. You're lucky to be assigned to Mess 2, not Mess 1 where she hangs out."

"Is she that bad? Tell me more."

Mary gave me a wry smile. "You'll find out soon enough."

Three days later, her prediction came true.

Confrontation With Captain Lord

Standing on the loading dock in the hot morning sun, I had checked in crate after crate of produce for Mess 2. Last off the truck came three boxes of cantaloupe swarming with fruit flies. When I poked a melon, my finger plunged through the rotten rind. Walter Reed training sprang into action. I refused to accept the melon.

Within ten minutes, Captain Lord summoned me to her office. Her steely eyes peered at me over her glasses. "Lieutenant, what gave you the idea that you could reject any item on the invoice? Don't you realize we are four hundred miles from another source of supply?"

"Yes Ma'am, but rotten melons are not edible."

She snapped, "That's not for you to decide. In the future, you accept whatever is delivered. Do you understand?"

"Yes, Ma'am."

Angry and confused, I stumbled back to work. The mess sergeant winked at me. "She got yah, didn't she? Just do as she says. She gets a kickback from the wholesaler in town for accepting bad stuff. There's nothing we can do about it, so, we ignore it." I knew I must accept his advice to survive.

It was a relief to be transferred to the locked psychiatric ward to substitute for the vacationing dietitian. Most people found it a depressing place to work but I liked it. Captain Lord never went there. Not once had she investigated the food service for two hundred mental patients.

Perhaps, the routine for admittance kept her away. I had to ring a bell on a locked metal door. After being admitted, I signed in. A long lonely corridor led to another locked door. Once again, I rang a bell and waited for an attendant with a key. Bang! The door clanged shut behind me cutting me off from the outside world.

One soldier ran the ward with the help of those patients capable of following instructions. Prepared food was delivered from the main hospital. All knives and sharp objects were forbidden to inmates. I carried a paring knife in my pocket and often used it to cut meat in smaller portions. It never entered my mind that one of the men could easily have overpowered me.

We began food service by sending trays to the worst cases in locked rooms. Troublemakers and unstable individuals came through the cafeteria line accompanied by guards. They carried their metal trays, spoons, and unbreakable metal cups to a walled-off area. The rest shuffled through the line and ate at long tables in the cavernous room.

A large percentage of those patients were younger than I. They shared one thing in common — a haunted look in their eyes. Many of them stared at the floor and never spoke. Others never stopped talking, some making sense, some not. The horrors they had witnessed hung over them like dark clouds. I wondered whether their mothers knew their sons had retreated from reality.

A noisy room filled with chatter was a good sign, a sudden silence meant trouble. I kept alert for those who might plunge their hands into the applesauce or grab canned peaches to throw at their buddies. I was not prepared for the fellow who dove head first into a hundred-ration pan of rice pudding. An attendant led him away leaving a trail of pudding across the floor. Those behind him in line received no dessert.

Every morning a colonel sat on the steps to the second floor waiting for me. His words, always the same, came with a sly smile, "And how's my little hummingbird today?" He sent chills down my spine. If I was a hummingbird, he was a vulture. I darted away to the kitchen as quickly as possible.

One of his buddies waited there to brag, "Lieutenant I wanted to help you. Got up at four o'clock to toast all the bread for breakfast." He had arranged the cold soggy toast in towering stacks. We had to serve it anyway.

Another fellow tugged at my sleeve and told me I reminded him of his mother. He pulled a tattered snapshot from his pocket. I stared at a disheveled toothless woman in a shapeless dress. She must have weighed two hundred pounds.

"That's your mother? I'm flattered that I remind you of her." He grinned happily the rest of the day.

I was delighted to be offered an escape from days of confinement in the locked ward for an evening outdoors. Dot Miller, the only dietitian with a car, suggested five of us join her for a picnic in a canyon. She drove up the mountain and parked when the road became too steep. We walked the last mile lugging boxes, salad bowls, and thermoses up a boulder-strewn path. Deep blue shadows settled on the harsh rocky landscape giving an ethereal beauty to the mountains.

As I spread out the tablecloth, I laughed. "Dot, now I know I'm in the Wild West. Look at that sign." It read, "NO HORSES ALLOWED TO EAT ON TABLE." A rising moon added to the dramatic impact of the mountain looming above our heads. The air grew chilly. What a delightful sensation to shiver for the first time in months.

The next afternoon I added another sign to my growing collection of western lore. Tired after shopping in town, Mary and I stopped for cherry cokes. In the smoky café, a hand-printed notice hung above the counter. "THIS IS NOT A SALOON. ONLY ONE BEER TO A CUSTOMER."

Over dinner in the hotel dining room, I told Mary about my father's last letter. He was excited to have found a pound of butter in the A&P for the first time in a month. It cost him eighty-two cents. "I'd better not tell him butter is served freely in Texas, and several pats melt on every oversized steak served in the restaurants."

The butcher had told Dad no meat would be available in Connecticut for another four weeks. The family ate well on

Sundays when Grandpa killed a chicken. Grandpa feared he might have to get rid of the whole flock for lack of chicken feed.

Mary sighed. " We're so spoiled. We forget that civilians in other parts of the country still deal with war time shortages."

Letters continued to keep me connected to my family and friends. I had a note from Edith Roberts, who had worked with me on the paraplegic wards at Kennedy. On our last day there, she had told me of her heartbreak.

Her brown eyes brimming with tears, she had confided, "My dear John lost his sight at Anzio Beach. I still wear his ring, although he refuses to see me and returns my letters unanswered. I've been waiting months but he insists his blindness would ruin my life. I'm afraid he'll never see me again."

The irony of her letter made me sad. She was now stationed at Avon Convalescent Hospital in Connecticut, where every recuperating patient carried a white cane. At her new post, all the patients, like her fiancé, were blind.

When I met up with Peg at a staff meeting, she made me forget my distress over Edith. I had seen little of Peg since our adventure-filled trip from Memphis to El Paso. She was still complaining, this time about an injustice done to us in the Nurses' Quarters.

Every month at Kennedy we had been assessed a five-dollar fee to pay for the purchase and maintenance of furnishings in the lounges of the Nurses' Quarters. Before the army pulled out, the nurses voted to send the mahogany furniture to a permanent army base. Their choice — Beaumont General Hospital, El Paso, Texas.

The sofas, chairs, and mirrors had beaten us to El Paso by three days and had already replaced the old furniture in the Nurses' Quarters. Peg bristled at the notice posted on the bulletin board.

"ALL RESIDENTS WILL BE CHARGED FIVE DOLLARS A MONTH TO PURCHASE VENETIAN BLINDS TO GO WITH THE FURNITURE FROM KENNEDY."

Peg said, "Dammit, I've already paid enough to own one of those chairs and now I have to pay for accessories."

I agreed. "Bet we'll go on paying the fee long after the blinds are hung." When I left a year later, the fee remained, although the residents had long since forgotten the reason for the charge.

My first confrontation with Captain Lord over the melons had made me mad. My second run-in with her, after I left the psychiatric ward to work in Mess 1, was humiliating. She accused me of insubordination in front of two hundred officers.

When the mess sergeant had asked my permission to serve the green beans southern style by adding leftover bacon from breakfast I said, "Great idea. Go ahead." Mary had warned me about the hazards of working for Captain Lord in Mess I. I should have realized she would not approve of the change.

When she chose that day to inspect the lunch service, she caught up with me in the center of the dining hall. "Lieutenant Morrison, what the hell happened to these beans? The menu says green beans. These look full of garbage. Who decided to change the menu? You?"

The room fell silent. I wished I could sink through the floor.

"Yes, Ma'am. Using the cooked bacon left from breakfast seemed a good way to add flavor to a bland vegetable."

Captain Lord's voice rose to a high pitch. Her words resonated across the mess hall. "I'm in charge here and I make the decisions. Report to my office in the morning." She stalked from the room without responding to my feeble. "Yes Ma'am."

After a restless night, I reported to Captain Lord's office, uncertain of the penalty for my crime. How stiff was the punishment for adding bacon to green beans? It was a letdown to be told the captain had left town for a long weekend.

As a result of her tirade, I made many new friends. Some expressed disapproval over my chastisement in public and others preferred green beans southern style. The matter never came up again.

Texas Hospitality

I jumped when the intercom in quarters blared out my name, "Phone call for Lieutenant Morrison, Lieutenant Morrison, phone call." I rushed to the hall phone clutching the letter I had been reading from Aunt Edith in Washington, D.C. She mentioned a friend of hers, Carol Heasley, would be calling me.

I picked up the receiver. "Carol? This is Carol Heasley. My husband's name is Carroll, too, but we call him Herbert." Her Texas drawl made me concentrate on her words. "I just received a letter from Edith Wilson about you. Herbert and I hope you'll join us for supper Sunday evening."

My spirits soared — my first invitation to someone's home in the ten months I'd been in the army. All week I looked forward to Sunday. The bus let me off on a residential street of older homes and three-story buildings. "Look for the only tree," Mrs. Heasley had said. "It stands in front of our apartment building."

Stairs carpeted in brilliant green leaves led from the spacious lobby to the upper floors. After a steep climb, I rested to catch my breath before ringing the bell at apartment 201. As the door opened, a faint scent of perfume wafted into the hall. Before me, arms spread wide in greeting, stood a woman more glamorous than the movie star Greer Garson.

Mrs. Heasley gazed at me with mascara-accented, deep blue eyes. "Blue as Texas blue bonnets," her husband told me later. Her shining chestnut hair, flawless complexion, and willowy figure did not fit my image of the mother of teenage sons. My beige army dress accented with gold buttons felt limp and dull compared to her flowered frock and high heels.

She took me by the arm and led me into the airy living room where Mexican art, deep comfortable chairs, and colorful striped rugs added to the informality of the large space.

"Let me introduce the men in my life. This is my husband, Herbert." A trim man, wearing a well-tailored suit and cowboy boots, gave me a hearty handshake. His weather-beaten face suggested much time spent outdoors in sun and wind.

A blond good-looking boy, taller than his father, stepped forward. Mrs. Heasley looked at him with pride.

"This is Kay. He's almost eighteen, a senior in high school. He's lonesome for his friends in Washington. We moved back to Texas just three weeks ago. We want the boys to graduate from high school here in El Paso."

Behind Kay, a gangly kid pushed the hair out of his eyes. Mrs. Heasley continued, "And this is Bob, our star athlete. He's fifteen. Now let's sit down, and drink some iced tea while we hear about you."

At supper the bright place settings intrigued me. Deep blue pottery plates accented by thick green blown goblets stood out on a striped tablecloth made from cactus fiber. I smiled to myself remembering Aunt Hannah's austere white damask cloth and demure Haviland dinner service.

The spicy Mexican foods made me uncomfortable. While Mr. Heasley told me about his life, I tried to put out the fire with glass after glass of icy tea.

"My family's been Texas born and Texas bred for several generations," he bragged. "Born on a ranch near here, I started life as a rancher, later became a business man." He had spent several years in the nation's capitol working for the War Production Board and advising the President's cabinet members on matters concerning the southwest.

Mrs. Heasley looked too young to have an eighteen-year-old son. Her words gave me a clue she must be about thirty-six. "Herbert and I have always been in love. We started grade school together and he stole my heart in first grade. We eloped on my seventeenth birthday."

After Kay's birth a year later, they had bought this apartment. It had always been home base. They had enjoyed the excitement in Washington but grew homesick for El Paso. Her next words made Texas a friendly place, no longer a lonely one for me.

"Being far from Connecticut, you must miss your family. We want you to feel you have a home here with us. Come as often as you like. Someday, we hope to meet your mother and father. We want to introduce them to our fabulous part of the country."

As I rose to go, Mr. Heasley gave me hug. "How about coming back Friday night for a quick supper and the symphony? The music is played outdoors, sounds much better under the stars."

I hoped I wouldn't wear out my welcome but found myself saying, "I'd love to."

Back at work, the afternoon temperatures hovered above one hundred degrees. The heat in the kitchen became almost unbearable. After the night of Mrs. Heasley's Mexican dinner, I could not eat. My stomach never calmed down. Friends assured me the heat caused my problems, but I wondered why I was the only one affected.

The thought of a cool evening under the stars gave me the impetus to keep my Friday commitment with the Heasleys. Mrs. Heasley, wearing a sheer white embroidered blouse, blue-cotton ruffled skirt, and sandals greeted me with a look of concern.

"Darlin,' you're so pale. Are you all right?"

I sighed. "This has been such a hot week in the kitchen. An evening outdoors should help. Tell me about your silver jewelry. It's beautiful."

I studied the silver links circling her slim waist and the turquoise necklace surrounded by hammered silver. She assured me she knew the best shop for silver jewelry in Juarez, Mexico. She planned to take me across the border to buy some for myself.

Sitting on a blanket under the huge, starlit Texas sky, I forgot my fatigue. The last strains of the orchestra faded away all too soon. On the bus ride back to quarters, I relived the evening.

Mr. Heasley had said, "Let's forget about calling us Mr. and Mrs. Heasley. We Texans like informality. From now on we're Carol and Herbert."

I liked the Texan way of doing things. Mother would have expected me to call them Mr. and Mrs. for years before switching to Aunt and Uncle. My brothers and I had found that confusing — so many aunts and uncles unrelated to us. By making a decision about what to call friends older than myself, I was becoming my own person.

After another restless night, I concluded something must be wrong. My lack of energy and queasy stomach had to be caused by something other than the soaring temperature. I promised myself I'd go on sick call Monday morning.

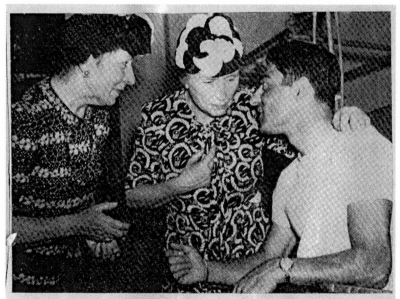

Miss Thomson, Miss Keller and Pfc Joe Zachariah

Helen Keller Leaves Unforgettable Impression of Courage and Faith

Photo appeared in the newsletter of Kennedy General Hospital, U.S. Army, the "Showboat", Vol. 1, No. 14, April 1, 1946.

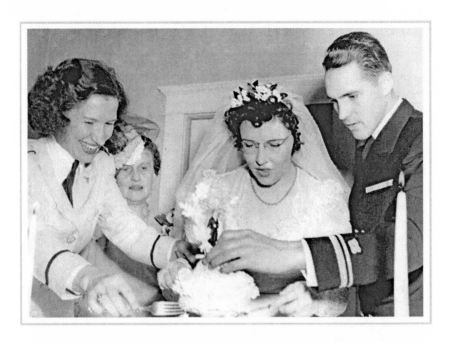

Cousin Polly's Wedding 1946.

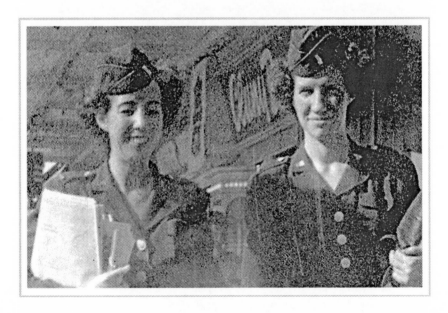

Peg Ward and Carol 1946.

Illness and Recovery 1946

We dietitians had joked about "ninety-day wonders." Those young doctors had been pushed through a speed-up medical program, commissioned in the army after ninety days of basic training, and sent out to learn on the job. They replaced experienced doctors eager to return to civilian practice.

When I went on sick call, the doctor's white coat still had creases from the packing box. Both doctor and coat impressed me as brand new. "Sir, I don't know what's wrong but I feel terrible. I'm losing weight, can't eat, have trouble sleeping, and have absolutely no energy." The doctor took my temperature, then peered at the thermometer a long time before giving me his diagnosis.

"Well, Lieutenant your temperature is only ninety-seven. I suspect your body has not yet adjusted to the high altitude and low humidity here. Drink plenty of water." He wrote a few words on my chart. Avoiding eye contact, he shouted, "Next."

Three days later, I again went on sick call. Much to my dismay, I found myself facing the same doctor in the same lab coat, now with a gray tinge. He ignored my weight loss of three pounds since Monday and again stared at the thermometer. Leaning back in his chair, he took off his glasses. "Lieutenant, I don't know whether you don't like Texas or whether you're trying to get out of the army. My advice to you is snap out of it. Next."

I stumbled down the hall, eyes blinded by tears. A sudden realization made me feel humiliated and angry. I couldn't keep food down. I had no fever. He thought I was pregnant!

I returned to Mess 2 visibly upset. After our run-in, Captain Lord had transferred me there. Dot Miller, the dietitian in charge, took pity on me. "You look as though you need a nap. We'll cover for you. Why don't you return to quarters?"

Back in my room, I collapsed on the bed. The intercom blared out my name. "Lieutenant Morrison, call on the hall phone. Lieutenant Morrison, phone call." Who would call me at this hour of the day? I lifted the receiver from the hook on the box on the wall.

"Lieutenant Morrison speaking."

The angry voice of Captain Lord made me tremble. "Lieutenant, what are you doing off duty without my permission?"

"Ma'am, I'm so sick. I had to take a break. Yes, Ma'am, I went on sick call this morning. What did the doctor say? He told me to snap out of it."

Captain Lord's chilling words cut through the pounding noise in my head. "Lieutenant, if you're not sick enough to be in the hospital, you're not too sick to work. I give you ten minutes to get back on duty."

"Yes, Ma'am."

I tried to follow her orders. In the one hundred and four degree heat, it took me twenty minutes to walk three blocks to Mess 2. That exertion caused a piercing pain in my side. Was I losing my mind? I must be. No, I didn't believe that. If only someone would listen to me.

In the stifling kitchen, the offensive odor of frying fish hung heavy in the air. As I tried to concentrate on inspecting pans of fried halibut, my body sagged against a stainless steel table. Behind me, heat blasted from the containers of bubbling oil on the coal ranges. My fingers gripped the edge of the table. If I should faint, I didn't want to fall backwards and land on a hot stove.

My anger at Captain Lord's lack of understanding kept me going through the afternoon. Back in quarters, determination alone kept me on my feet to wash my hair. Dietitians let nothing deter them from washing the odor of fried fish from their locks.

The next morning, afraid to disobey Captain Lord, I forced myself back on duty. At lunch I picked up my soupspoon, but gagged at the sight of the greasy vegetable soup. A major, whom I recognized as a surgeon, plopped his tray down next to mine.

"You shouldn't be eating that."

I stared at the bowl. "I've got to try to eat something."

He put down his sandwich. "Have you been on sick call? I've been watching you for a week wondering why you're working with food, sick as you are." I had not expected a major to come to my rescue but this one did.

"Sir, I keep going on sick call. The doctor tells me nothing's wrong. He says I should snap out of it."

The major pounded the table with his fist. "That son of a." He stopped short. "I'll find out who's responsible for this. You stay right there. Don't move and don't eat that greasy soup." He rushed from the room. Drained of all emotion, I slumped in my chair, my head in my hands.

Ten minutes later, he returned. "Lieutenant, I've been concerned about you — could see you were coming down with jaundice. I've talked to Captain Lord, called an ambulance. You're on the way to the hospital at the Annex. That doctor on sick call has some explaining to do. I'll deal with him later. Let's go."

He led me outside. I stared at the field ambulance, motor running. The driver, a large colored private jumped down from his high seat. "Lieutenant, Ah don't want yah to sit in the back with those sick fellas. You're goin' to sit up front with me." He scooped me up in his arms and deposited me in the cab.

Although only three miles separated the main hospital from the Annex in the desert, the ride seemed endless. We pulled up in front of a one-story shingled building next to a path lined with prickly cacti. While the driver hunted for a wheelchair, I sat alone in the truck feeling the last of my energy drain away.

On his return, as he picked me up, I put my arms around his neck, gaining comfort in his strength. He lifted me gently from the high seat and placed me in the wheelchair. His gleaming brown face reminded me of the horse chestnuts my brother used to carry in his jacket pocket — same color, same shine.

He patted my shoulder. "Yah goin' be just fine. The Lord goin' tah take care of yah." His broad smile was the last thing I remembered.

I awoke lying on a bed in a hospital ward, still dressed in my uniform. Empty beds lined each side of the room. An eerie silence hung heavy in the still air. I closed my eyes and fell into an exhausted sleep.

Breaking The News

After the ward doctor, Captain Cernock, completed the physical exam, he pulled no punches in giving me a diagnosis. "You're suffering from infectious hepatitis, a serious liver disease. After a series of tests, I'll know more about your condition. One thing I can promise you, you're in for a long, long rest. That means, stay in bed. No breakfast tomorrow until the blood tests are completed."

The appearance of the nurse, who guided me back to bed, surprised me. Her left shoulder and hip, four inches higher than the right, made her dumpy figure walk on the bias. She ran her hands through her thin hair.

"My name is Velma Specht. Like you, I'm a patient. I'm still recovering from polio I picked up in Iran. That's why I'm lopsided." She said she'd become bored with so much time on her hands. When the nursing staff was short-handed, she helped. She explained my bed was the one closest to the bathroom.

"Think you can walk that far? I'll help you undress."

"Velma, is that me?" I stared in the mirror at a thin yellow face. My haunted yellow eyes stared back. "I had no idea I looked so bad. Do people die from hepatitis?"

Velma pulled me away from the mirror. "Sometimes, but you won't. I'll see to that. With lots of rest, proper diet and good care you will get well."

She pulled back the bedspread. "Let's start by getting you in bed. Do you have a friend who could go to your room for the things you'll need? Robe, slippers, toothbrush, comb — anything else?"

"Writing paper. I have to write to Mother and Dad." Grateful to have someone do my thinking for me, I drifted off to sleep. I awoke disoriented by a bright light overhead and the chatter of several women. Velma had told me the other patients spent afternoons and evenings away from the ward. In no mood to talk to anyone, I closed my eyes.

In the morning, I awoke groggy and confused. Velma stood by the bed holding my robe and slippers. "Dot Miller sent your things on the bus from the main hospital. Your escort will be here in five minutes to take you to the lab." She giggled. "That pink housecoat really clashes with your buttercup complexion. You've turned deep yellow over night."

"Lieutenant Morrison, your chariot awaits you. Hop in for a trip to the Bloody Bar." A seedy corporal wearing a wrinkled uniform, hair uncombed, steadied my arm to keep me from falling. I collapsed into an ancient wood wheelchair, probably a relic of WW I. The sagging cane seat hurt my bottom and the awkward leg rests thrust my legs straight out in front of me.

"Bloody Bar. What's that?"

The corporal laughed. "That's where we're goin' while they drain all the blood out of yah. Hold on." The unwieldy wheelchair careened around the corner into the main corridor. As the chair raced faster and faster, I clutched the wooden arms in alarm.

"Corporal, slow down." My warning came too late. Weaving from side to side, the heavy chair grazed a fire extinguisher attached to the wall. Wham! The heavy metal cylinder fell to the floor. White foam escaped from the writhing, snake-like hose, spraying globs over my feet and my robe.

Bony fingers clutched my shoulder, "Lootenan' I'se sho shorry. Got married Saturday night. Thish first time I've been shober." After the corporal righted the fire extinguisher, he stopped the gushing foam and leaned the tank against the wall. We proceeded at snail's pace to the end of the hall.

A banner over the door proclaimed "Bloody Bar." The letters dripped with realistic drops of blood painted in bold vivid red. Inside a dozen soldiers sat on stools before a slanted plank covered in white paper. Each man rested his arm on the board while a technician drew blood.

"Let the lady go next," called the contrite corporal. As the men jumped to their feet, they looked at me in surprise. I felt as though I'd dropped in from a far off planet. My dainty pink robe looked inappropriate amid a group of men dressed in maroon exercise suits. It dawned on me my strange yellow complexion might have something to do with their reaction.

On the slow return trip to the ward, I said to the corporal, "You were right about one thing. There's no blood left in me. Wonder what the lab's going to do with all those vials." I never saw the Bloody Bar again. From that day onward, the lab technician came to my bed.

I worried about how I'd break the news to Mother and Dad. If I told them the truth about my illness, would they be unduly alarmed? I had promised to tell them anything that happened, but I didn't want to make them frantic with worry. In my weakened state, it took several days to write a letter one sentence at a time. I decided not to mention my collapse on duty.

Dear Mother and Daddy,

I don't quite know how to begin this letter. Since we agreed it would be best to keep each other informed, I want to let you know my life has changed. Instead of caring for patients, I have become one myself. Try not to worry. I am getting the best of care.

All last week I was ill — couldn't eat a thing and felt miserable. When I went on sick call the doctor told me my symptoms were heat related. Then I began to turn yellow. Last Saturday I was sent to the hospital. So far, the diagnosis is hepatitis. Jaundice is one of the symptoms of this disease. Guess so many things have gone wrong with me that my liver felt cheated and decided to assert its authority.

Glad you can't see me. I'm a gorgeous shade of yellow. My eyes are more colorful than a cat's at night. Every time I look at my feet, I think of an old stewing chicken hanging in the window of a store on Third Avenue in New York.

I have complete faith in the doctor, which is unusual in the army. He says I'm in for a long, long rest. I'm guessing four to six weeks in bed, but I won't know 'til the tests are completed.

After writing special diets for months, I'm on one myself —low fat, high carbohydrate. It isn't bad. No butter, no fried foods, no gaseous vegetables. I have to drink a banana formula three times a day, which I detest, and eat all the hard candy I can manage. Since my liver gets no fat, it needs a constant supply of carbohydrate.

I'm in a ward with twelve women. I'd prefer a room alone but I suppose, as the weeks drag on, I'll be glad of the company. The ward is in a barracks on the edge of the desert. We keep the shades pulled down all day to keep out the hot, hot sun. My friends find it hard to get down here from the main hospital three miles away. Anyway, I'm not ready for visitors. I'm getting used to resting all the time.

I promise to keep you up-dated on my progress. Glad your worries about gas are over. It must be great to whiz about in Sherman's convertible.

All my love,

Carol

One evening a patient from Ward 30, the psychiatric ward, where I had supervised meal service, appeared by my bed. A visitor, even an unbalanced one, broke the monotony. My roommates shook with laughter over his comment.

"Hey, Dietitian. I told my buddies you'll probably be a patient on our ward before you get out."

In my wildest nightmare, I had not imagined ending up behind bars on Ward 30.

Bed Rest and Diet

As I stepped on the scales, the nurse looked at her clipboard. "Ninety-eight pounds, three pounds less than when you came in. Are you sure you're following orders and eating your meals?"

"I try hard, really I do." Toast without butter, unseasoned noodles, and dry baked potato stuck in my throat. I did suck on hard candy on the hour, drank water on the half hour, and tried to choke down three glasses a day of the horrible banana mixture. Without any appetite, that was best I could do.

The days fell into a monotonous routine — blood tests before breakfast, take a rest, write a few lines of a letter, and take a rest. By noon, the groan of the antiquated air conditioner, outmatched by the sun beating down on the roof, grated on my nerves.

Along with the unappetizing lunch tray came the worst hour of the day. As temperature shot higher and higher, a popular radio program, "The Answer Man," blared forth from the intercom above my bed. I detested the inane questions called in to Mr. Know-It-All. If I fell asleep, I awoke soaked in sweat feeling worse than before the nap. The ambulatory patients were lucky — they could escape the ward.

Carol Heasley brought me books and magazines, which made the afternoons less tedious. Supper at four-thirty left many hours before lights out at ten. The first week I dreaded the evening return of the noisy patients to the ward. When I began to feel better, their conversation became a welcome diversion after my lonely days surrounded by empty beds.

When the sun went down, the lowered window shades went up. Sometimes, I caught a glimpse of a dramatic sunset. The air conditioner finally made progress cooling the air. I marked off another dull day on my pocket calendar.

I looked forward to 9:00 p.m. when the nurse turned off the air conditioner and opened the windows. Cool desert air crept across my bed. Those quiet comfortable hours gave me time to think.

I realized I had been losing ground for three months, ever since the disaster in the dental clinic. That colonel had not even washed his hands much less taken precautions to keep the instruments sterile. Those shots of Novocain, those needles must be the way I contracted hepatitis.

When I questioned Velma, her words confirmed my suspicions, "Yes, transfusions and contaminated needles are sometimes the cause."

How different my life would have been, had I chosen to go to Letterman in San Francisco instead of Kennedy in Memphis. What I had to do now was fight harder to overcome this downturn in my life.

Dr. Cernock's words ran through my mind like a mantra. Diet and bed rest. Diet and bed rest. The only means to recovery — diet and bed rest. I knew it would take more than that to make me well.

The words of the driver who brought me to the hospital, "The Lord's gonna watch over yah," gave me hope and peace.

My thoughts turned to the First Congregational Church in Danbury, Connecticut, where the family had sat together in the same pew every Sunday morning. Architectural students from Yale were sent there to study the proportions of the beautiful brick building with its white steeple piercing the sky. I pictured the white walls of the sanctuary and the glimpse of trees with green leaves in summer or bare branches in winter, though the paned windows.

I prayed. I recited the words to many hymns, including the first one I sang in Sunday school, "Jesus loves me, this I know." Again and again I recited the twenty-third psalm, "The Lord is my Shepherd, I shall not want."

Many memories crowded my mind and gave me inspiration — candlelight services on Christmas Eve, sunrise services on Easter, Ernie's flag-draped coffin surrounded by flowers, and the many churches Mary and I had attended in Greensboro. We had visited a different denomination every Sunday for a year. Faith, memories, and letters from home kept me from getting depressed.

One afternoon, Dr. Cernock spotted the glass of banana drink on my nightstand. The mixture of skim milk, egg whites, malt and mashed bananas, twenty-two hundred calories to the quart, turned sour within minutes of leaving the refrigerator. He gave me his daily lecture on the importance of drinking the concoction to help me gain weight.

I looked him in the eye. "Sir, I'd like to make a deal with you. If you can drink a glass of this dreadful mixture, I'll never complain about it again." He gave me the kind of condescending look Mother had displayed when pouring cod liver oil on a spoon.

"Sure, I can do that. Chug-a-lug." He tossed back his head, took a large gulp. Gagging, he covered his mouth with his hand before running from the ward toward the bathroom. The anguished look on his face gave me my first laugh in weeks. The detested banana drink disappeared forever. My first victory on Ward 85!

That day marked the beginning of my recovery. Although my eyes still glowed like a cat's, the yellow tinge to my skin became less intense. When I said, "I think I can walk to the bathroom without holding your arm," Velma looked doubtful. I took a few shaky steps on my own, which made both of us shout with joy.

Her next words came as a surprise. "Let's wash your hair. Think you're ready to stand in the shower?" That activity took more energy than I had anticipated. Exhausted, I clutched her arm on my way back to bed. After a long nap, I wrote a note to Mother and Dad. "Great news. I have a clean head."

Lying in bed day after day made it difficult to find items of interest to write to the family. Not everything I saw could be told. Looking to my right through the double doors into the hall, my view was restricted to the linen room door. The first time I saw a doctor glance around before slipping into the linen room, I wondered why he needed linen.

Soon a nurse's actions mirrored his. She emerged twenty minutes later, followed after a brief interval by the doctor. They were the first of many couples to take advantage of the privacy offered by the linen room — unaware an observer kept score.

An announcement boomed over the intercom made an amusing story to write home. "Attention. Private Burke lost his upper plate this noon between the mess hall and Ward 4. The plate is attached to a set of dog tags and should be returned to the ward immediately." Apparently, Private Burke did not find his uppers. The urgent message was repeated for twenty-four hours.

One morning, I watched two GIs in fatigues wrestle with the battered, baby grand piano that stood in the recreational area at the end of the ward. After much swearing and groaning, they hefted it onto a platform with wheels. They pushed the piano down a ramp, loaded it into a truck, and drove away.

Several days later, a Red Cross worker, looking puzzled, stared at the empty space. "What happened to the piano? I planned to play it at a sing-a-long." I told her I had watched two GIs cart it away and load it on a truck. This led to an investigation by three officers, who questioned me, the only eyewitness, three times. The culprits were never apprehended, the stolen piano never recovered.

Even on Ward 85, unexpected events broke the monotony.

Time Marches On

Mother's letters gave me the impression she looked on the army as a guardian angel, ready and willing to consider my welfare. She responded to my carefully worded letter about my diagnosis of infectious hepatitis with her usual optimism. "I am so glad the army is giving you the rest you have needed for so long. If you relax and enjoy it, there may a pleasant side to it after all."

She was convinced I would be discharged as soon as I felt better. Reminding her my tour of duty would not be up for another year made no impression. When she questioned whether I was telling her all I knew about my illness, I tried to explain.

"Mother, being in an army hospital is different from your experience as a patient. No one tells me anything. I'll be the last to know how I'm doing. I could be sent back on duty tomorrow or I could be dead."

Her next letter spoke only of the future. With her usual enthusiasm, she suggested my experience with food would make me successful running a tearoom. Dad's job was not working out as they had hoped. It was time to go in another direction. This could be a perfect solution for all of us. They were already looking for a good location.

Before I could think up an answer to that bombshell, another familiar pink envelope lay on my bed. She wrote on pink stationary left over from the gift shop at Bonita Grove. All pink letters automatically found their way to me. Before I finished reading the first sentence, I could feel her enthusiasm.

I shared the content with Velma. "Listen to this. Mother has located the perfect place for the tearoom — a charming two hundred year old house with seven fireplaces. Seven fireplaces! Does she expect me to chop the wood and lay the fires when I'm not in the kitchen?"

A special delivery letter from Dad relieved my mind. "That old house," he wrote, "would take more money to maintain than a tearoom could ever support." His next words gave me hope.

"Carol, I realize you have a long road ahead before deciding on your future. You just concentrate on getting well."

I wanted to follow his advice but every Monday morning brought a new, trembling, pathetic lab technician-in-training to my bedside. "Lieutenant, I've come to draw blood. I've never worked on a woman's veins before. They're small, aren't they?"

"Unfortunately private, they're the ones I was born with. Give it a try. You boys have already turned me into a human pin cushion."

The first pinprick indicated whether this would be a painful or super painful experience. An improperly sharpened needle meant trouble. The black and blue swath running six inches down my arm attested to many dull needles.

By Friday the procedure would go smoothly. "Private, tell your buddy who comes next week to practice on an orange and to be prepared for small veins."

Other tests proved more hazardous than blood tests. One morning a white lab coat stood by my bed. "Hope you haven't had breakfast. Take this pill, which will send dye through your liver. I'll be back later to take a blood sample. That will tell us how well your liver is functioning."

Within half an hour, pains in my stomach had me writhing in agony. Uncertain what to do, Dr. Cernock and the nurse hovered over me. They had put in a call for a gastro-intestinal expert. He rushed into the ward, struggling into his lab coat.

"How many glasses of water did you drink with the pill? Only a swallow? No wonder you have pains. You were supposed to be given two glasses of water. Drink as much as possible the rest of the day to flush the dye out of your system."

As I lay on my bed, water logged and exhausted, I wanted to cry but lacked the energy. Next morning at dawn, the lab technician handed me two of the now familiar pills and two glasses of water. When I protested I had eaten no food in twenty-four hours and wanted to postpone the test for a day, he showed no mercy.

"Hurry up and drink that water. I have other patients to see."

A few days later, a problem arose with a P.S.P. test for kidney function. This time, after I drank two glasses of water, a nurse injected dye into my arm. Every hour urine samples were collected to determine how fast the dye passed through my system. This went on all day — left me feeling miserable. As though that wasn't bad enough, I learned I had been given the wrong test. It should have been B.S.P. for liver function.

The following morning I had no breakfast, not even water. Without explanation, a doctor injected a solution into my left arm and later took out an equal amount of blood from my right arm. He never told me why.

Another test gauged the amount of yellow pigment in my system. Normal was eleven or below. Mine had topped out at seventy-five. No one told me how much it had dropped.

August nineteenth became a day of victory. The nurse let me walk unaided to the phone in her office to accept a telegram received by the signal corps from Mother and Dad. I had walked no farther than the bathroom in three weeks. There was no way I could send a telegram in return. They had no idea I had to depend on strangers to do me favors.

On September 5, Dr. Cernock gave me good news. "Today you have my permission to sit in a chair. Start with ten minutes." I was shocked to find myself exhausted after five minutes. The next day a new doctor set back my progress when he tried the B.S.P. test. He missed the vein, shot 5cc of dye into the muscle in my arm.

That caused a black and blue mark more offensive than the lab technician's. The pain lasted for hours. Even the next day, my fingers ached as well as the muscles in my back. Those fellows had to learn but I was tired of being their guinea pig.

September 10, 1946 — my twenty-fifth birthday. I felt depressed and old. I had never anticipated ending my first quarter century like this. While my friends were enjoying civilian life, I lay in an army hospital two thousand miles from home wondering what chance I had of recovery.

My cousin Bob had married Helen Plumb on Labor Day. My cousin Ted had given Betty Hainlin a diamond ring. Mary Kirschner, my college roommate, planned to wed Dave in April. My brother Sam, discharged from the navy, had moved to Boston with his wife, Betty. I was unaware that the fight to overcome hepatitis often brought on severe depression, but I knew their good fortunes made my situation look bleak.

Carol and Herbert Heasley changed all that. They brought their son Kay, a high school senior, for a surprise birthday visit. Herbert grinned at me, "Carol, do we have a birthday present for you. We're going to tell you on the count of three. One, Two, Three."

Carol, Herbert and Kay linked arms before shouting in unison, "We bought a car."

Carol Heasley took over, "We've never needed a car here. There's good transportation and nowhere to go outside of town for hundreds of miles. Now we have a convenient way to take you to our apartment."

She leaned over the bed and kissed me. "Happy birthday, Darlin." We hope you'll be well enough to join us in ten days to celebrate your birthday with our son Bob, when he turns sixteen."

Sick Leave Denied

The Heasleys' visit on my birthday made my spirits soar. Other patients gathered round my bed to hear my exciting news. They couldn't believe the Heasleys had bought a car just to whisk me away from the hospital to their apartment. A colorful bouquet of purple asters, yellow roses, and daisies from Mother and Dad lifted my mood even higher.

After my nap, Mary Schroeder pushed a wheelchair decorated with a huge pink bow to my bed. "Climb in. This is party time. Lieutenant Cernock has given permission for you to spend two hours in my room." She rummaged in the drawer of the nightstand for lipstick.

"Mary, I never expected to celebrate my birthday wearing robe and slippers, but this is fantastic. My first taste of freedom in six weeks."

Mary grinned. "Peg called at the last minute. Said to tell you she's sorry to miss your party but she's meeting someone special in Mexico. I'm sorry to tell you Captain Lord can't make it either." We both laughed.

At Mary's door, ten friends greeted me and led me to a seat of honor. After opening gag gifts, I ate every bite on my plate of juicy chicken and crisp salad. Planned with my diet in mind, angel cake and strawberries topped off the birthday meal.

Suddenly, like the bouquet of roses on the table, I drooped. Mary rushed me back to Ward 85 and tucked me into bed. My thoughts turned to Mother, Dad, and the joint celebrations in the past for my birthday and their anniversary. If only there were a way for me to call them and tell them about the Heasleys' magnificent gift. This day had brought me a taste of life away from Ward 85. I wanted more.

My slow recovery caused Mother and Dad concern. After Commanding Officer Colonel Reyer turned down my request for sick leave for the third time, Dad decided to act. Thank Goodness, he asked my advice before he carried out his plan to get me released from the army.

He wrote Mr. Osborne, his boss, an influential Connecticut Republican, was a friend of Claire Booth Luce. She had become a national figure, as well as being active in state politics. Her recent move to Newtown, ten miles from Bethel, made her readily accessible. Dad wanted to ask Mr. Osborne for an introduction. A word from Clare Booth Luce in the right circles might bring me a discharge.

Many celebrities had used their influence to get people out of the service, but my first response was horror. I was amazed my father would go against his principals of fair play to pull strings on my behalf. How could I ever hold up my head with pride, if he did that? My second response was overwhelming love for a father who would go to such extremes to protect his daughter.

In my letter to him, I tried to be diplomatic. Told him it was grand of him to want to help, but it would be best not to interfere. The doctor expected me to recover and return to duty. If I should suffer a relapse while in the army, I could return to the hospital. If I had to go to a Veterans' Hospital, the care, especially for a woman, might not equal that I now received.

A friend of mine had asked Senator Meade of New York to use his pull in her behalf. He had had no success trying to help her. The army was calling back discharged nurses and dietitians, which made it unlikely I could leave before my time was up. I just hoped I'd be a civilian before another war came along.

A week after my party, a group of patients and staff crowded round the bulletin board to cheer over a notice posted there. "As of October first, army personnel are granted permission to wear civilian clothes when off duty."

Women patients raced to town to shop. When they staged a parade through the ward in their new finery, I watched with envy. My only outfit remained the tired pink robe.

Three fourths of my time was spent in bed. At least, I no longer looked like a stewing chicken. My yellow eyes had not returned to normal but only a slight tinge of yellow colored my skin. Fighting fatigue with each step, I tried to walk farther each day. After meeting my goal to reach the PX, I called the Heasleys and accepted the invitation to the birthday party.

Carol Heasley responded with enthusiasm. "Darlin' your car has been sittin' here waitin' for you to take your first ride. Kay and Bob will pick you up on Friday evenin.' We're goin' to have a grand celebration for Bob's sixteenth birthday and your twenty-fifth."

The boys drove up to the barracks with horn blaring, which caused a few raised eyebrows. They were lucky the MPs were not around. Bob gave me his lopsided grin.

"I'm so glad you got sick. My parents would never have bought a car, 'cept for you. Now I've got my license, I want to drive all the way 'cross Texas. I want to keep goin' and goin,'"

At the apartment, I refused to be carried. Half way up the stairs, I wished I had accepted the boys' offer. Carol, irked that I had walked, put me to bed for half an hour. At dinnertime, Herbert seated me at the table in front of a beautiful bouquet of lavender ageratum, red roses, tiny white zinnias, and white chrysanthemums.

The birthday dinner began with grape juice followed by pear salad, the pears tinted red. Bob had requested hamburgers. Carol had prepared broiled fish for me. Maraschino cherries in Jell-O accompanied the three-layer birthday cake. It was the most colorful meal I had seen in months. With no thought of diet, I ate everything.

After dinner, I lay on the davenport and watched Bob open his gifts. Herbert expressed his disapproval that Colonel Reyer would not grant me sick leave.

"Why don't I wire some of my friends in Washington? I know many influential people. It makes me furious that you are not allowed to recuperate at home." I pleaded with him to do nothing. The consequences of going over the commanding officer's head would make my situation worse.

In my weeks on the ward, many patients had come and gone. The current group got on my nerves. Across from me, a WAC, forty-nine years old, reclined on her bed. She seemed determined to tell me every detail of her life. After a morning exam, she repeatedly related a description no one wanted to hear about her hemorrhoids.

"The doctor hurt me so much I thought he was trying to pull my appendix out through my rear end."

Next to her sat a gal from Savannah weighing two hundred and eighty pounds. While I was trying to choke down my Spartan diet, she liked to talk about her ten-pound tumors or rhapsodize about fried chicken, gravy, and beaten biscuits.

I had to defend Velma Specht, who had befriended me. The others considered her psycho. "No. She's a little eccentric. After what she went through contracting polio in Iran, who wouldn't be?" I did grow tired of Velma's lectures to me about the lack of men in my life.

"What do you expect me to do? The only man I see is the married doctor."

She suggested I go to the Red Cross room to play ping-pong. When I told her I wasn't up to that, she shrugged her high shoulder, the one not paralyzed. "Perhaps, it's just as well. There's no one playing but colored boys." In those days it would have been unacceptable, even though I had worked with many, to play a game with a person of color.

Ellen, in the bed next to mine, tried to keep me awake describing her arthritis pain. She started with her toes, put me to sleep by the time she reached her finger joints. When I awoke, she continued with elbows, shoulders, and back. She had not leaned to use her disease to her advantage like the two arthritis victims in the private rooms.

When the doctor made morning rounds, those sufferers held out their swollen hands and explained how miserable they felt. As soon as he left, they dashed off to the PX snack shop to line up dates for dinner in Mexico.

When they returned after midnight, they interrupted our sleep to brag about the dancing and drinking they had enjoyed. Still hung over in the morning, they complained to the doctor about their painful joints. Once rounds were over, they grabbed quick naps before preparing for another night on the town.

I had to get out of that madhouse. Captain Lord had never come to see me, but she was the only person to whom I could appeal for help. It was worth a try, even though I doubted she'd talk to Colonel Reyer. Rumor had it she hated him and he hated her.

Our interview got off to a bad start. She set her glasses on the desk. "Of course, you're weak after ten weeks in bed. You'll pick up once you get back to work."

"The doctor doesn't think I'm ready to work eight hours a day. He wants me to gain ten pounds before I return to duty. The liver function tests are not back to normal. He says I need rest I cannot get on the ward."

Captain Lord sighed in exasperation. "Come back tomorrow at ten. I'll take you to see the Adjutant."

Would he be willing to put in a good word for me? I hoped so.

Thirty Days Leave

In the presence of the Adjutant, Captain Lord displayed finesse I did not know she possessed. She smiled at the charming captain with his boyish grin.

"This is one of my special girls. She's been on Ward 85 for ten weeks with hepatitis. Captain Cernock, her doctor, wants her to go home where she can get some rest. Is there anything you can do to get around Colonel Reyer's order refusing sick leave?"

The captain turned to me. "Where are you from, Lieutenant? Connecticut? So am I. I'm from Bridgeport. How about you?"

"I was born in Bethel, grew up in Danbury. My family has returned to Bethel." I told him we had something in common. "P.T. Barnum, the circus man was born in Bethel and later established Bridgeport with money he made from his successful New York museum."

He laughed. "Yeah. I grew up with the story of how he hitched his elephant, Jumbo, to the plow whenever the train passed his Bridgeport estate on its way from Boston to New York. Advertising, as we know it today, all began with him."

Captain Lord snapped us back to reality. "Thank you Captain. We won't take any more of your time. I'd appreciate any help you can give Lieutenant Morrison." As she strode from his office, I thought the Adjutant gave me a brief wink. I tried to catch up with Captain Lord but she disappeared down the hall without a glance in my direction.

The following morning I sat on my bed writing to Mother. Since all attempts to get sick leave had failed, perhaps, she should come to Texas. Startled by a deep voice in the hall, I put down my pen.

"Where's Lieutenant Morrison?" Colonel Reyer, Commanding Officer of Beaumont General Hospital, strode into the ward.

I scrambled off the bed. "Here, Sir." As I saluted, I was aware of the incongruous sight of my skinny bare feet beneath my lace-trimmed pink robe. Towering over me, the middle-aged, rotund, red-faced officer puffed his cheeks in anger.

His tirade against me began with his first words. "What in the hell did you mean going over my head? When I give an order no one disputes it. Certainly not a pipsqueak like you." Following correct protocol, I stood silent with shoulders braced while he continued his harangue. I dared not say all I had done was talk to Captain Lord.

I interjected, "Yes Sir" and "No Sir" at the appropriate times, wiggling my toes in protest. Suddenly, like a popped balloon, the wind went out of him. He pivoted on his heel and headed for the door. Before disappearing from sight, he growled over his shoulder, "Thirty-day leave granted starting tomorrow."

Wondering whether I had heard what I thought I heard, I sank onto the bed. Tomorrow, how could I be ready that soon? Velma, who had listened to this exchange, rushed to my rescue.

"What a pompous fool. Of course, you'll be ready. I'll help you. Let's make a list of what needs to be done. First of all, I'll call Transportation to make an airline reservation."

She decided I should take the next bus to my quarters at the main hospital. If I finished packing before lunch, I could rest in the afternoon. While in the nurses' quarters, I put in an excited call to Mother from the pay phone.

"Mother, sit down before I tell you my great news. Colonel Reyer broke down and gave me leave. I'll be in New York tomorrow night. Can you meet me at LaGuardia Airport at seven? I know. I'm in shock myself."

Reality did not set in until I picked up my orders in late afternoon. I stared at my name underlined in yellow far down the list of changes in personnel. "2ᵈ Lt Caroline Morrison, R2432, MDD, is granted thirty <30> days sk lv eff 19 Oct 46. <MA>248 Greenwood Ave, Bethel, Conn." My future lay on that sheet of cheap gray paper. Of all the special orders issued that day, only mine granted sick leave.

When the plane soared into the sunrise, I felt like a bird freed from a cage. Too excited to relax, I watched the sere desert landscape of west Texas give way to green fields and trees. Never before had I taken a flight long enough to include breakfast, lunch, and dinner. No one in my family had ever had that experience.

Twelve hours later, as the plane's wing dipped, I glanced out the window. Far below, rays of gold from the torch of the Statue of Liberty pierced the night sky. On the horizon, twinkling lights in all directions reminded me of fireflies on parade. In one long day I had flown more than two thousand miles from Texas to New York.

The plane hit the runway hard and rolled to the gate. The stewardess, who had given me special attention on the flight, came to my aid.

"Let me take your handbag. You grab my arm and hold onto the railing. I'll help you down the stairs." On shaky legs, one step at a time, I descended to the ground.

Slowly, I made my way across the tarmac into Mother's waiting arms.

Welcome Home

"Welcome home." Mother's words swept away my resolve to be strong. Feeling her arms around me, hearing the voice I had waited so long to hear, forced my loneliness, fears, and struggle to the surface. I put my head on her shoulder and wept. I cried until tears dampened the sleeve of her coat and the front of my uniform.

She guided me to a bench, where we sat, her hands clasped over mine until I regained my composure. "This has been such a long day for you. Do you want something to eat?" I was relieved when she told me we were not going to Grand Central Station to catch a train to Bethel. We had hotel reservations in New York.

Mother had spent hours during the afternoon at Travelers' Aid. An understanding woman there had made dozens of calls to locate a room. She had found the last available room in the city, not fancy but clean.

The cab driver dumped our bags on the sidewalk under a narrow marquee sandwiched between two storefronts in a seedy neighborhood somewhere on the West Side. He shifted his cigar to the corner of his mouth. "This ain't no neighborhood fer youse girls to go wanderin' around."

"Oh, no, Sir." Mother gave him a cheery smile. "Today my daughter has come all the way from Texas on sick leave. This is the only room left in New York and she needs some rest."

We lugged our bags into a dingy lobby. As the desk clerk slapped a skeleton key on the counter, he kept his eyes on the horse racing results in the newspaper. "Third floor at the front, elevator to your right."

The antiquated elevator jerked, moaned, and groaned on its way up. On the third floor, Mother glanced at the threadbare carpet, greasy wallpaper and stark light bulb suspended above each door.

"Keep your fingers crossed." She fitted the key into the lock. "Hope the room is better than this hallway."

I stepped in first. Two iron beds covered in worn chenille spreads faced the window. One straight chair and a chipped veneer bureau with murky mirror completed the furnishings.

"Well, Mother, it's basic, not the Waldorf. It does have a special feature perfect for you with your love of color."

Outside the window, a neon sign blinked steady as a heart beat. A flash of red light, followed by one of green, illuminated the room with the intensity of a fireworks display. We burst into laughter. We laughed until our weak knees made us collapse on the beds.

Mother heaved on the warped sash until it opened, then stuck her head out the window. "Its a sign several stories high extending out from the side of the building. The red flash says 'Hotel' the green flash says 'Hudson.' We're opposite the red 'e,' followed by the green 'o.' I'm so sorry."

"I'm not. I couldn't have gone another mile tonight. The mattress doesn't sink in the middle. That's all that matters."

During our Technicolor night, pipes banged, the elevator groaned, and sirens wailed in the street below. Many sleepless hours later, I giggled. "Mother, this is the first time since college that I've talked from dark to dawn. We'll never forget this night. I can't decide whether you look better in a flash of red or green."

"Dear, I like you better red. Green reminds me of how you must have looked with hepatitis. I've saved some exciting news. Now is a good time to tell you."

She rambled on about the perfect house she and Dad had found. They planned to make an offer on it within days. She assured me the next time I came home I would have a room of my own.

The rumble of the garbage truck followed by the banging of the garbage cans grated on my taut nerves. "Mother, it's 5:00 a.m. Let's get out of here. We can eat breakfast in Grand Central Station and catch the seven o'clock train for Bethel. I bet the aroma of Lysol from our 'clean room' will follow us all the way home."

We tiptoed past the sleeping desk clerk and stepped out of the stuffy lobby into crisp chilly air. Standing arm in arm, we looked up at the flashing neon sign.

"Carol, take a good look. This is your last glimpse of this place. I'd be embarrassed to have anyone know we stayed here."

I winked at Mother. "Have you forgotten? We're the lucky gals who got the last hotel room in New York, not fancy, but clean." When the taxi crossed Fifth Avenue on the way to Grand

Central, we relaxed. It was comforting to be back in familiar territory.

We settled down on the worn plush seat in a coach of the New York, New Haven and Hartford train. The cups of strong coffee we'd enjoyed for breakfast could not keep us from dozing. Mother told me not to worry about missing our stop. Mr. Beaupain, conductor for the past thirty years, would watch out for us.

At Bethel, he even carried our bags and deposited them on the station platform. I inhaled the exhilarating October air. The few remaining red and yellow leaves on the trees gave me a rush of excitement I had not experienced in months. We strolled up Greenwood Avenue and the spring in my step lasted almost to Aunt Hannah's house.

Mother left me at the front door. "Hannah has gone to work. She has the early shift in the library today. Your room is ready for you. I know how much you need rest. I must get home to let Father know you are here safe and sound. Call me later."

I stepped into the imposing hall. The familiar old-house smell of furniture polish and floor wax with a hint of mothballs seemed comforting. The tick-tock of the clock echoed through the quiet rooms. I had forgotten how relaxing silence could be. On the towering hat rack, familiar dark felt hats foretold the approach of cold weather.

After reading Aunt Hannah's welcoming note on the walnut dining room table, I wandered from room to room. The green window shades had been drawn exactly three-quarters of the way down the long narrow panes to shield the rugs from the sun. Every chair stood primly in its proper place. Nothing had changed since my last visit.

I clutched the shiny banister and pulled my weary body up the steep carpeted stairs to the second floor.

As I filled the claw-foot bathtub almost to the brim with hot water, the Morrison creed of conservation almost caught up with me. I wondered how many years it had been since anyone had dared use that much water for one bath. I rationalized that this was my first tub bath in months.

Lying in the soothing water, listening to "the noise of the quiet," as some child in the family had described it, I felt at peace.

Changes On The Home Front

When I had stayed with Aunt Hannah in September 1945, I found it difficult to adjust to her set routine and cautious ways. Now in October 1946, I appreciated her concern and the strong family bond that tied us together. My outlook had been broadened by travel, by associating with people of different backgrounds, races, and economic levels. Her life had remained static, while I had moved on.

No longer did I feel compelled to let her control my actions. Working with everyone from critically ill patients to mess sergeants and prisoners of war had taught me how to think and act for myself.

I was sure she still considered drinking black coffee a bad habit I'd picked up in the army. At our first breakfast together, I poured a cup of coffee and stated my position. "Aunt Hannah, it's a good thing I like my coffee black for my diet doesn't allow cream."

Coping with Mother's high level of energy dragged me down. She thought she understood my illness, but she questioned me about my experiences long after my energy had waned. Dad had empathy for my problems. He faced a similar situation with his faltering heart. How often he must have longed for a quiet evening instead of guests for dinner.

Mother and Dad had been living with Grandpa Andrews for more than a year and were eager for a place of their own. Veterans had priority for the limited number of houses for sale. Then Grandpa sprang a surprise that made it imperative they move. When Mother told me about it, she shook her head in disbelief.

"I went in Father's room to make his bed. On the bureau stood a large framed picture of a woman I'd never seen. She had a plump face, dark hair, appeared to be in her sixties. I was stunned!"

It took Mother time to decide how to respond. When her father came in from the barn, she told him she had seen the nice looking picture on his bureau.

He replied, "You're gol darn right it is. She's a fine woman. Things are going to be different 'round here come spring. I'm gettin' married."

I held Mother's hand. "Mother, I can't believe it. My seventy-nine year old grandfather's getting married? I hope his fiancée is used to opinionated weather-beaten old Yankees. Where did he meet her?"

Mother sighed. "She came to visit Mrs. Edington next door. Her name is Louise. She and Father started talking over the fence. She's been a widow for forty years and has been companion to a woman on Park Avenue in New York."

Mother and Dad suspected she thought there was money in Grandpa's neat little white house. He could barely support himself. How could he take on a wife?

Mother's eyes filled with tears. "In my wildest dreams I never expected to have a stepmother. She's sixty-two, only six years older than I." That evening Mother and Dad hastened to sign the papers for their own house fifteen miles away at Timber Trails.

Timber Trails, a colony of summer homes, lay tucked away in the hills in the town of Sherman, Connecticut. My brother, like the village, had been named for Roger Sherman, signer of the Declaration of Independence from Connecticut. Roger Sherman was a distant ancestor of Mother's.

On our way to meet Mrs. Young, owner of the house, we drove along a narrow two-lane road full of curves, up hills and down. What were Mother and Dad thinking? That road would be a nightmare in ice or snow.

Mother caught up in the beauty of the fall evening exclaimed, "That old red barn has such character. I can hardly wait for spring when the apple trees blossom."

We turned off the paved road onto gravel. Dad pointed out a beaver pond in the swamp. At irregular intervals, neat brown-stained shingled houses, surrounded by groves of trees, blended into the landscape. The shuttered windows made them appear in hibernation for the winter ahead.

Mother exclaimed in rapture, "Carol, look. Here's our new home. Isn't this the most beautiful location you've ever seen?"

We stood on the edge of the road looking down the steep driveway and sloping lawn. Only the pitched roof of the small house nestled against the hill was visible. Far below lay the valley overshadowed by the graceful outline of the opposite mountain.

I wanted to cry out, "It seems so lonely to me." Instead, I murmured, "Yes, this is lovely." My thoughts were on the vertical driveway. It would be impossible to park in the garage under the house in the winter. And what about the snow? Who was going to shovel the snow? Not Dad, with his bad heart.

I had to admit the interior had charm. Mrs. Young welcomed us in the tiny hall and led us into a living room with windows on three sides. We stood before the picture window entranced by the dramatic view. In sharp contrast to the dark outline of the mountain, golden shafts of light shot through the orange sky. A crackling fire in the fieldstone fireplace echoed the color of the sunset.

To the right of the entrance we passed by the small dining area, a table and four chairs in front of a window with low sill. Outside a bird feeder filled with sunflower seeds hung above a brilliant patch of zinnias.

Mother gestured toward the compact Pullman kitchen, devoid of counter space. "Carol you'll enjoy cooking here."

As she stepped to an open door opposite the dining room, she sang out, "Here is the best room of all — our bedroom. The view is the same as from the window in the living room." The fading glow in the sky reflected on the white walls and her smiling face.

"You'll have that same view of the mountain from your room upstairs. Let's look."

The narrow stairs winding upwards reminded me of a lighthouse. To make the spiral, boards fanned out narrow at the center, wider at the outer edge. In the two bedrooms, knotty pine covered the walls and the low ceilings, which were pierced by dormer windows. I felt smothered.

Sipping sherry by the fire gave me a chance to ask Mrs. Young a question. "Does any one else spend the winter on this hillside?" She looked surprised.

"Oh, no, but I don't think you'll miss people. There are deer, foxes, raccoons, and birds for company. I wouldn't leave if my husband were still alive. The innkeeper in the valley is good about plowing the road. You won't be snowed in for more than a couple of days at a time."

Walking up the driveway toward the car in the chill night air, I shivered. Dad squeezed my hand. "We do need to get away from Grandpa's and have a place of our own. Mother has fallen in love with this house. It gives me pleasure to see her so happy."

I felt disconnected from this place and from Mother and Dad's life. The time had come for me to return to Texas.

Feeling Better

"Good news, Mother. I took the safety pins out of my waistband and my skirt stayed up. I'm gaining weight." After three weeks on sick leave, I was feeling better.

Mother smiled. "I can see the change in your face. I hate to think of you going back to Texas next week. It would do you so much good to stay here." She asked whether it was possible to extend my leave.

I sat by the phone a long time before I found the courage to call the adjutant to request an extension. A telegram brought his response. "Sick leave extension denied. Two weeks accrued regular leave time may be added to the five remaining days of sick leave. Please advise."

There were advantages to army life. Every month spent in that hospital had given me the same accrued leave time as on duty, two and one-half days per month. I extended my leave to cover Thanksgiving with the family, our first holiday together in two years.

As I gained stamina, every day became a holiday. Dad said the three of us should celebrate at one of my favorite places, the Spinning Wheel Inn. "Carol dear, remember the evening we brought you and Marie here before you left for the army? I had a lump in my throat the whole time. Tonight is a happy occasion for soon you'll be home for good." This time I was the one with a lump in my throat.

Aunt Pauline, Mother's sister, gathered the family together for a celebration of my recovery. I met Cousin Bob's bride, Helen, and his petite stepdaughter, Leslie Ann. Cousin Ted showed me dozens of pictures of his beloved Betty, a Florida gal he had found living near Mother and Dad's grove. Now there were two named Betty and two named Sherman in the family.

I saw Cousin Polly and her husband Sherman for the first time since attending their wedding. Although out of the navy, Sherman still carried himself with the ramrod erectness of an officer and talked endlessly of his naval career. My brother Sam had put his navy days behind him. He and his Betty talked of their plans for the future.

The din of many conversations at the long dining room table reminded me of the mess hall. This occasion was much more fun. Uncle Ed insisted I take his place at the head of the table.

Aunt Pauline's cooking proved a diet meal could be delicious. None of the guests noticed the difference. Following crustless pumpkin pie and coffee, we gathered in the living room around the upright piano.

During our childhood, a songfest had been the climax to every holiday. We six cousins used to make up in enthusiasm and volume what we lacked in harmony. Now older voices carried on the tradition of singing old favorites. For a short time, we felt young again.

Mother called out a song request. I chose "The Bird in The Gilded Cage." Sam made us laugh with his rendition of "The Man on the Flying Trapeze." Ted dedicated "Don't Sit Under The Apple Tree With Anyone Else but Me" to his Betty.

The songs of WWI and WWII were sung with nostalgia rather than longing and heartache. When I requested Christmas carols, everyone laughed. Even though it was November, I wanted to make up for Christmases I had missed. Finally, Aunt Pauline protested her stiff fingers could play only one more song. She ended the evening with the hymn, "Abide with Me."

The following week on Armistice Day, later called Veterans Day, the family lined up on Aunt Hannah's wide porch to watch the parade. Since 1885, the Morrisons had enjoyed a grandstand seat for parades passing by on Greenwood Avenue.

We could hear the shrill fifes and the muffled beat of drums long before the first parade unit came in view. As the color guard approached, I realized I, the only person in sight in uniform, was going to have a busy afternoon saluting the flag.

My first salute took on significance. In a convertible driven by a WWII veteran, sat a wizened frail veteran of the Civil War. Wrapped in a blanket for protection against the November chill, the one-time drummer boy wore his wide brimmed blue hat pulled low over his brow.

No parade would have been complete without the Bethel Fife and Drum Corps. Grandpa's brother, Uncle Stub, still marched in the back row playing his left-handed fife. Everyone in town knew he was positioned on the outside to make his unsteady gait less noticeable. He always arrived ready to march well fortified by a visit to the local tavern. I'd never met him. Grandpa refused to acknowledge his brother's existence.

A huge flag led the group of WWI veterans riding on a float draped in red, white, and blue bunting. "Dad, why aren't you up there with your comrades?"

"I tried a few meetings of The American Legion, the most popular group of WWI veterans, but I wasn't interested in rehashing stories of the past. I wanted to live in the present, much preferred doing things with Mother and you children."

The High School Marching Band preceded the large contingent of WWII veterans. Soldiers, Sailors, Marines and one lone Coast Guardsman marched tall and proud. They were new enough to civilian life to retain their erect bearing and military precision.

I saluted American flags, large and small, carried by Boy Scouts, Girl Scouts, Campfire Girls, Indian Guides and school children, as well as fraternal organizations and The League of Women Voters. My saluting arm ached by the time the deep rumble of fire engines signaled the end of the parade.

My final salute had gone to a horseman dressed in the garb of a Revolutionary War soldier. He struggled to control the long pole attached to the flag of the colonies, a circle of thirteen stars on a field of blue next to red and white stripes.

I stepped back inside the comforting warmth of the house and reflected on the past hour. People in the West did not understand the sense of history and responsibility ingrained in New Englanders by the centuries of continuity built from one generation to the next.

I thought about my ancestor Roger Sherman, who had rallied his Connecticut family and neighbors to the cause of freedom. The withered veteran of the Civil War reminded me of Grandpa's stories about his Uncle Thomas. Imprisoned by the Confederates in notorious Andersonville Prison, Thomas was never heard from again. His mother cried for her lost boy every day the rest of her life.

I could understand the sacrifice Mother and Dad had made in WWI to postpone their marriage until Dad's army enlistment had ended. He had refused to marry during the war for fear he might be severely wounded and become a burden to Mother.

Down through the generations the men had responded to the call to duty to protect the country. Now I continued the tradition — the first woman in the family to serve in the armed forces. In spite of the personal cost, I felt proud and privileged to be doing my part.

After Thanksgiving, I would be ready to return to Fort Bliss, El Paso, Texas to serve the seven remaining months of my army career at Beaumont General Hospital.

Return To Duty

For the first time in many years, the Morrison family celebrated Thanksgiving in the home where Dad had been born. Aunt Hannah, her culinary skill limited to baked potatoes, gave Mother and me free rein in the kitchen. Roasting one plump turkey in her gas oven was more fun than dealing with twenty birds in the army mess.

In the pantry, I reached for cut glass water tumblers on the top shelf. From a deep drawer, I selected the longest of several snow-white damask tablecloths to cover the three leaves added to the dining room table.

Opening the silver drawer, I admired a row of coin silver spoons, delicate and fragile. They had been a wedding gift to Mary Ann and David Morrison, my great-great grandparents, in 1828. "Aunt Hannah, I'd like to use Mary Ann's spoons for the coffee."

She hesitated. "I guess this once it will be all right."

When she saw the cranberry sauce shimmering in a cut glass dish, she nodded approval. "Mama used that dish for preserves on Sundays. When your father was a child, there were always nine of us at the table."

I wondered how many relatives had joined the family on holidays in the 1890's. We numbered twelve, including my cousin Mildred's two children, Shirley and Earl. "Let's call everyone to dinner." I opened the door from the kitchen flooding the dining room with the tantalizing odors of turkey, gravy, creamed onions, and turnips.

Guided by Mother's artistic place cards, hungry children and eager adults found their seats at the table. We joined hands for the blessing, kept short for the sake of the children.

When I appeared from the kitchen balancing the heavy bird on the large Haviland platter, little Earl gasped, "Are we going to eat all that?"

Dad picked up the bone-handled carving knife and sharpened the blade on the hone. When he pricked the skin of the bird, I relaxed. The burst of clear juice assured me the turkey had been cooked to perfection. During the meal the dining room, usually so quiet, resounded with chatter and laughter.

Before serving the pumpkin pie, Aunt Hannah padded round the table, a small metal tray in one hand and a soft-bristle brush in the other. She brushed away stray crumbs from the tablecloth, reminding me of my younger days. I had never eaten a roll to avoid the embarrassment of leaving crumbs by my plate.

Dad broke into my reverie. "Hate to bring this happy occasion to a close. Hazel, Carol, and I must leave you to attend the wedding reception for Bill Crill's daughter at the Hotel Green."

Bill, who had shortened his name from Ciccerelli to Crill, had been Dad's foreman on many highway construction projects. Dad relied on Bill's ability to handle the workmen and appreciated his ribald sense of humor. Bill's daughter had chosen Thanksgiving Day to marry the son of Joe Vaghi. Families in Bethel turned to Joe to make new furniture or repair the old.

This was my introduction to an Italian wedding reception, a colorful exuberant noisy affair compared to staid wedding receptions in the Congregational Church parlor.

Those in the service seemed to gravitate to others in uniform. Several military men asked me to dance. Another invitation came from an unlikely source, "One-arm Dominick." It must have been the red wine, which prompted gray-haired Dominick to ask the boss's daughter to dance.

He grasped me firmly around the waist. Unfazed by his prosthesis, after my experience with army patients, I grabbed the icy hook, a replacement for his right hand. Away we pranced across the dance floor at breakneck speed, to the applause of the appreciative audience.

Back in the thirties, artificial limbs for injuries had been a rarity. My friend, Alice Landis, and I, age fifteen, sat on the steps at our new lake cottage watching Dominick load debris into a dump truck. Intrigued by his competence at using the hook in place of a hand, we raced to the bathroom and stuck a camera out the window. The results were disappointing — one grainy shot. Neither he nor we questioned the propriety of calling him "One-arm Dominick."

Now, due to thousands of wartime injuries, a prosthesis was no longer a novelty. I wished Dominick could benefit from new technology developed at Walter Reed. I had seen the improvement in a soldier's morale after he was fitted with a natural-looking hand with improved mobility.

For a couple of hours, I had forgotten hepatitis and enjoyed my return to the social scene, but the fast paced dance drained away my energy. "Mother and Dad, I hate to leave but I'm exhausted." Dad took my arm and guided me toward the door.

"We're ready to go. Let's hurry. Here comes Dominick hoping for a repeat performance."

Safely out-of-sight, in the elevator Mother's question made me laugh. "What are you going to tell your Texas friends about your new boyfriend?"

Two days later Dad drove me to LaGuardia Field for my return flight to Texas. No tears on parting, for I'd soon be home again. As the plane gained altitude, I looked down on the Statue of Liberty standing proud and tall in the sunshine. She reminded me of the night six weeks before, when she had welcomed me, worn and weary, to New York.

I felt like a different person now. Although still tired and thin, I felt confident I could cope with the days ahead. The year had been difficult. I looked forward to 1947 when my life was bound to be better.

Back on Ward 85, the lonely rows of empty beds and blood tests before breakfast came as a shock. Dr. Cernock, as well as most of the patients, had vanished. This time I was an ambulatory patient with permission to leave the ward. In the afternoons, I escaped to Janet Fox's room for a nap. We had first met at basic training in San Antonio.

Captain Lord acted as though I had never been on sick leave. When I met her in the hall, she sneered, "Are you still a patient?"

Peg Ward, my traveling companion from Memphis to Texas the previous year, showed up by my bed. I had not set eyes on her in months. She put it to me bluntly, "I think you're afraid to go back to work. We've covered for you long enough."

A few days later Peg's wish was granted. Colonel Reyer ordered me back to duty. Lieutenant Leaf, my new doctor gave me the bad news.

"I told Colonel Reyer you're not strong enough to work eight hours a day. Your liver function tests aren't back to normal and you need lots of rest. I'm sorry. My words were no match for his vindictive attitude." I did not explain to the doctor that Colonel Reyer was getting back at me for the unfortunate incident over my sick leave.

Lieutenant Leaf suggested he ask Captain Lord to assign me an easy job. I begged him to say nothing. I had learned asking for favors had a way of backfiring.

Lieutenant Leaf and I felt satisfaction over a small victory, which we surmised irritated Colonel Reyer. My chart did not get to the registrar in time to cut the orders, delaying my return to duty for three days.

My new assignment seemed almost too good to be true — the station hospital at Biggs Field. Only two miles from the Annex, where I had been a patient, Mary Schroeder from Walter Reed, Janet Fox from basic training, and I would be the staff dietitians working under Lieutenant Louden.

Janet expressed our delight. "Aren't we lucky? We'll be five miles away from Captain Lord and the main hospital."

The Hospital Annex, including Ward 85, would become living quarters for German scientists working on the atom bomb and V-2 rockets. Some of them had defected to the United States others had been captured during the war.

We had been aware of the compound, visible in the distance, where the scientists had been held behind barbed wire. Both the scientists and their role in development of bomb had been top secret until the blast on Hiroshima.

Now in 1946, the government was setting them free. German families arrived daily to live at the Annex. It seemed strange to see clothes lines strung between the wards and children riding tricycles in the street.

I, too, felt liberated. After five long months, I was no longer patient Morrison. I could hold my head high, once again Lieutenant Morrison, Dietitian. Looking forward to my new assignment, I moved into the barracks expecting an improvement over the ward in the hospital.

The sickly green walls, a preferred army color, were depressing. The large window faced the bleak desert, not a tree in sight. A metal bureau, straight chair, and single bed furnished my new home.

Enthusiasm for my room in a one-story temporary building faded away.

Biggs Field

The first day on duty did not meet Lieutenant Leaf's criteria for an easy assignment. In eight hours, every patient remaining at the Annex had to be moved to Biggs Field station hospital. That chaotic day allowed me no time to "ease back" into the job.

The transfer of patients did not go smoothly. SNAFU, a favored GI expression, described the foul-ups. The diabetic patients showed up for lunch at Biggs Field while their weighed diets awaited them at the Annex. Four hundred pounds of potatoes disappeared. None of the pans arrived in the Biggs

Field kitchen. The chow line ran out of food at lunch leaving an irate line of hungry people unfed. The same thing happened at supper.

Dead tired, I was in no mood to talk to Lieutenant Loudon, the dietitian in charge, when she stopped me in the hall. "I hate to give you this news on a hell-of-a-day like this one, particularly, when you just moved last week. Tomorrow you move closer to Biggs Field."

The new quarters proved to be flimsier and draftier than the old. At least, the small room had not been painted army green. I stared out the window at the same desolate desert view — not a tree, not a blade of grass, not a cactus in sight, just a huge sky over a sea of sand.

Living only a quarter of a mile from the Biggs Field airstrip, our small medical group felt part of the Army Air Force. We fed all personnel on the base, as well as three hundred convalescent patients. Eating together in the mess hall, personnel and patients became one happy family.

One of the most active airfields during the war, Biggs Field remained a busy place. When the planes roared down the runway at 5:00 a.m., the building shook, the windows rattled. Their noisy departure followed by the precise notes of the bugle call made an alarm clock unnecessary.

Lieutenant Louden, a heavy-set, middle-aged woman with a cigarette always dangling from the corner of her mouth, tore around the kitchen like a whirlwind accomplishing little. Whenever she dashed by the huge steam-jacketed soup kettle, she peered in.

The kitchen help grinned when the long ash from her cigarette drifted downwards into the soup. One of the GIs exclaimed, "That ain't no soup kettle. It's Louden's giant ash tray."

The happy-go-lucky attitude of the air force crews who ate with us kept us laughing. Wearing cowboy boots, their headgear set at a jaunty angle, they defied all attempts to make them conform to the military dress code. Fearless and daring, they lived life at a fast pace.

Lieutenant Louden's ineptness at ordering food led to constant shortages of basic supplies. Appalled when the milk ran out, I said to Mary, "How did we ever learn so much in one year at Walter Reed? We're better trained to run a mess hall than people who've made the army their career."

Mary's departure on a twenty-one day leave left Janet and me to run the mess hall over the holidays. We made our own schedule and divided the workload between us. Both Easterners flung into this desert spot in Texas, we had much in common.

Janet had lost her mother two years previously. Her father, a doctor in Philadelphia, planned to visit her for the holidays. The evening before his arrival, Janet and I returned to the mess hall on our own time to help decorate for Christmas. We did not trust the mess sergeant and the night cooks to do a good job.

It took many cups of black coffee to keep me going until ten p.m. The cooks, reminding me of my brothers, showed little patience for separating the shiny strands of tinsel icicles. They tended to throw gobs of tinsel toward the tops of two massive Christmas trees. Strand by strand, Janet and I decorated the lower branches.

Janet appealed to the sergeant for help. "Sergeant, if you strung this red rope from beam to beam across the ceiling, we could hang red bells from it." He muttered to himself about the ideas of foolish women.

I teased, "Come on. It's Christmas."

As he teetered on the ladder, Janet, almost six feet tall, handed him the red paper bells. Soon the ceiling appeared to be a mass of color. The sergeant surveyed his handiwork.

"You're right. The patients will enjoy Christmas dinner in such a festive setting." Janet and I lingered to clink coke bottles with the cooks and the sergeant in celebration of a job well done.

On Christmas Eve, Dr. Fox, a tall, dignified man with a dry sense of humor, took Janet and me to The Tivoli, our favorite restaurant in Juarez, Mexico. While watching the spirited dances in a lively floorshow, I sipped a forbidden margarita.

Dr. Fox twirled the glass in his hand and peered over his spectacles. "I'm not sure Philadelphians would approve of a drink with salt on the edge of the glass."

Later we strolled past shops full of colorful wares. Persistent shopkeepers, desperate to make a sale, tried to lure us inside. Janet and I smiled at the incongruous sight of Dr. Fox strolling the crowded street, a bright pink and green donkey piñata tucked under his arm.

Janet pulled me aside. "I'm so happy to see my father having a good time. Wonder what his patients would say, if they could see him now?" The non-traditional Christmas Eve in a foreign land left the three of us in high spirits.

Back in El Paso, we parted in front of Dr. Fox's hotel. He gave Janet a lingering kiss before taking a step toward me. "I think you should have a kiss, too. Merry Christmas. Thank you, girls, for making this a memorable evening instead of a lonely one."

As the taxi sped us through the deserted decorated streets to Biggs Field, we planned for the workday ahead.

Back in my room, I lighted the tiny Christmas tree. "Janet, it's after midnight. It's Christmas day. While we're still keyed up, let's open our presents. I have a hunch when we get off duty we'll be too tired to care about gifts."

I began with a small box from my brother Sherman. It contained a leaf shaped pin washed with a thin coat of silver. His note said he bought it from a starving German artist on the dock in Bremerhaven. The fellow had used his ingenuity to turn bits of scrap metal into souvenirs.

Sherman's second gift caught me by surprise. At twenty, recently released from the merchant marine, he sent me a subtle message that I could no longer think of him as "little brother." Wrapped in many sheets of pastel tissue lay a sexy black slip lavishly decorated with lace.

By 2:00 a.m. I had to give up. "Janet, my eyes won't stay open. In four hours we have to go to work. Merry Christmas." I didn't even hear her leave the room. When she returned to knock on my door, the first streaks of dawn lit the sky.

Munching on coconut patties, Dad's gift from Jacquimoux, a candy store in Miami, we hurried toward the mess hall. The rays of the rising sun highlighted the red mountain peaks against a bright blue sky promising a clear Christmas day.

That peaceful dawn gave no hint of the chaos we'd face before the day ended.

Send in the MPs

On Christmas morning 1946, few people showed up in the mess hall for breakfast. Janet and I lingered over coffee before plunging into a busy day. We had agreed she would supervise the kitchen and I the mess hall. My first priority was to decorate twenty tables to accommodate two hundred diners.

Two volunteers, recruited from the breakfast chow line, assembled the honeycomb tissue paper bells left over from our earlier decorating. By the time I had scattered bells over fake greenery at the hundredth place setting, my enthusiasm for the project waned. I could understand why the impatient cooks had thrown the globs of tinsel at the Christmas trees.

The elaborate design on the large menu seemed too grand for meals served on metal trays. The cover displayed a cutout of a candle in a candlestick backed by silver foil and accented by a red satin cord with tassel. The traditional dinner menu printed inside varied little from previous years.

The mess sergeant surveyed the room, "Lieutenant, this looks great, almost like home. We've done a good job, haven't we?"

The cooks wrestled the hundred ration pans, heaped high with turkey, cornbread stuffing, yams, and vegetables, onto the steam table. Janet appeared from the humid kitchen. She pushed back her damp hair. "At last its time to serve our guests."

The loud voice of the mess sergeant resounded in the hall. "Chow Time. Patients first in line."

As the men entered through double doors, Janet and I handed out packages of cigarettes. We gave each man a cheery greeting, "Merry Christmas, Private. Don't skimp on the seconds."

The detachment men and hospital personnel followed the patients in the food line. Many of the detachment appeared to be drunk. Some couldn't carry their own trays, others slid off their chairs to the floor.

"Don't sit near me," shouted an angry voice.

"Try and stop me," snarled a drunken orderly.

Before we could react, a tray sailed over our heads and crashed on the opposite wall. Our carefully planned Christmas celebration turned into a brawl. Drunken men hurled metal trays across the room and startled patients cowered under the tables.

The mess sergeant tried to separate the instigators of the fight, but he was no match for the unruly crowd. "Call the MPs," he shouted.

I rushed to the office, ran my trembling finger down the list of emergency numbers on the wall. The angry shouts and catcalls in the dining room grew louder. "This is Lieutenant Morrison in the mess hall. We have a near riot on our hands. We need all the men you can spare."

The response from the guardhouse made me gasp. "Sorry, the MPs are too drunk to move. There's no one here fit to help you."

I studied the list again. Officer of the Day, I'd try him. What a relief to hear his positive response, "I'm on my way." I rushed back to the mess hall and edged my way along the wall to avoid the fray.

"MPs too drunk. The O.D. is coming." The out-manned sergeant gave a brief nod in my direction. Stunned, Janet and I stood helpless on the sideline. We watched as rolls were hurled across the room like missiles and Christmas dinners were dumped on peoples' heads. Food, mashed red bells, and torn menus formed a squishy mess underfoot.

"At-ten-shun." The Officer of the Day loomed tall in the doorway. He bellowed his orders in a tone approaching rage. The confused uproar died down. His icy stare dared anyone to challenge his authority. No one did.

The mob remained frozen in place. The O.D. ordered the ringleaders still on their feet out of the room. With the aid of the mess sergeant and a few sober men, he dragged away bodies passed out on tables and the floor.

The truce did not last long. The cooks were still brushing up debris when a free-for-all broke out in the hall. The sounds of splintering wood, as chairs crashed against the walls, mixed with the curses and angry shouts of the rioters, frightened those of us trapped in the room.

After the hubbub faded away, a dark mood descended on the mess hall. Our Christmas Day, so long in the planning, lay in ruins. Trying to put up a good front, Janet and I set fresh tables.

When the last person had been fed, Janet and I joined the rest of the dietitians for Christmas dinner at 3:00 p.m. in the main hospital. We were too upset to talk, too tired to eat.

My outlook improved when I opened an envelope from Mother and Dad. They had sent three, one for each meal on Christmas Day. The one for dinner contained an original poem and a generous check.

Janet and I ambled back to the mess hall to serve supper. "Janet, I know how anxious you are to get to town and see your father. Go ahead. Not many will show up tonight. I can manage alone."

She said she'd feel guilty to leave me. "Go ahead. This is my Christmas present to your father for the delightful time on Christmas Eve in Mexico." Had that been only the night before?

Back in quarters, after serving supper, I wondered why I had accepted the Heasleys' invitation for dinner at eight. As I stepped into their living room, feeling confident in my new black dress, my fatigue melted away.

The fragrance of pine and candles filled the air. I sat close to the Christmas tree, decorated with miniature piñatas, and nibbled on corn chips and salsa. I loved the distinctly Texas flair to the evening. A telegram to all of us from Dad added a touch of Connecticut and brought thoughts of home to me.

Carol Heasley grew indignant over my description of the mayhem in the mess hall. "Darlin'," how could this happen? Even the MPs drunk?"

Herbert nodded in agreement at my explanation. "The disciplined troops have been discharged. The new recruits are kids and riff-raff off the streets. No longer fighting a common cause to beat a common enemy, they remain an undisciplined group led by poorly trained officers. After this day, I'll be glad to leave the army."

Kay Heasley drove me back to quarters. My gift from the Heasleys, the largest, brightest red poinsettia I'd ever seen, added a welcome note of color to my drab room. In the following weeks, it served as a reminder of the lovely Christmas dinner with understanding friends. Slowly the disaster in the mess hall receded into the background.

Mother's comments made me smile. "I don't think much of your commanding officer. Wasn't he the one responsible for the men in the detachment?" Her mental picture of the army as a large happy family concerned about my welfare had not changed.

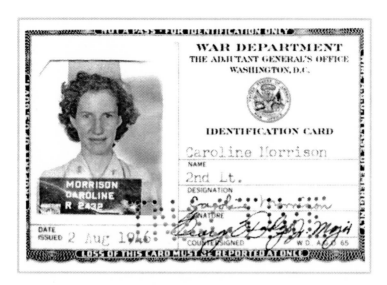

Stricken with Hepatitis in 1946.

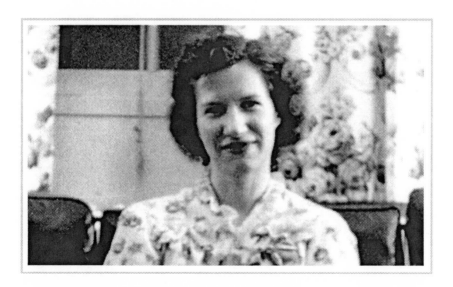

Feeling Better by 25th birthday.

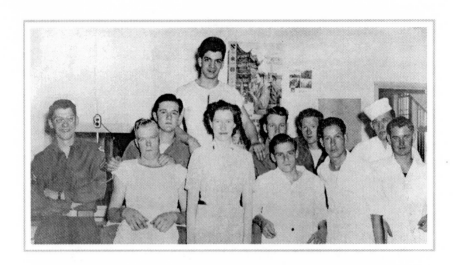

Return to duty.

Lt. Morrison 1947,
the lady in charge.

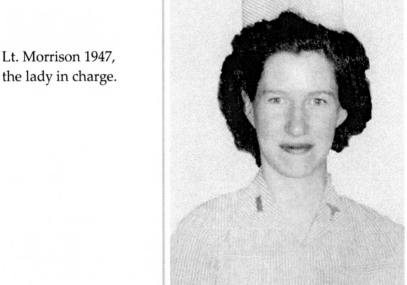

The Last Eight Months 1947

In exchange for working on Christmas day, Janet and I earned an extra day off. Twenty-four hours in bed did little to restore my energy after the debacle in the mess hall. For days, I slept whenever I wasn't on duty.

Near the end of that week, Janet knocked on my door. "Carol, wake up! Let's go outside. It's snowing."

"Snowing? Give me ten minutes to dress." We left the barracks and found the world transformed. The harsh desert had disappeared under a fluffy blanket of white. The light touch of snowflakes on my face felt soft as feathers.

Janet brushed the snow from her sleeve. "Even the snowflakes are bigger in Texas. This will spoil the image promoted by the Chamber of Commerce — Sunny El Paso, Winter Vacationland. Do you think they'll cancel the New Year's football game?"

"I doubt Texans would do that," I said. "They take too much pride in their toughness. They'd better not cancel, not when I plan to be there to root for Dad's alma mater, Cincinnati."

It did seem incongruous for the University of Cincinnati to be playing Virginia Poly Tech in the Sun Bowl in Texas on New Year's Day. Why would two eastern teams accept a Bowl bid far out in the Wild West?

On New Year's Eve, I gladly said goodbye to 1946. It had been a tough year. Getting to bed by 10:00 p.m. seemed a better way to celebrate than staying up late. I wanted to be ready for the game. Next morning the sun shone dazzling bright on the snow but a chill wind foretold a cold day.

Although off duty on this New Year's Day, I responded to a distress call from Freddie in the storeroom. "Lieutenant, there's an emergency in the mess hall. We need your help." Hoping this wouldn't be a repeat of the brawl on Christmas, I couldn't resist his plea. Freddie, an eighteen-year-old private, reminded me of my brother Sherman.

He waited at the door while I knocked the snow off my boots. "Happy New Year, Lieutenant. Step into the walk-in refrigerator and look behind the potatoes. That seemed the best place to hide your present." Curious, I stepped into the icy cubicle.

Behind a towering sack of potatoes, a lone glass of eggnog sat atop a paper sack. Judging from the strong fumes of alcohol, that New Year's treat did not meet my strict dietary requirements. Teeth chattering, I poured Freddie's gift of eggnog down the drain in the center of the walk-in refrigerator. However, I kept the bag containing a pint of whiskey.

I stepped back into the warm kitchen. The cooks gathered round me shouting, "Happy New Year, Lieutenant. We don't want you to be cold at the football game."

The ruse Freddie had used to lure me to the mess hall left little time to dress in my heaviest clothes for the game. Janet had to overcome the taxi driver's doubts before he agreed to hide our heavy olive-drab comforters in the trunk.

"We need the blankets to keep us warm at the game but we don't dare get caught taking army property off the base." He suggested we might need something stronger than blankets to fortify us against the bitter cold. We assured him we were prepared — Freddie and the cooks had taken care of that.

While most of the spectators turned blue in the frigid air, we remained cozy, wrapped up to our chins in army comforters. I told Janet I'd always known there must be a use for those things but never considered a football game. Sleeping under one felt like smothering under a load of bricks.

I seemed to be the only person in the stadium rooting for Cincinnati. When my team won 16-14, 1947 was off to a great start.

Later, I wrote Dad a long letter giving him details of the game and the colorful half time. I described the band, triple in size of any I had ever seen, plus a hundred girls in the color guard chancing pneumonia in skimpy outfits. Their eagerness to restore circulation to chilled bodies probably inspired the energetic performance and spectacular show.

Much to the chagrin of El Pasoans, sub-freezing temperatures continued for the next two weeks. Water pipes froze. Chill wind swept through our living quarters forcing sand through every crack of the old wooden buildings. We breathed and ate sand. At one meal, a liberal coating of sand turned chocolate cake with white icing into cake with brown icing.

Severe weather across the country brought airmail delivery to a halt. Never before had I gone two weeks without a letter from home. Back in Connecticut, no mail from Texas concerned Mother and Dad. They feared another calamity had befallen me. After fourteen days, the longest cold spell on record broke.

Freddie was not my only admirer. Yakanak, an Eskimo patient often waited outside the mess hall to walk me back to quarters. Only five feet tall with straight black hair, alert black eyes, and three missing teeth, he never complained about his bland ulcer diet. He seemed an unlikely soldier and an unlikely Baptist missionary, although to be one was his goal.

One noon, going down the chow line, he handed me a list of words on a wrinkled sheet of paper. "I teach you speak Aleut. Learn these words by next meal. Jamai — hello, stoolook — table, stoolchick — chair, whash buddy — Oh Lord."

The following day I tried out my new language, "Jamai, Yakanak."

He looked at me in disgust. "That's not way you say it. Repeat after me."

By the end of the week, the vocabulary list included boy, girl, and love. It seemed prudent to end this game. "Sorry, I'm too busy to learn any more words. We're holding up the cafeteria line."

His shoulders sagged. "But how you marry me and be missionary in the Aleutians, if you can't learn my language?"

"Yakanak, your country's too cold for me. I'd freeze. When you get home, you look for a pretty Aleutian girl to be missionary." He had taught me one useful phrase. Whenever anything went wrong, Janet and I looked at each other and exclaimed, "Whash buddy. Oh, Lord."

Throughout January, chill winds and blowing sand kept us confined to quarters. Hour after hour, we played bridge. Although the natives warned us March would bring the worst sandstorms of the year, spring-like weather in February gave us a break.

One Sunday morning Mary Schroeder, the dietitian from my class at Walter Reed, invited me to a waffle breakfast. She had warned me I'd have to walk three blocks from the bus stop to her isolated quarters in the desert. As the bus pulled away, her barracks loomed in the distance — a lonely outpost silhouetted against the sky.

A hint of spring filled the air. Buds on the desert plants gave a preview of the riot of color to come. Small birds hopped from cactus to cactus. I wondered how they avoided the sharp thorns. Warm sun on my back relaxed me.

I never remembered the fall, never knew whether I fainted or lost my balance. I came to, sprawled in the weeds beside the gravel road. Searing pain shot through my ankle. I gingerly sat up and looked in dismay at the blood running from my scraped elbow and at my torn nylons.

The silence across the vast desert settled over me like a heavy weight. On Sunday, the bus would not pass that way again for hours. I felt helpless, frightened, and frustrated. Hot and thirsty, I struggled to my feet, set my eyes on that distant building, and forced myself to limp along.

Step after painful step, I kept my eyes on my goal. An hour later, I stumbled, exhausted and irrational, into Mary's room.

She packed my ankle, twice its normal size, in ice and treated my scrapes and bruises. My throbbing foot would not move. When Mary called for an ambulance to transport me to the main hospital I panicked.

"This is so discouraging. I can't believe I'm going back to the hospital. Why did this happen now? I've been out of the hospital only two months. How long, do you suppose, I'll be a patient this time?"

Help Is On The Way

The technician in the emergency room did his best to lift my spirits. "You're lucky it's Sunday morning. We've already taken care of the Saturday night drunks. We have plenty of time for you. Wow! This ankle has to be x-rayed before you see the doctor."

Thinking back to my treacherous wheelchair ride to the Bloody Bar, I was dubious about a wheelchair trip to the lab. A serious non-talkative private hauled the squeaky chair up a long ramp through heavy double doors marked, "Hazardous Area X-ray Department."

A patient lay on a stretcher next to the cumbersome x-ray machine. "Help is on the way," the private assured us. "The technician should be here in five minutes. Good luck." The door slammed shut behind him. A crushing silence lay between the stretcher and my wheelchair.

When the young man on the stretcher moaned, I tried to forget my own distress by concentrating on him. "What happened to you?"

He gasped through clenched teeth, "Fell down a flight of stairs. Hell, if my ankles are broken, I'll miss my chance at making sergeant. Where's that damn technician? I've been here at least an hour."

Five minutes passed, ten minutes, half an hour. The moans of my companion increased in intensity. My swollen ankle looked like a multi-colored birthday balloon. "I'll try to get us some help." I pushed the heavy wood chair to the exit. Standing on my good foot, I ignored the throbbing pain in my injured ankle and threw my weight against the lead-lined door. It did not budge. We remained trapped.

An hour later, a corporal burst through the door putting on his lab coat. "Gee, I'm sorry. I've been lying on my bunk 'on call' all morning. No one told me I had two emergencies here. Who's first?"

"He is, but could you find us some water?" Waiting my turn on the x-ray table, I took slow sips from the tiny paper cup. Moving my foot into position sent pains to the top of my head. I crushed the cup in my hand but kept my ankle still.

"Did that fellow break his ankles?" The technician nodded. "He sure did. Wonder what kind of horsing around led to a fall like that? You may be luckier than him, maybe not. Your ankle's not broken but bad sprains take longer to heal than clean breaks." Tired, discouraged, and hungry, I wondered why I had had an accident on Sunday, the day the hospital was always short-staffed.

A nurse helped me stretch out on a bed in a two-bed room. "Your roommate is on leave. I'll be back with ice for your ankle." Three hours later, she kept her promise. She appeared in the doorway with an ice pack and a food tray. Although I had not eaten all day, ice to relieve the pain was what I craved.

Unlike my first hospital experience when I knew few people, my friends rallied round. Janet brought my robe, slippers, and toothbrush from Biggs Field to the main hospital. Velma came with books and, most important to me, writing paper, pen and stamps. I waited until my dark mood lifted to write home.

Dear Daddy,
I love my beautiful Valentine handkerchief. Just admiring the embroidered red heart has done so much for my morale, for I have once again met misfortune.
It seems as though, no matter how hard I try, just as I am getting back on my feet, something always

happens. This time I fell and sprained my ankle very badly. The x-ray shows my ankle is not broken, but the ligament is torn away from the bone.

The doctor says nothing can be done until the swelling goes down. After thirty hours "on ice" with my leg elevated, there is still a lot of swelling. Probably my foot will be put in a cast.

I try to look at the bright side, but I don't feel I have the patience to be bed-ridden for long. I am in a two-bed private room, a new experience for me — much more restful than the ward. Being flat on my back makes it difficult to write. The Red Cross is here with a movie. I'll write more tomorrow.

All my love,

Carol

The following Saturday brought an old army custom — doctors making rounds to assess the progress of each patient. Eight doctors hovered over my ankle to discuss the pros and cons of my case. They made me feel like a page in a medical book.

The Colonel said his technique had always been to shoot the ankle full of Novocain, strap the foot, and make the patient walk.

A major spoke up, "Maybe, with a mild sprain, but it stands to reason only rest will heal a torn ligament."

Another noted I would be getting along faster had I not broken the blood vessels. With a parting shot that a sprain, such as mine, was much worse than a simple fracture, they wandered off down the hall.

The arrival of a roommate put my situation in proper prospective. Although Judith had recently undergone surgery, her radiant smile charmed everyone. Tumbling brown hair and clear blue eyes added to her beauty.

For three years, she'd been a nurse in the South Pacific. Staff members there had been warned repeatedly to report any foot problems, but she ignored the sores on her feet. Aware of the shortage of nurses, she stayed on duty in the operating room tent until she collapsed.

The doctor's diagnosis included malaria, dysentery and, much more serious, jungle rot in her feet. Since being evacuated to Texas, Judith had undergone seven operations in efforts to straighten her toes. A viral infection had caused them to curl under.

Only a flimsy curtain separated us when the surgeon gave her his verdict. "My dear, I did my best. There is no improvement. I doubt whether you'll ever walk again."

I had seen much suffering and agony in the past two and a half years, things I would never forget. This seemed among the most tragic. After hearing her receive such devastating news, I realized I was the lucky one. Her display of faith and courage made my swollen ankle insignificant.

After the doctor left, she called through the curtain. "Did you hear what he said? To hell with him, I am going to walk again. We've seen the boys fight back from worse than this. If they can do it, I can too. As long as my fiancé sticks by me, I'll not give up the fight."

Along with my Sunday supper tray came a telegram. "Leaving New York 10 p.m. train. Arrive El Paso Wednesday 8 a.m. Love, Daddy"

I couldn't believe it. Dad planned to spend three nights and three days on a train just to give my morale a boost? I suspected he and Mother wanted assurance I had told them the whole story.

Whirlwind Week

Dad's strenuous train journey from New York ended in El Paso on a crisp, clear morning. Carol Heasley, the Texan friend who had made me part of her family, waited for him on the platform. As she rushed toward him, her hands outstretched in greeting, her smile put him at ease.

"I'm Carol Heasley. Welcome to Texas. I know you're Bob 'cause Carol looks so much like you."

While Carol Heasley drove Dad on the scenic route to the hospital, I waited impatiently in my wheelchair in the lounge. By the time they greeted me, they appeared to be life-long friends.

Dad dropped down on one knee to my level, his eyes looking into mine. "Dear, this is a dream come true to spend a week with you. My trip has been exhilarating. Your friend is charming. If only Mother could have come with me, this would be perfect. We felt we could not leave Hannah alone."

Carol said a hasty goodbye. Dad and I found a secluded corner where we could talk and talk. I longed to hear about home but Dad insisted we discuss my welfare and my recent accident. I tried to make light of my misery.

"For a week I lay in bed looking at my swollen rainbow-colored ankle. The doctor did nothing, except give me a few pain pills." I hesitated to tell Dad the doctor had been adept at running his hand up my leg farther than necessary. Much to my relief, he had been transferred. I expected to meet a new doctor the following day.

The next morning, I knew Dad had brought me good luck. Dr. McNeil, an efficient man of few words, ordered immediate treatment — physical therapy. Soaking my foot in a whirlpool bath twice a day, plus a few simple exercises, brought dramatic improvement. While I spent my time in therapy, Carol Heasley whisked Dad away to introduce him to the customs and foods of her beloved Texas.

Evenings, Dad pushed me in the wheelchair to the lounge in the nurses' quarters. We could always find singles eager to make up a foursome for bridge. After I graduated to crutches, we left behind the manicured lawns and spreading trees of the main hospital to ride the bus to Biggs Field in the desert.

I wanted Dad to see where I had lived and worked. In the mess kitchen, he shook hands with the cooks and glanced at the stainless steel tables

"You're doing a great job. I remember from WWI how much elbow grease it takes to keep a mess like this clean."

Freddie's remarks made him laugh. "Lieutenant Morrison's a good boss. This place ain't right without her. Maybe, if you go home, she'll come back to work."

Observing the chow line, Dad sighed, "The boys look so young. It's hard to believe I was their age when I took my basic training in South Carolina in 1917."

His eyes lit up in recognition as Yakanak pushed his tray past the beef stew. Dad gave me a wink. "I'm glad you turned down his offer of marriage. He's not exactly what I had in mind for a son-in-law."

In the afternoon, we attended the post movie in a Quonset hut. Like cars at a drive-in, row on row of wheelchairs formed lines in front of the screen. Ambulatory patients and guests clustered on a few chairs in the rear. When the picture ended, Dad maneuvered my wheelchair through the wide double-doors leading to a ramp.

Suddenly, racing wheelchairs whizzed by us at dizzying speeds. High-pitched whistles and loud Rebel yells filled the air. Swept along by the momentum of the crowd, Dad kept a firm grasp on my chair. Forced to run to the bottom of the ramp, he steered me away from the mob into the shade. He stopped to catch his breath and mop his brow.

"I'll never forget this experience. We're lucky to have escaped alive."

Although I had to stay behind for therapy, Carol Heasley treated Dad to a day in Juarez, Mexico. They returned with their arms full of packages. She said she'd never met a man who enjoyed shopping the way Dad did. Dad said he'd never eaten a better steak.

He spread out his colorful array of purchases. "Carol, I thought you and Mother should have these jackets. It will be a thrill when I can see the two of you wearing them."

The jackets, one light blue felt, the other brighter blue, were embroidered with Mexican motifs on back and front — sombreros, donkeys, cacti, and peasant women.

I laughed. "Dad, when Mother and I walk down Greenwood Avenue in Bethel, Connecticut wearing these bright outfits, we'll cause a sensation. What fun that will be."

The last evening of Dad's visit, my friends put on a bountiful buffet in his honor in the nurses' lounge. Each dietitian had prepared her favorite recipe. Dad remarked after such a delicious meal he would not need to eat again until he was back home.

On Sunday, I insisted on seeing him off at the station. As the train appeared in the distance, I tried to hide my unhappiness over his departure by concentrating on my crutches.

Dad brushed a lock of hair from my forehead. "It makes me so happy to see you looking so well. Except for your ankle, you have not appeared this healthy, or this happy, since your college days. You have such grand friends including those dear, dear Heasleys. I know you're going to enjoy the rest of your time here." A quick kiss and he was gone.

The next morning I received a letter he had written Saturday night, his last night at the hotel in El Paso.

It is eleven o'clock and I have finished packing. When I came in tonight, a special delivery had just arrived from Mother. She sent two snapshots of our new home at Timber Trails. I want you to have them to show to your friends.

What a grand time we are going to have there when your army days are over. I hope you will not even think of a job for a year, but will feel you can just be lazy and relax in that dear little house at Timber Trails.

Tomorrow, when I squeeze your hand, you will not know what a wonderful week I have had, for probably at the last minute words will fail me. I am going home so full of energy and enthusiasm for the work of the coming summer, inspired with memories of every minute with you.

A thousand times I will wonder why we did not have at least one more wheelchair trip, but every one we did have will be a cherished memory to tell to Mother.

I just love you with all my heart Little Honem,
Daddy

"Little Honem," had been Dad's pet name for me when I was a baby. How I longed to be with him on that train speeding east. I had had enough of the army. I wanted to go home.

Marking Time

Two days after Dad's departure for Connecticut, Freddie's wish that I return to work came true. Captain Lord, Chief Dietitian, ordered me to resume my usual duties. She had never bothered to visit Biggs Field and I doubted whether she knew what my work entailed.

Lieutenant Louden, my boss, blew her top. "That's crazy. I'm not goin' to be responsible for you slippin' on a wet floor while you're on crutches. To hell with her! You do the desk work in the office until I decide to let you supervise in the kitchen."

Once again, Janet and I divided the workload between us. We had lost Mary Schroeder, the third member of our team, to the psychiatric ward. When she had begun to order huge quantities of unneeded supplies for the kitchen and to write special diets for non-existent patients, she had been ordered to seek help.

Six weeks after my accident, the shortage of staff forced Lieutenant Louden to send me back to the kitchen. Hobbling about on crutches proved awkward and exhausting. I bound extra layers of ace bandage around my ankle and stuck the crutches in the corner. That change led to rapid progress in my recovery.

Soon I could pay a visit to my former hospital roommate, Judith Crook. I found her in our old room huddled under untidy blankets, her eyes red from weeping. She grabbed my hand and held on tight.

"Last week, when the doctor told me he must operate on my feet for the tenth time, I thought the worst had happened. Now my fiancé has written that it's all over for us." Between sobs, she choked on her words. "He plans to marry someone else."

I thought of Dad's comments after he met Judith. "If the going ever gets tough for me, I think remembering Judith's cheery smile and happy disposition would be a tower of strength. Surely, she is wonderful." Now no words of mine could offer her comfort.

I often shared my letters from home with my friends. "Better than a novel," someone said. Mother's father, my Grandpa Andrews, planned to marry on June 17. We found it ludicrous that a seventy-nine year old man had found a woman seventeen years younger than he eager to become his wife. Only I realized the pain Mother experienced over his decision.

Grandpa had given her little warning about the ceremony. He'd called on Thursday to say Tuesday would be his wedding day. Mother drove him to the florist to order corsages, to the grocery to stock up on food, and to the church to finalize plans with the minister.

With a sinking heart, she tackled the house where she had spent her childhood. She scrubbed, dusted, and vacuumed every room for her future stepmother. After she pressed Grandpa's wedding suit, he made one more demand.

"Gosh hazel, I need you to cut my hair." He had given up the barber fifty years before when haircuts went up to twenty-five cents.

On the day of the wedding only three people accompanied the bride and groom to the Methodist parsonage. Mother and Dad, acting as witnesses, and Mrs. Edington, Grandpa's neighbor, who had introduced him to Louise.

Standing before the minister, Louise, a head taller than Grandpa and almost twice his weight, dwarfed the small erect man by her side. For the next thirteen years, her towering presence would prove symbolic of her dominance of their relationship.

Soon after the wedding, Grandpa wrote to me in his old-fashioned shaded script. "I guess you know that Louise and I were married on the 17th by the Methodist minister. Now I'll have to go to church. Louise is a great Methodist. We've been once in Danbury and twice in Bethel. I hope you are going to like her."

Meeting the newest member of the family would have to wait. I missed not only Grandpa's wedding, but also that of my college roommate, Mary Kirschner. That damned sprained ankle kept me from being her maid-of-honor. During our four years in college, we had looked forward to taking part in each other's weddings. After being off duty for weeks, I dared not ask for leave to fly to York, Pennsylvania.

That was a bitter blow to Mary as well as to me. She had counted on my support to deal with her mother's opposition to the marriage. Her letter describing the difficulties on her special day made me feel guilty that I had not been there. Mary had even decorated the church hall herself with no help from her family.

By the time she and Dave, her groom, drove to New York after the reception, he had developed a high fever and a rash. Due to a smallpox scare in the City, he and Mary were isolated in their room. Dave had chickenpox!

Their planned one night at the Waldorf Astoria turned into a week. Instead of Bermuda, they ran up a monumental bill quarantined in the hotel on their honeymoon. When Dave was well enough to travel, he and Mary departed by way of the freight elevator and the back door.

Mary's mother had the last word. "You might have known he'd pull a stunt like that."

Throughout March, tumbleweed tumbled and sandstorms swirled. I often stood by the window to watch the blowing sand sweep across the desert. The coarse particles filtered through cracks around the windows leaving a white film on clothes in the closet. When I gave my uniform a hard shake, grains of sand littered the floor.

In the hospital, nurses distributed sheets to the patients. "Cover your heads. Another sandstorm's on the way."

Easter brought warmer weather and a burst of color in the desert. Hoping to make up for the trouble in the mess hall at Christmas, Sergeant Murphy, the mess sergeant, helped me plan a festive day for the patients.

He lounged against my office door. "Lieutenant, we've cleaned all the turkeys. Let's make the night crew decorate the eggs. I'm in no mood to play Easter bunny to six crates of eggs."

"That's only fair. You deserve a break after cleaning those twenty-pound birds. Take a few hours off. Lieutenant Louden hitched a plane ride to California for the weekend. With her away, we can do as we please. Let's make the most of it."

Sergeant Murphy and I had a good working relationship. We often traded shifts. I worked the early shift for him. He worked the late shift for me. That way I could go off duty when my foot began to swell and he could sleep in to make up for late nights spent with his girlfriend.

I had his sympathy the morning of the next inspection. The diet cook failed to show up forcing me to cook breakfast. Lye used to scrub the floors splashed on my nylons making them a network of runs. Even before a chocolate milkshake splattered the front of my uniform, my hair had uncurled in the heat. At the approach of the inspecting officer, I hid in the closet. If he had seen my untidy appearance, we'd have flunked the inspection.

Lieutenant Louden returned from California in a foul mood. She had been unable to find a military flight headed our way. All commercial flights were booked solid due to rumors of a price hike to take place the next week. The GIs thought it a huge joke that she was AWOL for twenty-four hours. She fumed about the kitchen in a cloud of cigarette smoke strewing ashes in the food.

After a shopping trip in town, Janet and I rode back on the bus with the mess sergeants. They regaled us with their description of a trick they'd played on Lieutenant Louden. "We wanted to see her go on the rampage, so we cooked all the peas for dinner at 8:00 a.m. She nearly blew a gasket over that one."

Janet and I knew it paid to be on good terms with the mess sergeants. They could make us or break us.

Desert Spring

When Sergeant Murphy announced plans for his wedding, Janet and I discovered our cooperation with the mess sergeants had paid off. Much to our surprise, Sergeant Murphy obtained permission from the commanding officer for us to attend the reception in the NCO Club. To our knowledge, Janet, Lieutenant Louden, and I were the only lieutenants to ever set foot in the non-commissioned officer's club.

The attention Janet and I received equaled that of film stars at the Academy Awards. Cooks and KP workers lined up at the door. Most of the GIs had seen us in our workday garb — brown and white striped seersucker uniforms with caps to match. They whistled their approval of our civilian outfits — short skirts and high heels.

Aware of their admiring glances, I knew they appreciated my dramatic blue and white print dress, white gloves, and spectator shoes. After I had made my way down the receiving line, the pot washer tapped me on the shoulder.

"Hey Dietitian, wanna' dance?" I danced until my ankle screamed for mercy. In spite of the line of cooks waiting to dance with an officer, I limped to a bench on the sidelines.

Even Lieutenant Loudon headed for the dance floor on the arm of a bald old sergeant. After the reception ended, she invited seven of us to pile in her car to go night clubbing. In spite of letting down her guard for one night, she did not change her opinion that officers and enlisted personnel should not mix. Janet and I hoped she'd never find out that later we dated fellows we met that night at the NCO.

A couple of sergeants enticed us with an invitation to take a seven-mile taxi ride to a popular nightspot, The Westerner Inn.

We ate the usual enormous charcoal broiled steaks in a dining room decorated in western décor of ropes, steers, and saddles. Seeking cooler air, we headed to a table on the patio under starry skies.

"Seems strange to call you Carol instead of Lieutenant," said Sergeant Jim. "How about a dance? The Westerner Inn calls this 'Dancing under a Blanket of Blue.' Sounds corny, doesn't it?"

"Gorgeous starlit night seems more like it. Jim, I'd love to dance. It sounds great to be called Carol here, but don't let that slip out on the base." We agreed we'd both be in big trouble if Lieutenant Louden found out we were together. I told him we didn't need to worry about that now, but I might be in trouble with him if I tried to dance the rumba.

May brought ninety-eight degree weather with news, both good and bad.

The good news made me shout for joy. "My separation from the army is official. I'm going home in August." I rushed to the phone to spread the good word. After two long years in the army, the end was in sight. Forty-four days of accumulated leave came in handy. It changed the date from October 1 to August 12.

The bad news — Biggs Field was closing. All personnel were being transferred back to the main hospital. Biggs Field had been the most enjoyable experience of my army career. It had been a carefree time with none of the pressures associated with gravely ill patients, none of the "spit and polish" protocol expected by top brass. All that was about to change.

For the last time I shook the desert sand from my uniform. My previous run-ins with Captain Lord made me dread the move. Grass, trees, air conditioning, even a washing machine, would not compensate for the casual life Janet and I enjoyed at the airfield.

We agreed we weren't the only ones who would have to change their ways. If ashes from Lieutenant Loudan's cigarette fell in the soup in the main kitchen, she'd be in trouble.

When Captain Lord snapped, "Your new assignment will be working with Peg Ward in Mess I," elation over my discharge vanished. Ever since our flight the previous year from Memphis to El Paso, I had avoided Peg whenever possible. I found she had not changed. She spent most of her time hanging out in the officer's club, a technique to avoid work she had picked up from Captain Lord.

In the morning, when I was busy writing food orders and supervising the cooks, she sat in the office doing nothing. After smoking a few cigarettes, she disappeared for the day. I wilted under the tension. The worst flare-up of hepatitis in weeks sent me to bed for three days.

The doctor on sick call offered to put me back in the hospital. I shook my head. "No, I can't face being a patient again. With only six weeks to go until discharge, I'll find a way to stay on my feet."

The move back to Main coincided with Mary Schroeder's return from Ward 30. The psychiatrist had been baffled by her behavior. My next-door neighbor, she talked to me but refused to communicate with others. In spite of my concern, her strange ramblings wore on my nerves. Each of us was responding in a different way to the stress under which we lived.

During those trying days, the GIs in the kitchen did their best to keep up my morale. We had a good laugh over an article in Time magazine quoting General Eisenhower. He said he hoped he would be remembered as the Chief-of-Staff who did something about the army's cooking.

When the gravy burned, I reminded the cooks of the General's remark. Freddie shot back, "He didn't say whether the something would be good or bad."

How I was going to miss the repartee with the GIs.

Down To The Wire

Back home in Connecticut, Dad urged Mother to plan a visit to Texas to coincide with my discharge from the army. He wanted her to understand the life I had led in the military. He knew she would revel in the dramatic cloud formations over the desert and the bold colors in Mexico. Best of all, she would meet my friends, the Heasleys.

As we made plans for mid-August, letters flew back and forth. When ten days passed without a letter from home, I became uneasy. My worst fears came true. Dad had suffered a heart attack, almost five years to the day after the first one.

When I called Mother, she tried to make light of his condition. "Please don't worry. The doctor calls this a mild heart attack. Dad will be in bed only three weeks." I felt she was not as honest with me as I had been with her about my illness. The subject of a trip never came up again.

At my last dinner with the Heasleys, Herbert kept the mood light. "Carol, will you explain these new fashions to me? One of the few good things coming out of the early days of the war was the government order limiting the length of women's skirts."

He told how much he enjoyed looking at shapely legs, particularly his wife's. He wondered why women seemed determined to drop the hemline to the ankles in what he called the "Salvation Army style."

I looked down at my shimmering nylons and stylish spectator pumps. "Blame Christian Dior, not me. I assure you this 'New Look' isn't my idea." Herbert looked pleased when I told him I preferred the western look of jeans for informal wear. I had to admit I doubted whether Mother, or anyone in Bethel, was ready to see me in tight pants.

After army personnel were allowed to wear civilian clothes off the base, I had purchased two dresses. In a matter of weeks both were too short to be fashionable. I was lucky that I needed to start from scratch to build a civilian wardrobe.

At the end of the evening, I could not hold back the tears. Words seemed inadequate to thank the Heasleys for their generosity and love. The phone calls, flowers, dinner parties, and words of encouragement had brightened many a dreary day. Most of all, the car they had bought to whisk me away from the hospital had aided my recovery.

They tried to make me feel they were the ones who benefited most from our friendship. We agreed that Dad's visit had been a highlight of the year. Carol grabbed my hand, "Darlin,' we still have to find a way to get your Mother to Texas."

How I was going to miss the way she called me "Darlin."

Since Mother could not come to El Paso, I wanted to surprise her with a set of Mexican blue pottery dishes like Carol Heasley's. In return for a steak dinner in our favorite Juarez restaurant, my friends, Janet Fox and Alice Strong, agreed to lug pieces of the heavy earthenware over the border. I bought as many bowls, plates, cups and saucers as three of us could carry.

For the next week, whenever my friends went to Mexico, they returned with more pottery. The excelsior used to protect honeydew melons made excellent packing material. Soon a complete dinner service nestled in the wood shavings in several boxes added to my growing pile of possessions. The army would ship everything for free.

One hurdle stood in the way of discharge — the dreaded physical exam. I'd lost weight working in Mess and a deep pain constantly knocked in my right side. If I failed to pass the liver function tests, I'd be sent back to the hospital.

Four days after the exam, the doctor called me back to his office to give me the results. He came right to the point.

"Lieutenant, as you know, to qualify for discharge your health must be as good as when you entered the army. Otherwise, we must treat you until you meet that standard." His next words came as no surprise. "You flunked every liver function test I ordered."

While he paused to let his words sink in, he picked up a paper clip on his desk. "I'm concerned about your future. Diet and rest are the only known treatments for hepatitis. You're getting neither here."

His next words sent shock waves down my spine. "Frankly, in my estimation, if this goes on much longer, your chance of survival is not good." When I remained silent, he continued.

"However, I have a plan that might help you escape from the army."

I straightened up in the chair. What could that be?

His serious expression emphasized his next words. "Before I go on, regardless of your decision, you must agree to keep this conversation confidential."

I nodded. He explained that he could destroy the lab slips and give me a clean bill of health on the report. He figured both of us would be long gone before anyone discovered the discrepancy. He doubted anyone would ever notice. However, there was a problem.

I took a deep breath and waited for him to continue. "In the future, you may experience severe health problems caused by hepatitis. If you're discharged as being in good health, you'll probably be ineligible for treatment by the Veterans Administration. Think it over and let me know your decision tomorrow." He again underlined the trouble we'd both be in if anyone found out about our discussion.

"Sir, I don't need time to think this over. I have made up my mind. Your willingness to take this risky step overwhelms me. You are right. I know I can't keep going without proper rest and diet. I'd rather take a chance on recovery at home than stay here and die."

He nodded. "I think you've made a wise choice. Two weeks from today, you'll be out of the army. Good luck."

Although I longed to brag that I had met a doctor willing to risk his reputation for me, my lips remained sealed. His future and mine depended on my silence.

Looking Ahead

My army career ended as it had begun — filling out forms and signing papers. Without reservation, I stated that I had not stolen government property. I eagerly signed the pay voucher for the largest check I had ever received, eighteen hundred dollars including pay for accumulated leave time.

My hand gripped the pen and did not waver as I signed the line stating that I remained in good health. "Do or die," the doctor had said. It struck me as ironic that I had received my appointment to Walter Reed under false pretences without a physical. I was leaving the army the same way, thanks to destroyed lab slips.

The highlight of the day came with my promotion to first lieutenant. Janet replaced the gold bars on my shoulders with silver. I thought about the article in the college newspaper back in '42, which gave the girls advice on ranks in the military.

One rule had struck us as hilarious. "When it comes to lieutenants, go off the gold standard for silver ranks higher than gold." At that time, I had not considered joining the army. Now I knew how much hard work went into attaining that silver bar.

A command performance brought my days in the service to an end. All personnel received orders to appear in dress uniform at a reception for the Surgeon General. I polished my shoes, pressed my uniform, and, in a desperate measure, trimmed my hair. The air conditioning had quit, and my limp hair dragged on my collar.

In the Officers' Club, the receiving line moved across the lounge at snail's pace. Janet nudged my arm. "Look at 'our leader' over there in the corner. Even a formal reception cannot keep Captain Lord away from the slot machines."

I straightened my tie. "On cooler days the men would have joined her, but in this heat a Tom Collins takes priority over playing the slots." As soon as the officers finished shaking the General's hand, they headed for the bar like lemmings plunging into the sea.

The following evening, Alice, Janet, Mary, and I had a celebration of our own. Mary and I had received our orders for separation. Alice and Janet expected theirs by the end of the week. Wearing sundresses and sandals, we gathered in the cool lounge for our favorite supper — waffles prepared in the tiny snack kitchen.

Mary's psychological problems had not kept her from being discharged. Had the doctor, who smoothed my way out of the army, done the same for her? I dared not ask. She raised her iced tea glass in salute, "Here's to you, Carol. When we met at Walter Reed, I was such a greenhorn. Your description of New York and other places you'd been impressed me and made me wonder how I'd fit in. Thanks for all the encouragement you gave me."

Those days seemed a lifetime ago rather than three years. Back then I had been closer to Marie and Emma, but Mary and I had ended up in Texas with many shared memories. We had experienced the tough times at Walter Reed, Mary's first lobster in a fancy Washington restaurant, and my first taco in a joint in San Antonio. As we said goodbye, I wondered whether our paths would ever cross again.

By morning, my plan to hitch a ride on an army plane to save airfare had lost its appeal. I lacked the energy to wait hours for a plane heading east. Rather than an extravagance, a hundred twelve dollars and eighty-six cents for a ticket on American Airlines seemed a bargain.

As I waited for my taxi by the manicured lawns at the gate to William Beaumont General Hospital, the flag on the high pole fluttered in farewell. I returned the sentry's salute and realized with a jolt this was the last time anyone would salute me.

At the airport, Janet, Alice, and I stood near the windy runway making small talk. The day, which I had anticipated with such eagerness, now seemed one of sadness. Overwhelmed by the finality of leaving my friends, I gave them quick hugs before hurrying across the tarmac to the plane. At the top of the stairs, I turned for one last wave. I could no longer hold back the tears.

"Lieutenant, you need a cup of coffee. Cream and sugar?" The words of the smiling stewardess brought me out of my somber mood. The plane soared into the cloudless sky. Peering out the tiny window, I had one last glimpse of El Paso, the Rio Grande River, and Juarez, Mexico.

Dozing fitfully to the drone of the propellers, I thought about the seven years I has spent away from home. Throughout all that time living in the South, I remained a New Englander at heart, my northern accent still intact. Would I be content in the poster size state of Connecticut after the billboard size of Texas?

New Englanders of Grandpa Andrews' and Aunt Hannah's background, steeped in generations of tradition, were set in their ways and wary of strangers. I owed my life to people whose backgrounds and values were so different from those I had known as a child. My horizon had been broadened by exposure to circumstances my parents could not imagine.

I had learned to love the vast sweep of blue sky and the wide-open spaces of Texas. I would miss the people there. They matched their land — friendly, outgoing, and vibrant — larger than life. Herbert Heasley had told me he felt smothered in Connecticut. The hilly terrain and the small patches of sky peeking through the dense green leaves depressed him. Perhaps, I was about to share his point of view.

The 1940's had been shaped by the most cataclysmic war in history, a war in which I played one individual's small part. That chapter of my life had come to an end. I doubted the future would equal the drama and excitement of the past seven years.

During those years, a title had always defined my role. Four years at the Woman's College as Freshman, Sophomore, Junior, and Senior had been followed by one year at Walter Reed, as a Student and Apprentice Dietitian. The last two years I had answered to the name Lieutenant Morrison. Who would I be when I took off my uniform for the last time?

Bright light filling the cabin brought me out of my reverie. I sat up and gazed at the flaming sky. Sunset, the day had slipped away. The long journey had been a much-needed buffer separating the army life I had left from the civilian life looming ahead.

Below, the landscape basked in the warm glow of twilight. It seemed to reflect the upbeat mood of the nation. Thousands of soldiers, sailors, and marines had returned home to a country at peace. The GI Bill was paving their way to new and exciting possibilities.

For some of us the future appeared less optimistic. I felt weighted down by the prospect of the struggle ahead to regain my health. I had no job, no income, and no friends living near home.

The plane hit the runway with a thump. Entering the terminal, I spied Mother and Dad waiting arm-in-arm to welcome me home, as they had done so many times. Dad appeared pale and thin. Mother, bounding with energy, rushed toward me. She gave me a hearty hug and kiss. Her words washed over me but I lacked the energy to respond.

"Carol, we're going to have such a good time now that you're home. Everything always works out for the best. Don't you agree?"

I wanted to cry out, after the suffering I've seen and all I've been through, how can I think everything works out for the best?

Her words confirmed my suspicions. Returning to civilian life and resuming my role, as daughter in the family, would be a challenge equal to any I had faced in the army.

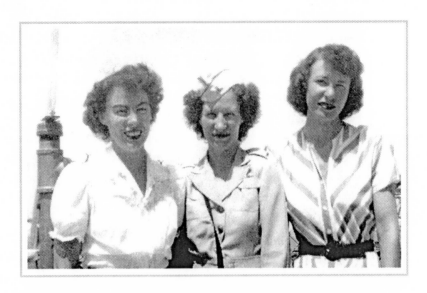

Alice Strong, Carol Morrison, and Janet Fox.
Carol's last day in the army.

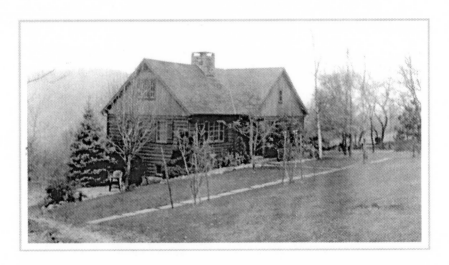

Timber Trails cottage in a snowfall.

359

About the Author

Caroline Garrett remains true to her New England heritage after forty-two years in California. Old furniture scrounged from Connecticut attics and stories about her Yankee grandfather contributed to the success of classes she taught for fifteen years at Antiques and Collectables in San Jose, California.

She and her husband, Eliot raised a son, Rob, and a daughter, Pam, before Eliot's death in 1985. At that time, Caroline's life changed direction. Her mother, Hazel Morrison, left her home in Bethel, Connecticut, to live with her daughter. Years of travel, entertaining, and laughter culminated in the publication of Hazel's book of poetry, "A Fluttering of Wings," on her one hundred fourth birthday. She retained her zest for life until her death at the age of one hundred seven.

Caroline is surprised to have accomplished her goal, of writing a book about her experiences during the years of WWII, in her eighty-sixth year.

Circles

Pebbles we throw in the steam of life
In widening circles blend,
Mingling with those that have gone before,
For circles have no end.

Thus our living will surely be
Blended with eternity.

Hazel A. Morrison
"A Fluttering of Wings"

CPSIA information can be obtained at www.ICGtesting.com
Printed in the USA
BVOW021143141011

273649BV00002B/6/A